Clinical Electrocardiography
Review and Study Guide

Clinical
Electrocardiography
Review and Study Guide

Second Edition

Franklin H. Zimmerman, M.D.
Assistant Clinical Professor of Medicine (Cardiology)
Columbia University College of Physicians and Surgeons
  New York, New York
Senior Attending Cardiologist
Phelps Memorial Hospital
  Sleepy Hollow, New York
Westchester Medical Center
  Valhalla, New York
St. Luke's-Roosevelt Hospital Center
  New York, New York

McGraw-Hill
Medical Publishing Division

New York   Chicago   San Francisco   Lisbon   London
Madrid   Mexico City   Milan   New Delhi   San Juan
Seoul   Singapore   Sydney   Toronto

Clinical Electrocardiography: Review and Study Guide, Second Edition

Copyright © 2004 by **The McGraw-Hill Companies, Inc.** All rights reserved. Printed in the United States of America. Except as permitted under the United States Copyright Act of 1976, no part of this publication may be reproduced or distributed in any form or by any means, or stored in a data base or retrieval system without the prior written permission of the publisher.

1 2 3 4 5 6 7 8 9 0   QPD/QPD   0 9 8 7 6 5 4

ISBN 0-07-142302-8

This book was set in TimesTen Roman by International Typesetting and Composition.
The editors were Darlene Cooke and Shelley Reinhardt.
The production supervisor was Phil Galea.
Project management was provided by International Typesetting and Composition.
Quebecor Dubuque was printer and binder.
This book was printed on acid-free paper.

Library of Congress Cataloging-in-Publication Data

Zimmerman, Franklin H.
    Clinical electrocardiography: Review and Study Guide / Franklin H. Zimmerman.—2nd ed.
        p. ; cm.
    Rev. ed. of: Clinical electrocardiography. c1994.
    Includes bibliographical references and index.
    ISBN 0-07-142302-8
    1. Electrocardiography—Examinations, questions, etc. 2. Electrocardiography—Problems, exercises, etc. I. Zimmerman, Franklin H. Clinical electrocardiography. II. Title.
    [DNLM: 1. Electrocardiography—Examination Questions. 2. Heart Diseases—diagnosis—Examination Questions. WG 18.2 Z72c 2005]
    RC683.5.E5Z543 2005
    616.1'207547—dc22
                                                        2003064614

• •

To

My wife, Laurie, and our children, Stacey and Ricky,

for their love, support, and sacrifice

• •

Contents

Introduction

Clinical Electrocardiography: Review and Study Guide has been designed to provide physicians with a clinically relevant, academic approach to the interpretation of electrocardiograms. This test should be useful to any physician who interprets electrocardiograms, including cardiologists, internists, family practitioners, anesthesiologists, critical care specialists, medical students, or any health care provider who wishes to maintain a high competency in the interpretation of electrocardiograms. The board-review format should provide a particularly useful instrument for candidates taking the cardiology board or electrocardiography proficiency examinations. Use of the review text should help the reader to (1) recognize common and uncommon electrocardiographic diagnoses, (2) learn the principles of interpreting cardiac arrhythmias, (3) identify areas of weakness, and (4) correlate electrocardiographic data with clinically relevant information.

This text contains a total of 200 electrocardiograms. All use a full-sized, three-channel format with a concomitant lead II rhythm strip. Both a narrative and a board-examination type of format are used for interpretation. The narrative interpretation is designed to simulate that used in a hospital's electrocardiographic laboratory. The board-review format is designed to resemble that which appears on the electrocardiographic portion of the cardiology board examination and that of the electrocardiography proficiency test of the American College of Cardiology.

The 200 electrocardiograms are divided into five tests of 40 tracings each. A brief clinical history appears with each electrocardiogram. Answers, explanations, and material for further reading are provided. A section of diagnostic criteria for standard electrocardiographic diagnoses precedes the first test.

Acknowledgments

Special appreciation is given to Dr. Arthur E. Fass, Assistant Clinical Professor of Medicine (Cardiology) at New York Medical College and Chief of Cardiology at Phelps Memorial Hospital Center. Dr. Fass reviewed and interpreted each electrocardiogram and was the major contributor to and editor of the section on diagnostic criteria that opens this text.

I wish to thank Dr. James Levy, Director of the Electrocardiography Laboratory, Westchester Medical Center; Dr. Carmine Sorbera, Director of the Electrophysiology Laboratory, Westchester Medical Center; and the late, Dr. Julian Frieden, former Chief of Cardiology, Sound Shore Medical Center, for their review of the electrocardiograms for the first edition of this book.

The clerical and nursing staffs of Phelps Memorial Hospital Center, Westchester Medical Center, and Sound Shore Medical Center were instrumental in collecting the electrocardiographic tracings.

I also wish to thank Darlene Cooke and the staff at McGraw-Hill for their efforts during this project.

Test Instructions

The reader should first interpret the electrocardiograms in a narrative format. Analyze the tracing in terms of the cardiac rhythm and identify the atrial and ventricular rates. Measure the PR, QRS, and QT intervals and determine the electrical axis within 15 degrees. Identify the electrocardiographic abnormalities and synthesize the findings into an integrated interpretation.

A board-review format may also be used. You may wish to practice using a time limit of 4 hours for each of the five tests of 40 tracings in order to simulate the format of the actual board examination. Cover the answers with a blank sheet of paper as you interpret each electrocardiogram. The following section provides a table of electrocardiographic diagnoses to be used with the sample tracings. The reader should select the best diagnoses that

apply to each electrocardiogram. Multiple diagnoses are likely for each example. There may not be an exact diagnosis to conform with the narrative interpretation; however, choose those that best apply. The author has listed the preferred selections in the answer section. Potential, unconfirmed, or alternative diagnoses appear in parentheses.

The selection of test answers is derived from standard electrocardiographic diagnoses. The test is similar but not identical to the cardiology board examination. All of the electrocardiograms are included not just to help you pass the boards, but also to help you become a master electrocardiographer. The author makes no claim that the American Board of Internal Medicine or the American College of Cardiology would interpret the enclosed tracings exactly as the author has done.

Abbreviations

AFIB   *Atrial fibrillation*
APC   *Atrial premature complex*
AV   *Atrioventricular*
bpm   *beats per minute*
CCU   *Coronary care unit*
CHF   *Congestive heart failure*
COPD   *Chronic obstructive pulmonary disease*
ECG   *Electrocardiogram*
ER   *Emergency room*
ICU   *Intensive care unit*
JPC   *Junctional premature complex*
LBBB   *Left bundle branch block*

LVH   *Left ventricular hypertrophy*
MAT   *Multifocal artial tachycardia*
MI   *Myocardial infarction*
PAT   *Paroxysmal atrial tachycardia*
RBBB   *Right bundle branch block*
RVH   *Right ventricular hypertrophy*
SA   *Sinoatrial*
SVT   *Supraventricular tachycardia*
VA   *Ventriculoatrial*
VPC   *Ventricular premature complex*
VT   *Ventricular tachycardia*
WPW   *Wolff-Parkinson-White pattern (or syndrome)*

Table of Electrocardiographic Diagnoses

I. RHYTHM ABNORMALITIES

A. Supraventricular Rhythms and Complexes

- ☐ 1. Sinus rhythm
- ☐ 2. Sinus arrhythmia
- ☐ 3. Sinus bradycardia
- ☐ 4. Sinus tachycardia
- ☐ 5. Wandering atrial pacemaker within the sinus node
- ☐ 6. Wandering atrial pacemaker to the AV junction
- ☐ 7. Sinus arrest or pause
- ☐ 8. Sinoatrial exit block
- ☐ 9. Ectopic atrial rhythm
- ☐ 10. Atrial premature complexes, normally conducted
- ☐ 11. Atrial premature complexes, aberrantly conducted
- ☐ 12. Atrial premature complexes, nonconducted
- ☐ 13. Multifocal atrial rhythm
- ☐ 14. Multifocal atrial tachycardia
- ☐ 15. Atrial tachycardia, regular 1:1 conduction, sustained
- ☐ 16. Atrial tachycardia, regular 1:1 conduction, short paroxysms
- ☐ 17. Atrial tachycardia, with non-1:1 conduction (with block)
- ☐ 18. Supraventricular tachycardia, unspecified
- ☐ 19. Atrial flutter
- ☐ 20. Atrial fibrillation

B. AV Junctional Rhythms and Complexes

- ☐ 21. AV junctional rhythm
- ☐ 22. AV junctional escape rhythm
- ☐ 23. AV junctional rhythm, accelerated
- ☐ 24. AV junctional escape complexes
- ☐ 25. AV junctional premature complexes

C. Ventricular Rhythms and Complexes

- ☐ 26. Ventricular premature complex(es), uniform
- ☐ 27. Ventricular premature complex(es), multiform
- ☐ 28. Ventricular premature complexes, paired
- ☐ 29. Ventricular parasystole
- ☐ 30. Ventricular tachycardia
- ☐ 31. Accelerated idioventricular rhythm
- ☐ 32. Ventricular fibrillation
- ☐ 33. Torsades de pointes

D. Pacemaker Function, Rhythms, and Complexes

- ☐ 34. Single-chamber atrial pacing
- ☐ 35. Single-chamber pacemaker, ventricular pacing on demand
- ☐ 36. Single-chamber pacemaker, ventricular pacing with complete control
- ☐ 37. Dual-chamber pacemaker, atrial sensing with ventricular pacing
- ☐ 38. Dual-chamber pacemaker, atrial and ventricular sensing and pacing
- ☐ 39. Pacemaker malfunction, failure to capture atrium or ventricle appropriately
- ☐ 40. Pacemaker malfunction, failure to sense atrial or ventricular complexes appropriately
- ☐ 41. Pacemaker malfunction, failure to fire appropriately on demand (inappropriate sensing of stimuli or complex)

II. AV CONDUCTION ABNORMALITIES

- ☐ 42. AV block, first-degree
- ☐ 43. AV block, second-degree, Mobitz type I (Wenckebach)
- ☐ 44. AV block, second-degree, Mobitz type II
- ☐ 45. AV block, second-degree, 2:1
- ☐ 46. AV block, high-grade
- ☐ 47. AV block, third-degree or complete
- ☐ 48. Accelerated AV conduction (short PR interval pattern with normal QRS duration in sinus rhythm)
- ☐ 49. Ventricular preexcitation (WPW pattern)
- ☐ 50. Physiologic AV conduction delay associated with supaventricular tachyarrhythmias
- ☐ 51. Nonphysiologic AV conduction delay associated with supraventricular tachyarrhythmias

III. MISCELLANEOUS AV RELATIONSHIPS

- ☐ 52. Ventriculophasic sinus arrhythmia
- ☐ 53. AV dissociation
- ☐ 54. Reciprocal (echo) complexes
- ☐ 55. Retrograde atrial activation from a ventricular focus
- ☐ 56. Fusion complexes
- ☐ 57. Ventricular capture complexes
- ☐ 58. Interpolation of ventricular premature complexes

IV. P-WAVE ABNORMALITIES

- ☐ 59. Right atrial abnormality
- ☐ 60. Left atrial abnormality
- ☐ 61. Biatrial abnormality
- ☐ 62. Nonspecific atrial abnormality
- ☐ 63. PR depression

V. ABNORMALITIES OF QRS AXIS OR VOLTAGE

- ☐ 64. Left-axis deviation
- ☐ 65. Right-axis deviation
- ☐ 66. Poor R-wave progression
- ☐ 67. Low voltage, limb leads
- ☐ 68. Low voltage, precordial leads
- ☐ 69. Electrical alternans

VI. INTRAVENTRICULAR CONDUCTION ABNORMALITIES

- ☐ 70. Right bundle branch block, complete
- ☐ 71. Right bundle branch block, incomplete
- ☐ 72. Left anterior fascicular block
- ☐ 73. Left posterior fascicular block
- ☐ 74. Left bundle branch block, complete
- ☐ 75. Left bundle branch block, incomplete
- ☐ 76. Intraventricular conduction delay, nonspecific (includes IVCD associated with chamber enlargement)
- ☐ 77. Probable aberrant intraventricular conduction associated with supraventricular arrhythmia

VII. VENTRICULAR HYPERTROPHY OR ENLARGEMENT

- ☐ 78. Left ventricular hypertrophy by voltage criteria, with or without associated ST-T-wave abnormalities
- ☐ 79. Right ventricular hypertrophy
- ☐ 80. Combined ventricular hypertrophy

VIII. Q-WAVE MYOCARDIAL INFARCTION

- ☐ 81. Anteroseptal, acute or recent
- ☐ 82. Anteroseptal, old or of indeterminate age
- ☐ 83. Anterior, acute or recent
- ☐ 84. Anterior, old or of indeterminate age
- ☐ 85. Anterolateral, acute or recent
- ☐ 86. Anterolateral, old or of indeterminate age
- ☐ 87. Extensive anterior, acute or recent
- ☐ 88. Extensive anterior, old or of indeterminate age
- ☐ 89. Lateral or high lateral, acute or recent
- ☐ 90. Lateral or high lateral, old or of indeterminate age
- ☐ 91. Inferior or diaphragmatic, acute or recent
- ☐ 92. Inferior or diaphragmatic, old or of indeterminate age
- ☐ 93. Posterior, acute or recent
- ☐ 94. Posterior, old or of indeterminate age
- ☐ 95. Suggestive of ventricular aneurysm

IX. ST-, T-, U-WAVE ABNORMALITIES

- ☐ 96. Normal variant, isolated J-point elevation (early repolarization pattern)
- ☐ 97. Isolated J-point depression
- ☐ 98. Normal variant, RSR' pattern lead V1
- ☐ 99. Normal variant, persistent juvenile T-wave pattern
- ☐ 100. ST- and/or T-wave abnormalities suggesting acute or recent myocardial injury
- ☐ 101. ST- and/or T-wave abnormalities suggesting either reciprocal change or myocardial ischemia in the setting of acute myocardial injury
- ☐ 102. ST- and/or T-wave abnormalities suggesting myocardial ischemia in the absence of acute myocardial injury
- ☐ 103. ST- and/or T-wave abnormalities associated with ventricular hypertrophy
- ☐ 104. ST- and/or T-wave abnormalities associated with ventricular conduction abnormality
- ☐ 105. ST- and/or T-wave abnormalities suggesting early, acute pericarditis
- ☐ 106. Nonspecific ST- and/or T-wave abnormalities
- ☐ 107. Postextrasystolic T-wave abnormality
- ☐ 108. Peaked T waves
- ☐ 109. Prolonged QT interval for heart rate (QTc)
- ☐ 110. Prominent U waves
- ☐ 111. Inverted U waves

X. TECHNICAL PROBLEMS

- ☐ 112. Incorrect electrode placement
- ☐ 113. Artifact secondary to tremor

Clinical
Electrocardiography
Review and Study Guide

Diagnostic Criteria

Arthur E. Fass, M.D., Editor

The following are suggested diagnostic criteria for the items listed in the test section. These are not intended to be comprehensive, and minor variations of these criteria exist in textbooks of electrocardiography. The suggested test answers in this text, however, use the following basic criteria.

OUTLINE

I.   Rhythm Abnormalities

  A. Supraventricular rhythms and complexes
  B. AV junctional rhythms and complexes
  C. Ventricular rhythms and complexes
  D. Pacemaker function, rhythms, and complexes

II.   AV Conduction Abnormalities

III. Miscellaneous AV Relationships

IV. P-Wave Abnormalities

V.   Abnormalities of QRS Axis or Voltage

VI. Intraventricular Conduction Abnormalities

VII. Ventricular Hypertrophy (or Enlargement)

VIII. Q-Wave Myocardial Infarction

IX. ST-, T-, U-Wave Abnormalities

X.   Technical Problems

ELECTROCARDIOGRAPHIC DIAGNOSES

I.   Rhythm Abnormalities

  A. Supraventricular Rhythms and Complexes

  1. Sinus rhythm
    A physiologic rhythm initiated in the sinus node and characterized by a heart rate of 60 to 100 bpm. The configuration of the P wave is upright in leads I, II, and aVF and inverted in lead aVR.

  2. Sinus arrhythmia
    Sinus rhythm in which the PP interval varies by 0.16 s or more.

  3. Sinus bradycardia
    Sinus rhythm with a heart rate less than 60 bpm.

Note: For clinical purposes, many cardiologists consider sinus bradycardia to be less than 50 bpm.

  4. Sinus tachycardia
    Sinus rhythm with a heart rate greater than 100 bpm.

  5. Wandering atrial pacemaker within the sinus node
    Sinus rhythm with minor variations in P-wave morphology remaining upright in leads I and II and inverted in aVR. The PR interval is variable but remains 0.12 s or greater.

  6. Wandering atrial pacemaker to the AV junction
    Sinus rhythm with progressive alteration in P-wave configuration, eventually becoming inverted (retrograde). The PR interval of the AV junctional focus characteristically becomes less than 0.12 s.

  7. Sinus arrest or pause
    A failure of the SA node to initiate an impulse, which results in absence of P waves and QRS complexes. The pause is not a multiple of the intrinsic PP interval.

  8. Sinoatrial exit block
    An abnormality of transmission of the sinus impulse, which results in a delay or failure of production of a P wave. Only second-degree SA block can be identified on the surface electrocardiogram. It may manifest in two patterns, type I and type II.
    ☐ Type I second-degree SA block is characterized by progressive shortening of the PP interval prior to an absent P wave.
    ☐ Type II is characterized by a pause in the PP cycle that is an exact multiple of the intrinsic sinus rate.
    Note: In some individuals with underlying sinus arrhythmia, the duration of the longest pause may be slightly less than an exact multiple of the sinus rate.

9. *Ectopic atrial rhythm*

A rhythm initiated by an atrial pacemaker other than the sinus node. It is characterized by a rate less than 100 bpm with a P-wave morphology different from that of the sinus node. The PR interval is within normal limits.

10. *Atrial premature complexes, normally conducted*

A premature complex originating in the atrium and characterized by a P-wave morphology different from the normal sinus complex. The PR interval of the premature beat may be shorter, longer, or no different from the sinus complex. The PR interval characteristically is ≥0.12 s, which helps distinguish it from a premature complex of AV junctional origin.

11. *Atrial premature complexes, aberrantly conducted*

An atrial premature complex that, because of partial refractoriness of the conduction system, is conducted to the ventricles in an abnormal fashion and results in an alteration in the normal morphology of the QRS complex.

12. *Atrial premature complexes, nonconducted*

An atrial premature complex that, because of complete refractoriness of the conduction system, fails to conduct to the ventricles and is therefore not followed by a QRS complex.

13. *Multifocal atrial rhythm*

An atrial rhythm at a rate less than 100 bpm, characterized by absence of one dominant pacemaker, P waves of at least three different morphologies, and varying PR and PP intervals.

14. *Multifocal atrial tachycardia*

An atrial rhythm at a rate 100 bpm or greater, characterized by absence of one dominant pacemaker, P waves of at least three different morphologies, and varying PR and PP intervals.

15. *Atrial tachycardia, regular 1:1 conduction, sustained*

A supraventricular arrhythmia characterized by abnormal P waves and an atrial rate of 100 to 200 bpm. The term *sustained* indicates a rhythm that lasts 30 s or more, or for standard electrocardiographic interpretive purposes, the entire tracing.

16. *Atrial tachycardia, regular 1:1 conduction, short paroxysms*

An atrial tachycardia that is at least three complexes or more but is not sustained.

17. *Atrial tachycardia, with non-1:1 AV conduction (with block)*

Atrial tachycardia characterized by an atrial rate of 150 to 250 bpm with non-1:1 conduction. An isoelectric interval is characteristically present between the abnormal P waves in contrast to the *sawtooth* baseline of atrial flutter.

18. *Supraventricular tachycardia, unspecified*

A supraventricular tachyarrhythmia in which the mechanism cannot be determined.

19. *Atrial flutter*

An atrial rhythm characterized (classically) by an atrial rate of 250 to 350 bpm with flutter waves exhibiting a *sawtooth* appearance in leads II, III, aVF, and V1.

20. *Atrial fibrillation*

An absence of organized P waves with replacement by irregular atrial fibrillatory waves of varying morphology.

B. AV Junctional Rhythms and Complexes

21. *AV junctional rhythm*

A regular rhythm characteristically at a rate of 35 to 60 bpm that originates in the AV junction, with inverted (retrograde) P waves in leads II, III, and aVF. The P waves may occur prior to, within, or after the QRS complex. In the absence of retrograde block, the PR interval is characteristically less than 0.12 s.

22. *AV junctional escape rhythm*

An AV junctional rhythm that emerges as a result of a failure of conduction or slowing of a normally faster physiologic pacemaker (e.g., sinus node).

23. *AV junctional rhythm, accelerated*

An AV junctional rhythm that is more rapid (generally between 70 and 130 bpm) than the usual rate of the AV junction. It is secondary to enhanced automaticity of the AV junction and lacks a paroxysmal onset and termination. An equivalent term for this rhythm is *nonparoxysmal junctional tachycardia.*

24. *AV junctional escape complexes*
Isolated AV junctional complexes that emerge as a result of a failure of conduction or slowing of a normally faster physiologic pacemaker.

25. *AV junctional premature complexes*
Isolated AV junctional complexes that occur prematurely relative to the basic sinus cycle.

C. Ventricular Rhythms and Complexes

26. *Ventricular premature complex(es), uniform*
Premature depolarizations that originate in the ventricles. They are characterized by a wide, abnormal QRST morphology.

27. *Ventricular premature complex(es), multiform*
Ventricular premature complexes that demonstrate more than one morphology.

28. *Ventricular premature complexes, paired*
Two ventricular premature complexes in a row.

29. *Ventricular parasystole*
Ventricular complexes that are independent of the intrinsic rhythm. These complexes are characterized by varying coupling intervals and fusion beats. The interectopic intervals are constant or are multiples of a common denominator.

30. *Ventricular tachycardia*
Three or more ventricular complexes in succession at a rate greater than 100 bpm.

31. *Accelerated idioventricular rhythm*
Three or more ventricular complexes in succession at a rate of 100 bpm or less.

32. *Ventricular fibrillation*
A disorganized rhythm originating in the ventricles characterized by absence of discernible QRS complexes and by fibrillatory waves of variable rate and amplitude.

33. *Torsades de pointes*
A polymorphous ventricular tachycardia with an alternating amplitude and polarity.

D. Pacemaker Function, Rhythms, and Complexes

34. *Single-chamber atrial pacing*
A pacemaker stimulus captures the atrium. In the absence of conduction abnormality, a native QRS complex follows (the presence of a ventricular lead cannot be excluded).

35. *Single-chamber pacemaker, ventricular pacing on demand*
A pacemaker stimulus captures the ventricles after a pause in the native rhythm.

36. *Single-chamber pacemaker, ventricular pacing with complete control*
A ventricular pacemaker captures the ventricles without evidence of intrinsic ventricular depolarization.

37. *Dual-chamber pacemaker, atrial sensing with ventricular pacing*
A ventricular pacemaker captures the ventricles following a normally sensed P wave.

38. *Dual-chamber pacemaker, atrial and ventricular sensing and pacing*
A pacemaker rhythm with evidence of both atrial and ventricular sensing and pacing.

39. *Pacemaker malfunction, failure to capture either the atrium or ventricle appropriately*
A pacemaker stimulus that fails to capture the appropriate chamber when nonrefractory.

40. *Pacemaker malfunction, failure to sense either atrial or ventricular complexes appropriately*
A pacemaker stimulus that fails to be appropriately inhibited by an intrinsic depolarization of either the ventricles or atria.

41. *Pacemaker malfunction, failure to fire appropriately on demand*
A pacemaker stimulus that does not appear when it would normally be expected.

II. **AV Conduction Abnormalities**

42. *AV block, first-degree*
In sinus rhythm, a consistent PR interval of greater than 0.20 s.

43. *AV block, second-degree, Mobitz type I (Wenckebach)*
In sinus rhythm, classic Wenckebach is characterized by progressive lengthening of the PR interval until a P wave fails to conduct to the ventricles. There is associated progressive shortening of the RR interval until a beat is dropped. The resulting pause is the sum of two PP intervals.
  □ Mobitz type I second-degree AV block may also be present without the Wenckebach phenomenon. In this instance, there is prolongation of the PR interval prior to the dropped beat but without a gradual progressive increase in the PR interval and shortening of the RR interval.

44. *AV block, second-degree, Mobitz type II*
In sinus rhythm, a constant PR interval is identified in consecutively conducted beats

with intermittent failure of the P wave to conduct to the ventricles.

45. *AV block, second-degree, 2:1*
In sinus rhythm, there is a 2:1 relationship of the P waves to QRS complexes. Mobitz type I and type II cannot be differentiated.

46. *AV block, high-grade*
In sinus rhythm, conduction of the P waves to the ventricles in a ratio of 3:1 or more. The atrial rate must be greater than the ventricular rate. This is also applicable when the majority (but not all) of the P waves fail to conduct to the ventricles and the rhythm is maintained by a subsidiary pacemaker. Conduction must be expected and not interfered with by the subsidiary pacemaker. The identification of occasional conduction to the ventricles defines the conduction abnormality as high-grade rather than complete AV block.

47. *AV block, third-degree or complete*
Absence of AV conduction. The atrial rate must be greater than the ventricular rate.

48. *Accelerated AV conduction (short PR interval pattern with normal QRS duration in sinus rhythm)*
Characterized by a PR interval of less than 0.12 s, a normal P-wave morphology, and normal QRS duration.

49. *Ventricular preexcitation (WPW pattern)*
Characterized by a PR interval of less than 0.12 s, a normal P-wave morphology, an initial slurring (delta wave) prior to a wide QRS complex of 0.11 s or more, and secondary ST-T-wave changes.

50. *Physiologic AV conduction delay associated with supraventricular tachyarrhythmias*
A manifestation of physiologic delay in AV conduction associated with a supraventricular tachyarrhythmia (responses at heart rates listed are approximations and are dependent on autonomic tone). Included are:
a. Prolongation of the PR interval with 1:1 conduction at atrial rates of 150 bpm or more.
b. The Wenckebach phenomenon at atrial rates of 130 to 200 bpm.
c. Uniform, 2:1 AV conduction at atrial rates greater than 200 bpm in atrial tachycardia and atrial flutter.

d. Atrial fibrillation with an average ventricular response of 100 to 180 bpm.

51. *Nonphysiologic AV conduction delay associated with supraventricular tachyarrhythmias*
A nonphysiologic impairment of AV conduction secondary to either intrinsic disease or pharmacologic agents (responses at heart rates listed are approximations and are dependent on autonomic tone). Included are:
a. PR interval prolongation with 1:1 conduction at atrial rates of 100 to 149 bpm.
b. The Wenckebach phenomenon at atrial rates of 100 to 129 bpm.
c. A greater than 2:1 AV conduction ratio (either uniform or variable) at atrial rates greater than 200 bpm in atrial tachycardia and atrial flutter.
d. Atrial fibrillation with an average ventricular response of less than 100 bpm.

III. Miscellaneous AV Relationships

52. *Ventriculophasic sinus arrhythmia*
A form of sinus arrhythmia in which the sinus cycles that contain ventricular depolarizations are shorter than those cycles that do not.

53. *AV dissociation*
Independent atrial and ventricular rhythm mechanisms.

54. *Reciprocal (echo) complexes*
A reentry complex that results from an impulse depolarizing the chamber of its origin and returning to depolarize the same chamber. The impulse may arise from the SA node, atria, AV junction, or ventricles.

55. *Retrograde atrial activation from a ventricular focus*
Activation of the atria in a retrograde fashion from an independent depolarization in the ventricles.

56. *Fusion complexes*
A complex or complexes arising from the simultaneous transmission of impulses from more than one focus. The resulting hybrid complex demonstrates a morphology intermediate between the usual, undisturbed pattern of the two depolarizations.

57. *Ventricular capture complexes*
The presence of conducted beats from supraventricular impulses during a period of

AV dissociation. This generally refers to sinus capture during a period of ventricular tachycardia.

58. *Interpolation of ventricular premature complexes*
Ventricular extrasystoles that are interposed between two sinus beats and do not disturb the sinus rhythm. A prolongation of the subsequent PR interval is characteristic secondary to concealed retrograde conduction to the AV junction.

IV. P-Wave Abnormalities

59. *Right atrial abnormality*
   □ The P-wave amplitude is 2.5 mm or more in leads II, III, and aVF. The P-wave duration is less than 0.12 s.
   □ The initial positive component of the P wave in lead V1 is 1.5 mm or more.
   Supporting criteria: The P-wave axis in the frontal plane is +75 degrees or more.

60. *Left atrial abnormality*
   □ The P-wave duration is prolonged (0.12 s or more) and notched in leads I, II, and aVL.
   □ There is an abnormal P-terminal force in lead V1 with the product of the depth and duration equal to or greater than 0.04.
   Supporting criteria: The P-wave axis in the frontal plane is leftward of +15 degrees.

61. *Biatrial abnormality*
   □ An abnormal P-terminal force combined with an initial positive P-wave component of 1.5 mm or more in lead V1.
   □ Combined wide (greater than 0.12 s) and tall (greater than 2.5 mm) P waves in the limb leads.

62. *Nonspecific atrial abnormality*
   A wide P wave (duration 0.12 s or more) without other criteria for abnormality.

63. *PR depression*
   A depressed PR segment below the baseline of more than 0.8 mm.

V. Abnormalities of QRS Axis or Voltage

64. *Left-axis deviation*
   A frontal plane QRS axis between −30 and −90 degrees.

65. *Right-axis deviation*
   A frontal plane QRS axis between +90 and +270 degrees.

66. *Poor R-wave progression*
   R waves are present in leads V1–V3, but the R-wave magnitude is 3.0 mm or less in V3, and the R wave in V2 is equal to or smaller than the R wave in V3. Reverse R-wave progression is as above except that R-wave voltage decreases from V1–V3. Excluded are patients with low voltage in the precordial leads (see below), left bundle branch block, or preexcitation (WPW).

67. *Low voltage, limb leads*
   The sum of the R- and S-wave voltage in each of the limb leads is less than 5 mm.

68. *Low voltage, precordial leads*
   The sum of the R- and S-wave voltage in each of the precordial leads is less than 10 mm.

69. *Electrical alternans*
   A regular alternation of the amplitude of the P, QRS, or T waves, either alone or in combination. The complexes must originate from a single pacemaker.

VI. Intraventricular Conduction Abnormalities

70. *Right bundle branch block, complete*
   □ A QRS duration of 0.12 s or greater.
   □ A secondary R' wave in the right precordial leads with the terminal R' greater than the initial R wave.
   □ Secondary ST-T-wave abnormalities in the right precordial leads.
   Additional supporting findings: Slurred S waves in leads I and aVL and in the left precordial leads.

71. *Right bundle branch block, incomplete*
   Criteria for right bundle branch block, but with a QRS duration of 0.09 to 0.11 s.

72. *Left anterior fascicular block*
   □ Left-axis deviation between −30 and −90 degrees.
   □ A positive terminal deflection in aVL and aVR with the peak of the terminal R wave in aVR occurring later than in aVL.
   □ QRS duration less than 0.12 s (uncomplicated by other diagnoses that prolong the QRS).
   □ No other cause of left-axis deviation.

Additional supporting findings: A qR complex in leads I and aVL; an rS complex in leads II, III, and aVF; and an S wave in lead III larger than that in lead II.

73. *Left posterior fascicular block*
    ☐ Right-axis deviation between +90 and +180 degrees.
    ☐ An rS pattern in lead I and aVL and a qR pattern in leads II, III, and aVF. (Q waves less than 0.04 s in duration.)
    ☐ QRS duration less than 0.12 s (uncomplicated by other diagnoses that prolong the QRS).
    ☐ No other cause of right-axis deviation.
    Additional findings: The R wave in lead III should equal or exceed that in lead II.

74. *Left bundle branch block, complete*
    ☐ QRS duration of 0.12 s or more.
    ☐ Broad, notched, or slurred R waves in leads I, aVL, and V5–V6.
    ☐ Secondary ST-T-wave abnormalities in leads I, aVL, and V5–V6.
    ☐ Absence of Q waves in leads I and V5–V6.
    ☐ R-wave peak time (intrinsicoid deflection) prolonged to 0.06 s or greater measured in leads V5–V6.

75. *Left bundle branch block, incomplete*
    Three of four criteria are required:
    ☐ QRS duration of 0.10 to 0.11 s.
    ☐ Absence of Q waves in leads I and V5–V6.
    ☐ Broad, notched, or slurred R waves in leads I, aVL, and V5–V6.
    ☐ R-wave peak time (intrinsicoid deflection) prolonged to 0.06 s or greater measured in leads V5–V6.

76. *Intraventricular conduction delay (IVCD), nonspecific (includes IVCD associated with chamber enlargement)*
    Prolongation of the QRS duration to 0.11 s or more in the absence of criteria for either left bundle branch block or right bundle branch block.

77. *Probable aberrant intraventricular conduction associated with a supraventricular arrhythmia*
    Transient abnormal intraventricular conduction secondary to partial refractoriness of the intraventricular conduction system.

VII. Ventricular Hypertrophy (or Enlargement)

78. *Left ventricular hypertrophy by voltage criteria with or without associated ST-T-wave abnormalities (acceptable in patients over 40 years of age)*
    ☐ Sum of S wave in leads V1 or V2 and R wave in leads V5 or V6 is greater than 35 mm, or
    (greater than 40 mm for age 30–40 years)
    (greater than 60 mm for age 16–30 years)
    ☐ R wave in lead aVL is greater than 11 mm, or
    ☐ Sum of R wave in lead I and S wave in lead III is greater than 25 mm, or
    ☐ Sum of R wave in lead aVL and S wave in lead V3 is greater than 28 mm in men or 20 mm in women.
    Additional supporting findings: ST-T-wave abnormalities (see criteria no. 103); prolongation of the R-wave peak time (intrinsicoid deflection) to 0.05 s or more in the left precordial leads; left atrial abnormality.

79. *Right ventricular hypertrophy*
    ☐ Right-axis deviation (in the absence of other causes).
    ☐ R-wave voltage greater than S wave in lead V1.
    ☐ R wave in lead V1 is greater than or equal to 7 mm.
    ☐ qR pattern in lead V1.
    ☐ rSR' pattern (with normal QRS duration), with R' greater than 10 mm.
    ☐ The R/S ratio in lead V5 or V6 is less than or equal to 1.
    Additional supporting findings: Delay in the R-wave peak time (intrinsicoid deflection) measured in lead V1 to greater than or equal to 0.04 s; ST depression and T-wave inversion in the right precordial leads; and S wave in lead V1 is less than 2 mm.

80. *Combined ventricular hypertrophy*
    The criteria for left and right ventricular hypertrophy occur together.

VIII. Q-Wave Myocardial Infarction

1. *Old or of Indeterminate Age*
   Old or indeterminate infarction should be identified when there are diagnostic Q waves on the electrocardiogram without associated

ST-segment or T-wave abnormalities to suggest acute or recent injury. Q (or QS) waves are considered diagnostic when they have a width of 0.04 s or more. Diagnostic accuracy is increased when the depth of the Q wave is equal to or greater than 25 percent of the R-wave amplitude in that lead.

2. *Acute or Recent*

Acute infarction is characterized by diagnostic Q waves (or developing Q waves) in conjunction with ST abnormalities of acute myocardial injury. Horizontal or concave down (coved) ST elevation is present in the affected leads (ST depression in leads V1–V2 for posterior infarction). Recent (subacute) infarction is characterized by resolving ST-segment abnormalities associated with T-wave inversion in the infarction leads (upright T wave for posterior infarction). It is often impossible to definitively assess the timing of the infarction without clinical correlation or serial tracings. Multiple patterns as well as those that do not conform exactly to the following diagnoses may be seen.

81–82. *Anteroseptal*
Leads V1–V3.

83–84. *Anterior*
Leads V2–V4.

85–86. *Anterolateral*
Leads V4–V6 (with or without I, aVL).

87–88. *Extensive anterior*
Leads V1–V5 (V6).

89–90. *Lateral or high lateral*
Leads I, aVL.

91–92. *Inferior or diaphragmatic*
Leads II, III, aVF.

93–94. *Posterior*
Tall R waves of 0.04 s or more with R > S leads V1–V2.

95. *Suggestive of ventricular aneurysm*
ST elevation in leads containing Q waves that persists for at least 2 weeks following myocardial infarction.

IX. ST-, T-, U-Wave Abnormalities

96. *Normal variant, isolated J-point elevation (early repolarization pattern)*
Upward displacement of the ST segment at the J junction from 1–4 mm above the isoelectric line. The ST segment demonstrates upward concavity associated with tall, broad, symmetrical upright T waves.

97. *Isolated J-point depression*
Upsloping ST depression at the J junction found in an otherwise normal person.

98. *Normal variant, RSR' pattern lead V1*
☐ The RSR' complex is of normal duration.
☐ A primary R wave in lead V1 is 8 mm or less.
☐ A secondary R' is less than 6 mm.
☐ An R'/S ratio is less than 1 in any right precordial lead.

99. *Normal variant, persistent juvenile T-wave pattern*
Characterized by asymmetrical T-wave inversion in two or more of leads V1–V3 in an otherwise normal adult. T waves remain upright in leads I, II, V5, and V6.

100. *ST- or T-wave abnormality or both suggesting acute or recent myocardial injury*
Horizontal or concave downward (coved) elevation with or without associated T-wave inversion. (Horizontal ST depression with an upright T wave in leads V1–V2 for posterior wall injury.)

101. *ST- or T-wave abnormality or both suggesting either reciprocal change or myocardial ischemia in the setting of acute myocardial injury*
Horizontal or downsloping ST depression with or without T-wave abnormalities in leads opposite to those with ST elevation.

102. *ST- or T-wave abnormality or both suggesting myocardial ischemia in the absence of acute myocardial injury*
Horizontal or downsloping ST depression with or without T-wave inversion in the absence of concomitant ST elevation in additional leads.

103. *ST- or T-wave abnormality or both associated with ventricular hypertrophy*
☐ In left ventricular hypertrophy: ST depression with downward concavity and T-wave inversion in leads where the QRS is mainly positive (e.g., leads V5, V6). Also leads I and aVL with a horizontal axis and leads II, III, and aVF with a vertical axis. Slight ST elevation with upright T waves in leads where the QRS is mainly negative (e.g., leads V1, V2).

- ☐ In right ventricular hypertrophy: ST depression with downward concavity and T-wave inversion in leads V1, V2. Sometimes present in leads II, III, and aVF.

104. *ST- or T-wave abnormality or both associated with ventricular conduction abnormality*
    - ☐ In left bundle branch block: ST depression and T-wave inversion in the left precordial leads.
    - ☐ In right bundle branch block: ST depression and T-wave inversion in the right precordial leads.

105. *ST- or T-wave abnormality or both suggesting early, acute pericarditis*
    Characterized by diffuse ST elevation that is concave upward. The findings are often in multiple leads but are most common in leads I, II, and V5–V6. The absence of reciprocal changes and concomitant T-wave inversion helps to distinguish this from acute myocardial injury. The T wave remains concordant with the direction of the ST segment in early pericarditis.

106. *Nonspecific ST- or T-wave abnormality or both*
    Slight ST depression or elevation or isolated T-wave inversion or other abnormality that cannot be characterized as secondary to a specific abnormality.

107. *Postextrasystolic T-wave abnormality*
    An alteration in the T-wave morphology in the complex following a ventricular premature depolarization.

108. *Peaked T waves*
    The T-wave amplitude is greater than 6 mm in the limb leads or 10 mm in any precordial lead.

109. *Prolonged QT interval for heart rate (QTc)*
    - ☐ The QT interval varies inversely with the heart rate. A number of formulas have been proposed for correcting the QT interval for heart rate variability. All have been called into question. The most commonly used formula for correcting the QT interval for the heart rate (QTc) is Bazett's formula:

    $$QTc = QT \text{ interval (s)/square root of RR interval (s)}$$

    The upper limit of normal for the QTc that has been used for clinical studies is 0.44 s.
    - ☐ The use of Bazett's formula is not always feasible in routine interpretation. A brief approximation for determining the normal limits for the QT interval (uncorrected) has been suggested. This method is to assign an upper limit of 0.40 s for a heart rate of 70 bpm. For every increase or decrease in the heart rate of 10 bpm, subtract 0.02 s from or add 0.02 s to the QT interval, respectively. Measurements that are greater than these values suggest a prolonged QT interval.

110. *Prominent U waves*
    The maximum amplitude of the U wave is usually 1.0 mm, but it may rarely reach 2.0 mm. The amplitude of the U wave is proportional to that of the T wave but should be no greater than 25 percent of the height of the T wave.

111. *Inverted U waves*
    The U wave generally follows the vector of the T wave. U-wave inversion in leads with a normally upright T wave should be considered abnormal.

X. Technical Problems

112. *Incorrect electrode placement*
113. *Artifact due to tremor*

TEST A

A-1

NARRATIVE INTERPRETATION

Rhythm:	**Sinus**
Rate:	**82**
Intervals:	**PR 0.16, QRS 0.08, QT 0.36**
Axis:	**−30 degrees**

Abnormalities

P-wave voltage greater than 2.5 mm, leads II, III, aVF. Limb-lead voltage less than 5 mm. R-wave voltage V1–V3 less than 3 mm.

Synthesis

Sinus rhythm. Low voltage limb leads. Right atrial abnormality. Poor R-wave progression.

TEST ANSWERS: 1, 59, 66, 67.

Comment: Low voltage (the total amplitude of the R and S waves is less than 5 mm in any limb lead) is present in this tracing. Low voltage may be seen in patients with pericardial effusion, myxedema, amyloidosis, profound obesity, chronic obstructive pulmonary disease, and extensive loss of functioning myocardial tissue as might occur after multiple myocardial infarctions. Poor R-wave progression is identified when R waves are present in the anterior precordial leads, but R-wave magnitude is less than 3.0 mm in lead V3. Causes include anterior wall myocardial infarction, left ventricular hypertrophy, right ventricular hypertrophy, left anterior fascicular block, chronic obstructive pulmonary disease (COPD), or normal variants. In this case, the most likely cause of both low voltage and poor R-wave progression is COPD. The tall peaked P waves represent right atrial enlargement secondary to elevated right heart pressures.

FURTHER READING

Kilcoyne MM, Davis AL, Ferrer MI: A dynamic electrocardiographic concept useful in the diagnosis of cor pulmonale. *Circulation* 42:903–924, 1970.

Selvester RH, Rubin HB: New criteria for the electrocardiographic diagnosis of emphysema and cor pulmonale. *Am Heart J* 69:437–447, 1965.

Zema MJ, Kligfield P: ECG poor R-wave progression. *Arch Intern Med* 142:1145–1148, 1982.

A-1

Clinical History

A 79-year-old man with chronic dyspnea. He is a heavy smoker.

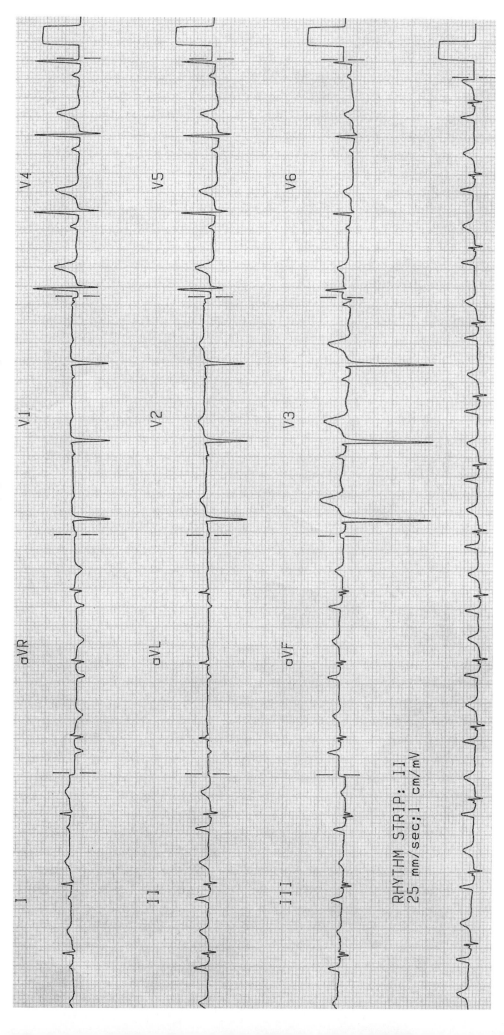

A-2

NARRATIVE INTERPRETATION

> **Rhythm:** Sinus
> **Rate:** 94
> **Intervals:** PR 0.20, QRS 0.08, QT 0.36
> **Axis:** −45 degrees

Abnormalities

APC. VPC. Axis leftward of −30 degrees. R wave V1–V3 less than 3 mm. R wave lead aVL + S wave lead V3 greater than 28 mm in a male. R wave in lead aVL greater than 11 mm. R wave lead I + S wave lead III greater than 25 mm. ST depression, leads I, V6. T-wave inversion, leads I, aVL, V6. T-wave biphasic lead V5.

Synthesis

Sinus rhythm. VPC. APC. Left-axis deviation. Left anterior fascicular block. LVH. Poor R-wave progression. ST-T-wave abnormalities associated with ventricular hypertrophy.

TEST ANSWERS: 1, 10, 26, 64, 66, 72, 78, 103, (106).

Comment: Even though "classic" precordial voltage criteria are absent, the gender-specific Cornell criteria call for a diagnosis of LVH. In addition, multiple limb lead criteria for LVH are present. Remember that left anterior fascicular block (LAFB) tends to mask precordial voltage for LVH in the chest leads while it increases voltage in the limb leads. Criteria for LVH in the presence of LAFB are met in this tracing (S wave lead III greater than 15 mm, R wave lead aVL greater than 13 mm).

The ST-T-wave abnormalities are likely secondary to ventricular hypertrophy, but may also be considered nonspecific.

FURTHER READING

Casale PN, Devereux RB, Kligfield P, et al: Electrocardiographic detection of left ventricular hypertrophy: Development and prospective validation of improved criteria. *J Am Coll Cardiol* 6:572–580, 1985.

Gertsch M, Theler A, Foglia E: Electrocardiographic detection of left ventricular hypertrophy in the presence of left anterior fascicular block. *Am J Cardiol* 61:1098–1101, 1988.

Milliken JA: Isolated and complicated left anterior fascicular block: A review of suggested electrocardiographic criteria. *J Electrocardiol* 16:199–212, 1983.

A-2

Clinical History

A 60-year-old man with long-standing hypertension.

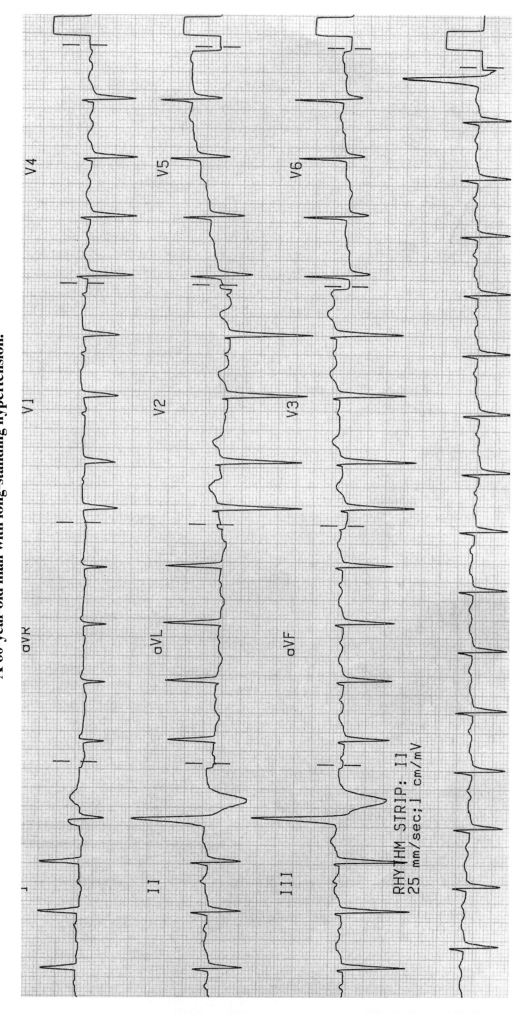

A-3

NARRATIVE INTERPRETATION

Rhythm:	**Sinus with complete AV block; AV junctional escape rhythm**
Rate:	**Sinus rate 98; AV junctional escape rate 43**
Intervals:	**PR −, QRS 0.08, QT 0.44**
Axis:	**+75 degrees**

Abnormalities

P waves nonconducted. AV dissociation. ST elevation leads II, III, aVF. ST depression leads I, aVL, V1–V6. T-wave inversion leads I, aVL, V2–V3. Biphasic T waves leads V4–V6.

Synthesis

Sinus rhythm with complete AV block. Junctional escape rhythm. AV dissociation. Inferior wall myocardial infarction with ST elevation suggestive of acute myocardial injury. ST depression with T-wave inversion in leads I, aVL, and precordial leads compatible with either reciprocal change, myocardial ischemia, or possible posterior myocardial injury.

TEST ANSWERS: 1, 22, 47, 53, 91, (93), 100, 101.

Comment: Remember that AV dissociation is not synonymous with complete heart block. In this example, heart block and AV dissociation are both present. Patients with acute inferior wall myocardial infarction may develop complete AV block as a result of profound vagal influences. In contrast to patients with anterior wall myocardial infarction, this is not a sign of extensive necrosis of the cardiac conduction system. Unless there is hemodynamic compromise, temporary pacemaker therapy is usually not required. Complete AV block in the setting of acute inferior myocardial infarction is usually transient and resolves within several days.

FURTHER READING

Berger PB, Ruocco NA Jr, Ryan TJ, et al: Incidence and prognostic implications of heart block complicating inferior myocardial infarction treated with thrombolytic therapy: Results from TIMI II. *J Am Coll Cardiol* 20:533–540, 1992.

Nicod P, Gilpin E, Dittrich H, et al: Long-term outcome in patients with inferior myocardial infarction and complete atrioventricular block. *J Am Coll Cardiol* 12:589–594, 1988.

A-3

Clinical History

A 52-year-old man with chest pain and hypotension.

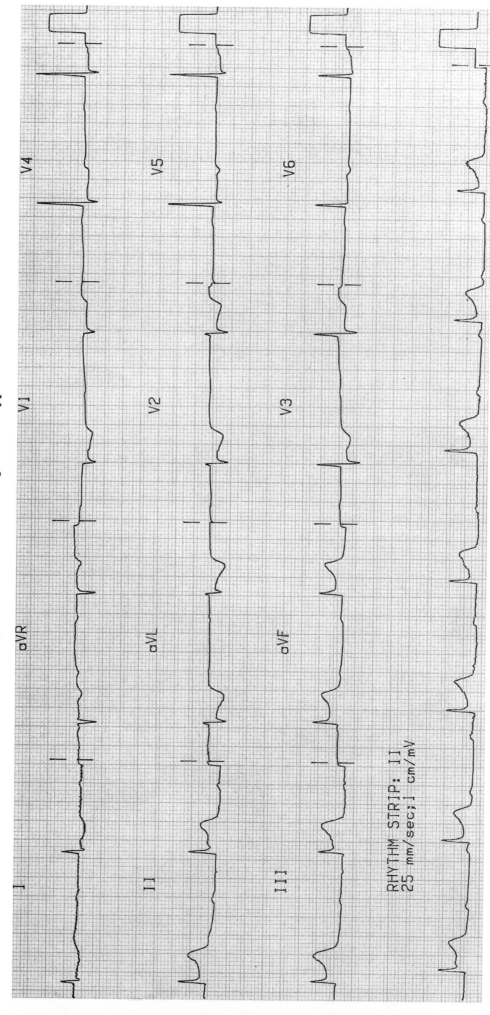

15

A-4

NARRATIVE INTERPRETATION

Rhythm:	**Sinus**
Rate:	**98**
Intervals:	**PR 0.18, QRS 0.08, QT 0.36**
Axis:	**+15 degrees**

Abnormalities

Increased P-wave voltage leads II, III, aVF, V1. R wave lead V5 + S wave lead V1 greater than 60 mm. ST depression I, aVL, V4–V6. T-wave inversion I, aVL. Peaked, "tent-shaped" T waves most prominent in precordial leads. QT interval prolonged for heart rate.

Synthesis

Sinus rhythm. Right atrial abnormality. LVH by voltage criteria. Nonspecific ST-T-wave abnormalities. Peaked T waves suggestive of hyperkalemia. Prolonged QTc interval.

TEST ANSWERS: 1, 59, 78, (103), 106, 108, 109.

Comment: The tall, narrow, peaked T waves noted in this example are characteristic of hyperkalemia. This patient had a serum potassium of 7.6 mEq/L. Other electrocardiographic abnormalities may be observed in patients with hyperkalemia including a prolonged QRS duration and a decreased P-wave amplitude. This patient had a P pulmonale pattern despite hyperkalemia. Interestingly, the P pulmonale pattern may occasionally represent left atrial enlargement. Such was the case in this patient.

When considering LVH in young patients, remember that different precordial voltage criteria must be used. In patients 16 to 30 years of age, precordial voltage up to 60 mm may be seen. This patient had values exceeding this.

FURTHER READING

Manning GW, Smiley JR: QRS voltage criteria for left ventricular hypertrophy in a normal male population. *Circulation* 29:224–230, 1964.

Walker CHM, Rose RL: Importance of age, sex, and body habitus in the diagnosis of left ventricular hypertrophy from the precordial electrocardiogram in childhood and adolescence. *Pediatrics* 28:705–711, 1961.

A-4

Clinical History

A 21-year-old man with end-stage renal disease.

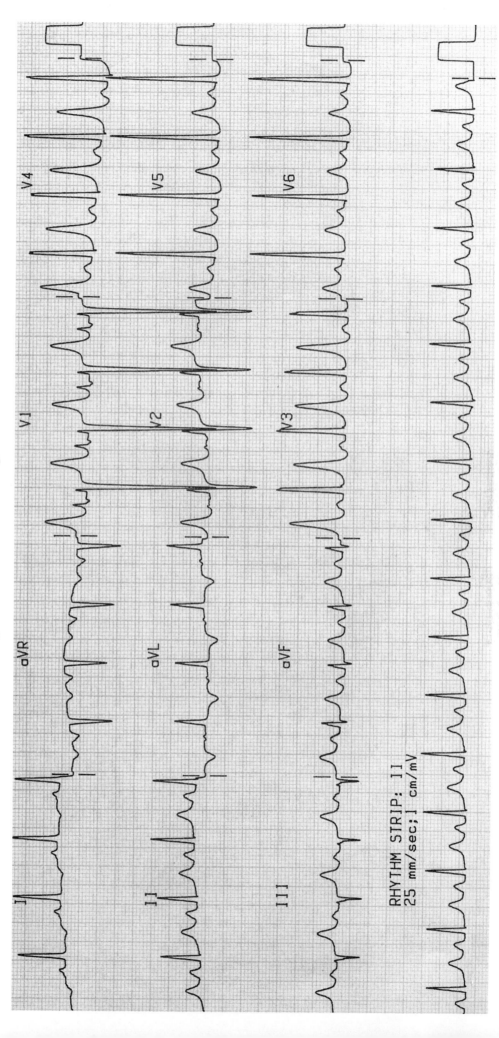

NARRATIVE INTERPRETATION A-5

> **Rhythm:** **Sinus with first-degree AV block**
> **Rate:** **75**
> **Intervals:** **PR 0.26, QRS 0.06, QT 0.40**
> **Axis:** **+105 degrees**

Abnormalities

Prolonged PR interval. Axis rightward of +90. R wave greater than S wave leads V1–V3. T-wave inversion leads V1–V3. ST depression leads II, III, aVF, V3–V6. Biphasic T wave leads V4–V5. Ventricular pacemaker complexes, rate 60, with occasional capture. Ventricular pacemaker malfunction with failure to sense. Pacemaker fusion complexes.

Synthesis

Sinus rhythm with first-degree AV block. Right-axis deviation. RVH with associated ST-T-wave abnormalities. Additional nonspecific ST-T-wave abnormalities. Ventricular pacemaker complexes with intermittent capture. Pacemaker fusion complexes. Pacemaker malfunction, failure to sense.

TEST ANSWERS: 1, 40, 42, 56, 65, 79, 103, 106.

Comment: This tracing suggests a diagnosis of cor pulmonale secondary to obstructive airways disease. An axis rightward of +90 degrees is unusual in patients over the age of 40 and suggests RVH, particularly in view of the tall R waves in the right precordial leads. The ST depression and T-wave inversion in the right precordial leads are also associated with RVH. The ST-T-wave findings in other leads may be considered nonspecific.

The pacemaker demonstrates complete sensing failure and is functioning independently of the native rhythm. It captures the ventricle when it does not fall within the ventricular refractory period, but it is not functioning "on demand." This activity results in occasional pacemaker fusion complexes, seen best in the rhythm strip. Note the occasional pacemaker capture beats interpolated between two sinus complexes. The next two complexes show a prolonged PR interval due to concealed retrograde conduction into the AV junction.

FURTHER READING

Kilcoyne MM, Davis AL, Ferrer MI: A dynamic electrocardiographic concept useful in the diagnosis of cor pulmonale. *Circulation* 42:903–924, 1970.

Schmock CL, Mitchell RS, Pomerantz B, et al: The electrocardiogram in emphysema with and without chronic airways obstruction. *Chest* 60:328–334, 1971.

Schmock CL, Mitchell RS, Pomerantz B, et al: The electrocardiogram in chronic airways obstruction. *Chest* 60:335–340, 1971.

Selvester RH, Rubin HB: New criteria for the electrocardiographic diagnosis of emphysema and cor pulmonale. *Am Heart J* 69:437–447, 1965.

A-5

Clinical History

An 83-year-old man with a recently implanted pacemaker. He has a history of heavy smoking.

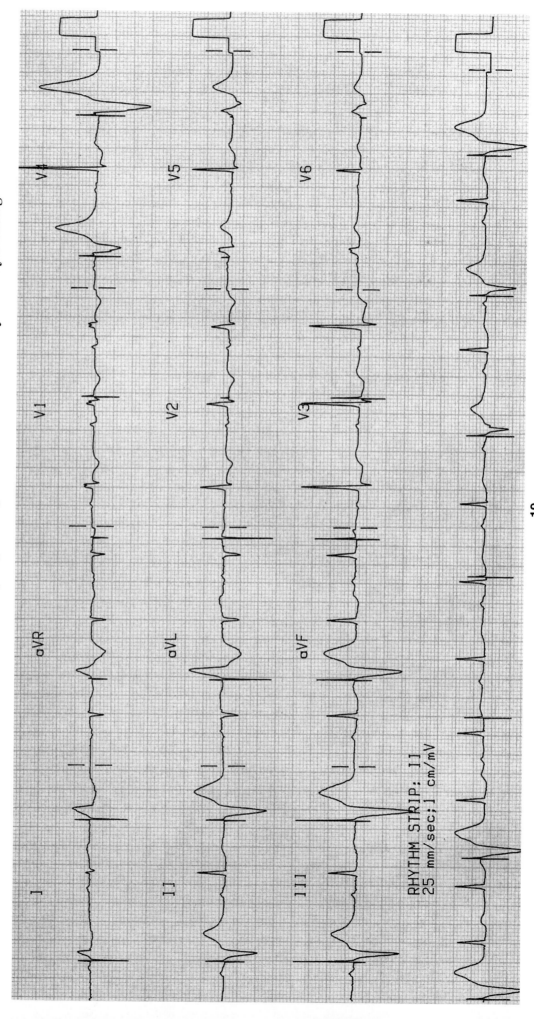

A-6

NARRATIVE INTERPRETATION

Rhythm:	**Sinus with second-degree AV block, Mobitz type I**
Rate:	**90**
Intervals:	**PR 0.20, QRS 0.07, QT 0.34**
Axis:	**−30 degrees**

Abnormalities
Progressive increase in PR interval with eventual failure to conduct P wave. R wave less than 3 mm leads V1–V3.

Synthesis
Sinus rhythm with second-degree AV block, Mobitz type I. Poor R-wave progression.

TEST ANSWERS: 1, 43, 66.

Comment: This patient demonstrates second-degree AV block, Mobitz type I (Wenckebach). In classic Wenckebach, there is progressive lengthening of the PR interval until the P wave fails to conduct to the ventricles. Additional features include a shortening of the RR interval, with the RR interval containing the blocked P wave less than twice the sum of two PP intervals. As seen in this example, Mobitz type I, second-degree AV block can occur without all the features of the Wenckebach phenomenon. Note that the RR intervals at first shorten and then lengthen prior to the blocked P wave. The PR interval increases in the second complex after the pause but does not progressively lengthen prior to the dropped QRS.

The site of origin of the conduction abnormality in patients with second-degree AV block, type I, and a narrow QRS complex is usually the AV node.

FURTHER READING

Hecht HH, Kossmann CE, Childers RW, et al: Atrioventricular and intraventricular conduction: Revised nomenclature and concepts. *Am J Cardiol* 31:232–244, 1973.

Zipes DP: Second-degree atrioventricular block. *Circulation* 60:465–472, 1979.

A-6

Clinical History

A 68-year-old woman with a history of palpitations.

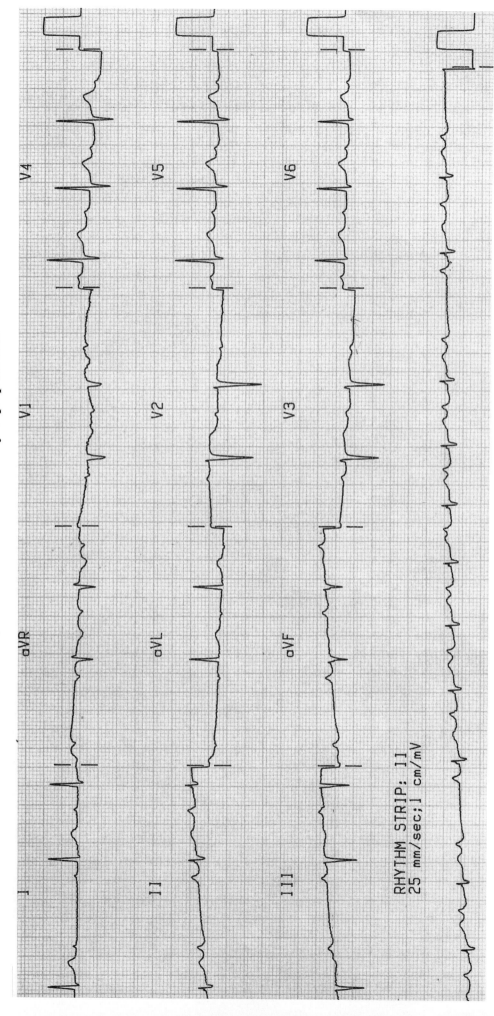

NARRATIVE INTERPRETATION A-7

Rhythm:	**Accelerated AV junctional rhythm**
Rate:	**77**
Intervals:	**PR 0.10, QRS 0.07, QT 0.34**
Axis:	**+30 degrees**

Abnormalities

Inverted P waves leads II, III, aVF with short PR interval. R wave less than 3 mm leads V1–V4. T-wave inversion leads II, III, aVF, V5–V6.

Synthesis

Accelerated AV junctional rhythm. Poor R-wave progression. (Probable anteroseptal wall myocardial infarction, old or indeterminate age.) Nonspecific T-wave abnormalities.

TEST ANSWERS: 23, 66, (82), 106.

Comment: The poor R-wave progression in this patient is most likely from a prior anteroseptal wall MI. This diagnosis is supported by a history of coronary artery disease and the absence of significant R-wave voltage in the anterior precordium. It is the author's practice to add *probable* when making this diagnosis on the basis of poor R-wave progression alone in the absence of Q waves. The additional ST-T-wave abnormalities suggest potential coronary artery disease; however, they are nonspecific and not diagnostic. This patient was known to have sustained a prior anterior wall MI and was prescribed verapamil to control angina and supraventricular arrhythmias.

Remember that in an AV junctional rhythm, the inverted P wave can occur either before, after, or within the QRS complex. By definition, the higher than expected rate of the AV junctional rhythm qualifies it as *accelerated.*

FURTHER READING

DePace NL, Colby J, Hakki A, et al: Poor R-wave progression in the precordial leads: Clinical implications for the diagnosis of myocardial infarction. *J Am Coll Cardiol* 2:1073–1079, 1983.

Warner RA, Reger M, Hill NE, et al: Electrocardiographic criteria for the diagnosis of anterior myocardial infarction: Importance of the duration of precordial R waves. *Am J Cardiol* 52:690–692, 1983.

Zema MJ, Kligfield P: Electrocardiographic poor R-wave progression. I. Correlation with the Frank vectorcardiogram. *J Electrocardiol* 12:3–10, 1979.

Zema MJ, Kligfield P: Electrocardiographic poor R-wave progression. II. Correlation with angiography. *J Electrocardiol* 12:11–15, 1979.

A-7

Clinical History

An asymptomatic 70-year-old man who has been treated with a calcium channel blocking agent for a history of angina.

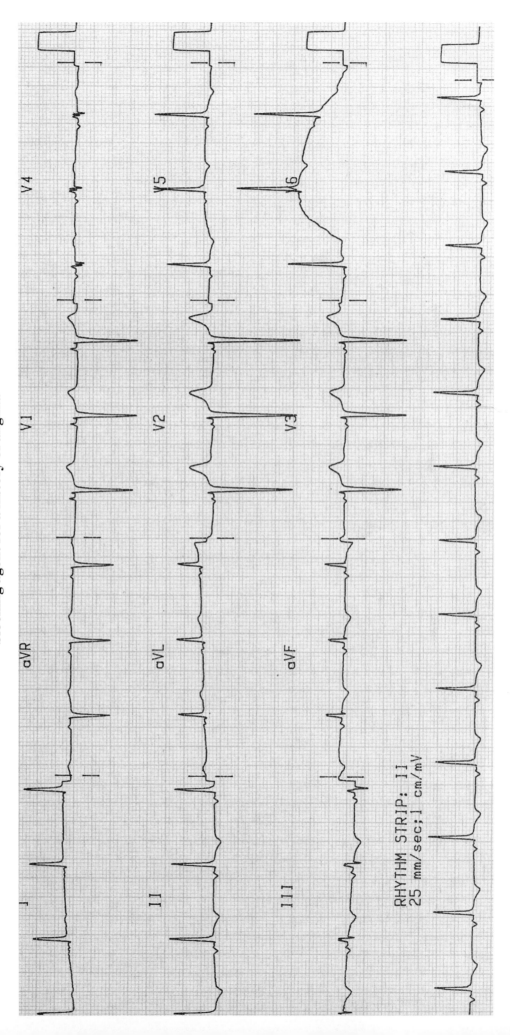

A-8

NARRATIVE INTERPRETATION

Rhythm:	**Sinus**
Rate:	**98**
Intervals:	**PR 0.14, QRS 0.08, QT 0.32**
Axis:	**+45 degrees**

Abnormalities
T waves inverted V1–V4.

Synthesis
Sinus rhythm. Normal variant, persistent juvenile T-wave pattern.

TEST ANSWERS: 1, 99.

Comment: In infants and children, the T-wave vector in the horizontal plane is oriented leftward and posterior; hence, T-wave inversion is normally seen in the right and midprecordial leads. With increasing age, the T-wave vector becomes anterior and T waves become upright. In the frontal plane, the normal T-wave vector is leftward and inferior, therefore T waves are always upright in leads I and II. In adults, the T wave is upright in the precordial leads. Lead V1 is an exception, where T-wave inversion is normal. Normal individuals who demonstrate T-wave inversion in two or more of leads V1–V3 are described as having a persistent juvenile pattern.

FURTHER READING
Blackman NS, Kuskin L: Inverted T waves in the precordial electrocardiogram of normal adolescents. *Am Heart J* 67:304–312, 1964.

A-8

Clinical History

A 16-year-old healthy female with atypical chest pain.

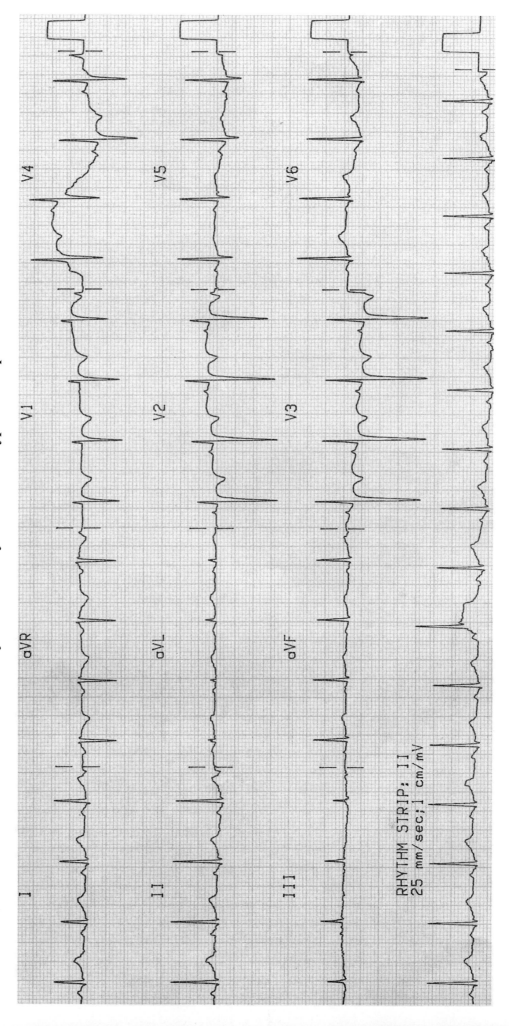

RHYTHM STRIP: II
25 mm/sec; 1 cm/mV

A-9

NARRATIVE INTERPRETATION

Rhythm:	**Sinus bradycardia**
Rate:	**50**
Intervals:	**PR 0.16, QRS 0.08, QT 0.42**
Axis:	**+60 degrees**

Abnormalities

Heart rate less than 60 bpm. APCs. Abnormal P terminal force V1. Biphasic T-wave lead II, T-wave inversion leads III, aVF.

Synthesis

Sinus bradycardia. APCs normally conducted. Left atrial abnormality. Nonspecific T-wave abnormalities.

TEST ANSWERS: 3, 10, 60, 106.

Comment: Note the U waves in the precordial leads. The U wave is a low-amplitude deflection that follows the T wave. Its amplitude is normally 5 to 25 percent that of the preceding T wave. It is considered abnormal if the amplitude of the U wave is 1.5 mm in any lead. The U waves in this example are within normal limits. Common causes of prominent U waves include bradycardia, hypokalemia, LVH, central nervous system abnormalities, and mitral valve prolapse.

FURTHER READING

Lepeschkin E: The U wave of the electrocardiogram. *Mod Concepts Cardiovasc Dis* 38:39–45, 1969.

A-9

Clinical History

A 75-year-old man with a history of palpitations.

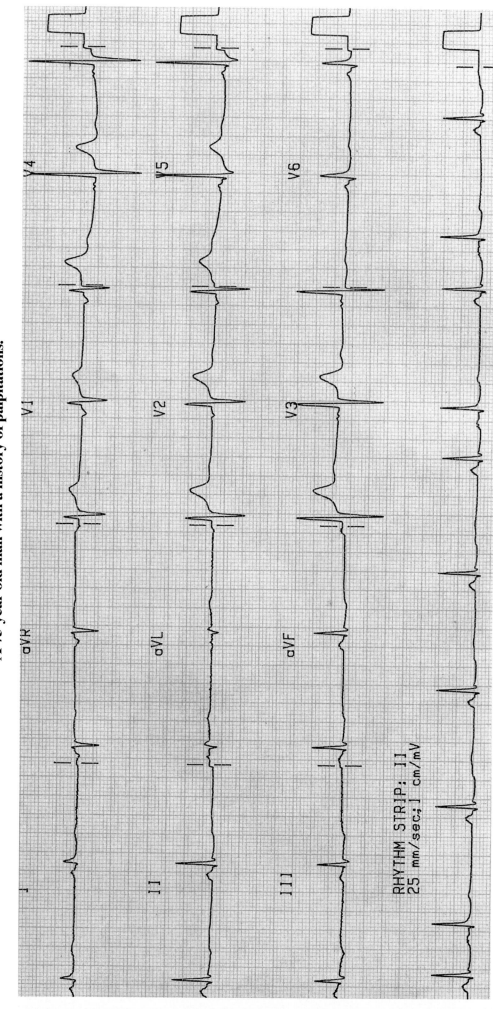

A-10

NARRATIVE INTERPRETATION

Rhythm:	**Sinus, with first-degree AV block**
Rate:	**65**
Intervals:	**PR 0.26, QRS 0.08, QT 0.38**
Axis:	**+75 degrees**

Abnormalities
Prolonged PR interval. VPC. APC.

Synthesis
Sinus rhythm with first-degree AV block. VPC. APC.

TEST ANSWERS: 1, 10, 26, 42.

Comment: First-degree AV block is the most common cardiac conduction abnormality. It is frequently seen in older patients in the absence of clinical cardiac disease. In patients with a narrow QRS complex, the conduction abnormality usually lies within the AV node. Asymptomatic first-degree AV block is usually clinically insignificant. Pharmacologic agents such as digoxin, beta-blockers, diltiazem, and verapamil may further depress cardiac conduction and produce more significant heart block.

Do not forget to carefully review the rhythm strip of each tracing. The APC seen in the second complex of the rhythm strip could easily be overlooked.

FURTHER READING

Mymin D, Matewson FAL, Tate RB, Manfreda J: The natural history of primary first-degree atrioventricular heart block. *N Engl J Med* 315:1183–1187, 1986.

A-10

Clinical History
A 78-year-old asymptomatic woman.

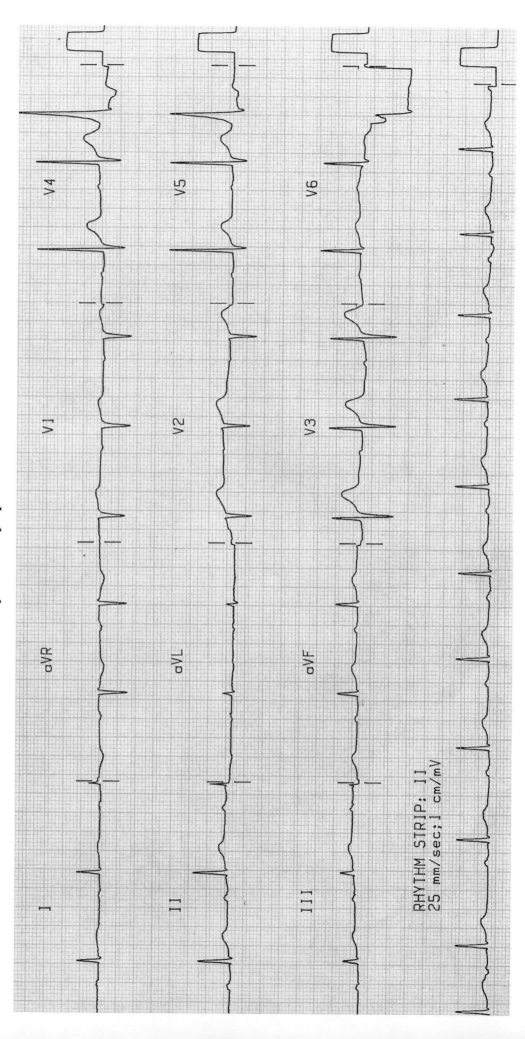

NARRATIVE INTERPRETATION A-11

Rhythm:	**Atrial tachycardia with variable conduction**
Rate:	**Atrial rate 175, average ventricular rate 75**
Intervals:	**PR variable, QRS 0.16, QT 0.40**
Axis:	**+15 degrees**

Abnormalities

Progressive prolongation of PR interval in conducted beats with eventual loss of conduction. Wide, notched QRS with associated ST-T-wave abnormalities leads I, aVL, V5–V6. (S wave lead V2 + R wave lead V6 greater than 45 mm.)

Synthesis

Atrial tachycardia with variable conduction. Wenckebach phenomenon. LBBB with associated ST-T-wave changes. (Marked increased precordial voltage in the presence of LBBB, consider LVH.)

TEST ANSWERS: 17, (50, 51), 74, (78), 104.

Comment: The diagnosis of atrial tachycardia with "block" would have been very difficult in this patient had there not been a period of increased block (decreased conduction). This uncovered the P waves buried in the QRS complex during 2:1 AV conduction. One could have easily mistaken this rhythm for sinus with first-degree AV block. There is a gradual prolongation in the PR intervals of the conducted beats until a P wave fails to conduct to the ventricles, an example of the Wenckebach phenomenon.

There is a variable conduction ratio in this example. An AV conduction ratio of 2:1 is a physiologic property of the AV node at atrial rates approaching 200 bpm. The superimposed Wenckebach phenomenon seen here produces a higher conduction ratio and is nonphysiologic. First-degree AV block should not be diagnosed in this example because of the presence of higher degrees of block. The combination of conduction abnormalities and rhythm disturbance seen here is often due to digitalis toxicity.

An additional finding in this example is the markedly increased precordial QRS voltage. Some studies suggest that LVH may be diagnosed in the presence of left bundle branch block if the sum of the voltage of the S wave in V2 and the R wave in V6 exceeds 45 mm. In the author's opinion, it is better to consider this as suggestive, but not diagnostic of LVH.

FURTHER READING

Kafka H, Burggraf GW, Milliken JA: Electrocardiographic diagnosis of left ventricular hypertrophy in the presence of left bundle branch block: An echocardiographic study. *Am J Cardiol* 55:103–106, 1985.

Klein RC, Vera Z, DeMaria JA, Mason DT: Electrocardiographic diagnosis of left ventricular hypertrophy in the presence of left bundle branch block. *Am Heart J* 108:502–506, 1984.

Vandenberg BF, Romhilt DW: Electrocardiographic diagnosis of left ventricular hypertrophy in the presence of bundle branch block. *Am Heart J* 122:818–822, 1991.

A-11

Clinical History

A 65-year-old woman taking digoxin for congestive heart failure.

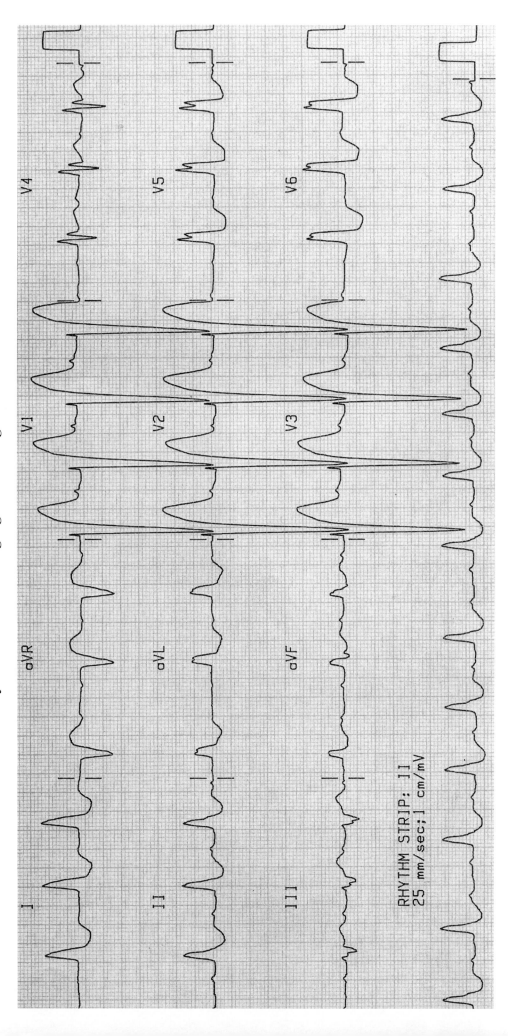

RHYTHM STRIP: II
25 mm/sec; 1 cm/mV

A-12

NARRATIVE INTERPRETATION

Rhythm:	**Atrial tachycardia, regular 1:1 conduction, sustained**
Rate:	**158**
Intervals:	**PR 0.14, QRS 0.06, QT 0.24**
Axis:	**+75 degrees**

Abnormalities
Rapid heart rate. Electrical alternans.

Synthesis
Atrial tachycardia, sustained. Electrical alternans.

TEST ANSWERS: 15, 69.

Comment: Note the alternating heights of the QRS complexes, a finding known as electrical alternans. This finding is highly suggestive that the arrhythmia utilizes an atrial-ventricular bypass tract. One review found that such a bypass tract was present in 92 percent of narrow complex tachycardias that exhibited QRS alternans. The presence of electrical alternans is very helpful in distinguishing the rhythm in this tracing as a supraventricular tachycardia, rather than simply a sinus tachycardia. Electrical alternans may also be seen in pericardial tamponade.

FURTHER READING

Green M, Heddle B, Dassen W, et al: Value of QRS alternation in determining the site of origin of narrow QRS supraventricular tachycardia. *Circulation* 68:368–373, 1983.

Kalbfleisch SJ, El-Atassi R, Calkins H, et al: Differentiation of paroxysmal narrow QRS complex tachycardias using the 12-lead electrocardiogram. *J Am Coll Cardiol* 21:85–89, 1993.

Kremers MS, Miller JM, Josephson ME: Electrical alternans in wide complex tachycardias. *Am J Cardiol* 56:305–308, 1985.

A-12

Clinical History

A 26-year-old woman with palpitations. Chest x ray and echocardiogram are normal.

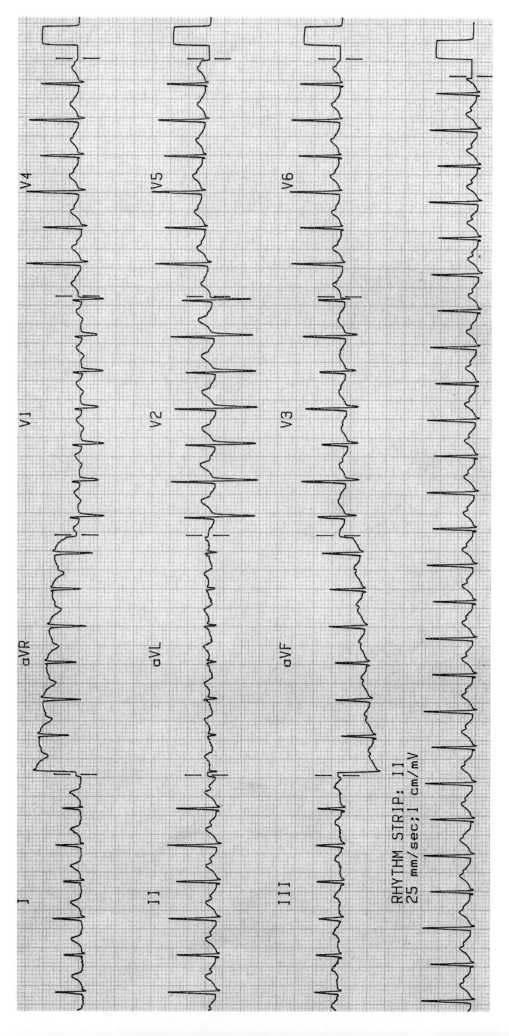

A-13

NARRATIVE INTERPRETATION

Rhythm:	**Atrial fibrillation**
Rate:	**105 (average)**
Intervals:	**PR −, QRS 0.08, QT 0.28**
Axis:	**−30 degrees**

Abnormalities

S wave lead V2 + R wave lead V5 greater than 35 mm. R wave lead aVL + S wave lead V3 greater than 20 mm in a female. ST-segment depression leads I, II, aVF, V4–V6. T-wave inversion leads I, aVL, V6.

Synthesis

Atrial fibrillation with a moderate ventricular response. LVH by voltage criteria and associated ST-T-wave abnormalities. (ST-T-wave abnormalities suggestive of possible myocardial ischemia.)

TEST ANSWERS: 20, 50, 78, (102), 103.

Comment: Note the horizontal ST depression in leads V5 and V6. This is not the classic *strain* ST-segment pattern of LVH, which is a depressed ST segment with upward concavity associated with T-wave inversion in the left precordial leads. The ST-configuration in the present example is different and the interpreter should consider LVH with superimposed ischemia. Serial tracings and clinical history would be necessary to determine the diagnosis.

Note that a ventricular rate of approximately 100 to 180 bpm is a normal, physiologic response in a patient with atrial fibrillation.

FURTHER READING

Hurst JW: Abnormalities of the S-T segment Part I. *Clin Cardiol* 20:511–520, 1997.
Hurst JW: Abnormalities of the S-T segment Part II. *Clin Cardiol* 20:595–600, 1997.

A-13

Clinical History

A 75-year-old asymptomatic woman with a long history of hypertension.

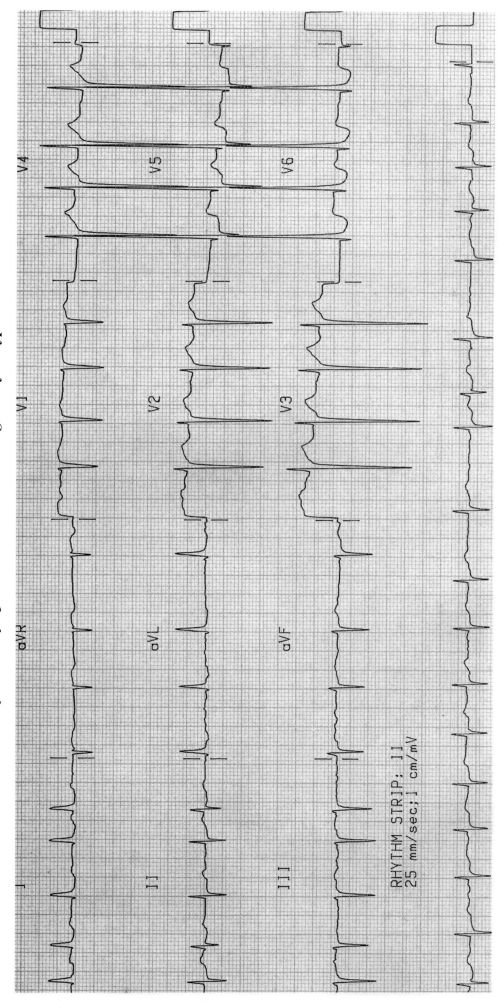

RHYTHM STRIP: II
25 mm/sec; 1 cm/mV

A-14

NARRATIVE INTERPRETATION

Rhythm:	**Sinus with wandering atrial pacemaker to the AV junction**
Rate:	**Sinus rate 74, AV junctional rate 76**
Intervals:	**PR 0.14, QRS 0.08, QT 0.34**
Axis:	**+60 degrees**

Abnormalities
Change in P-wave configuration with development of inverted P waves in lead II with short PR interval.

Synthesis
Sinus rhythm with wandering atrial pacemaker to the AV junction. Otherwise within normal limits.

TEST ANSWERS: 1, 6, (23).

Comment: This is a clinically insignificant rhythm in this young, athletically trained patient. Note that the rate of the ectopic pacemaker is slightly faster than the sinus rate and *usurps* control for a period of time. The first three complexes in leads II and III of the tracing best demonstrate a *wandering* to the AV junction. Note that the second P-wave configuration is intermediate between the normal P wave and the inverted AV junctional morphology. In this athlete, the sinus node is most likely suppressed by vagal influences from physical training, and a subsidiary pacemaker in the AV junction temporarily takes over.

FURTHER READING
Zehender M, Meinertz T, Keul J, Just H: ECG variants and cardiac arrhythmias in athletes: Clinical relevance and prognostic importance. *Am Heart J* 119:1378–1391, 1990.

Clinical History

A 16-year-old asymptomatic female high school basketball player.

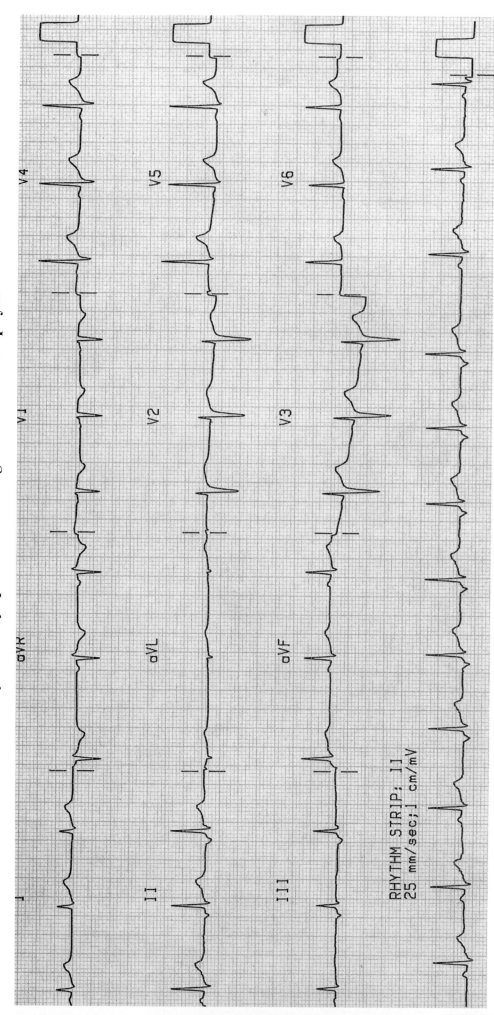

A-15

NARRATIVE INTERPRETATION

Rhythm:	**Sinus**
Rate	**70**
Intervals:	**PR 0.11, QRS 0.12, QT 0.40**
Axis:	**−45 degrees**

Abnormalities
Short PR interval with delta waves and wide QRS complex and generalized ST-T-wave abnormalities.

Synthesis
Sinus rhythm. Ventricular preexcitation (WPW pattern).

TEST ANSWERS: 1, 49.

Comment: The WPW pattern has been observed in approximately 0.2 percent of otherwise healthy individuals. Preexcitation may be confused with other electrocardiographic diagnoses. Note the pseudoinfarction pattern in leads III and aVF, that "imitates" inferior wall MI. The configuration in lead V1 might also be confused with RBBB. In otherwise healthy persons, the incidence of symptomatic tachyarrhythmias is estimated to be approximately 12 percent. Studies of hospitalized patients with WPW show an incidence of arrhythmias between 40 and 80 percent. There is evidence to suggest that preexcitation may disappear over time. In some subsets of asymptomatic patients, electrophysiologic testing and ablation may be beneficial.

FURTHER READING

Barrett PA, Peter CT, Swan HJC, et al: The frequency and prognostic significance of electrocardiographic abnormalities in clinically normal individuals. *Prog Cardiovasc Dis* 23:299–319, 1981.

Krahn AD, Manfreda J, Tate RB, et al: The natural history of electrocardiographic preexcitation in men. *Ann Intern Med* 116:456–460, 1992.

Horowitz LN: Electrophysiologic evaluation of patients with preexcitation syndromes. *Cardiol Clin* 4:447–457, 1986.

Pappone C, Santinelli V, Rosanio S, et al: Usefulness of invasive electrophysiologic testing to stratify the risk of arrhythmic events in asymptomatic patients with Wolff-Parkinson-White pattern. *J Am Coll Cardiol* 41: 239–244, 2003.

A-15

Clinical History

A 34-year-old man with Down's syndrome who complains of chest pain.

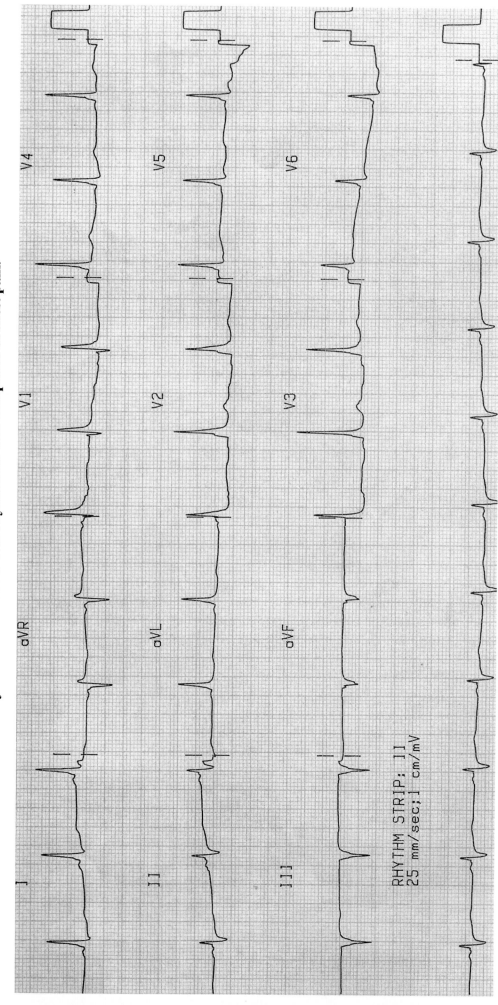

A-16

NARRATIVE INTERPRETATION

Rhythm:	**Sinus**
Rate:	**72**
Intervals:	**PR 0.18, QRS 0.08, QT 0.38**
Axis:	**−15 degrees**

Abnormalities
VPCs. QS waves leads V1–V2. Small R wave lead V3. Fusion beats.

Synthesis
Sinus rhythm. Anterior wall MI of indeterminate age. VPCs uniform. Fusion complexes.

TEST ANSWERS: 1, 26, 56, 82.

Comment: The rhythm strip provides an excellent example of fusion of supraventricular conduction with "late," uniform VPCs. The fusion complexes have a variable morphology because of slight variations in the sinus rate and extent of AV conduction prior to the VPC.

A-16

Clinical History

An 80-year-old man with dyspnea on exertion.

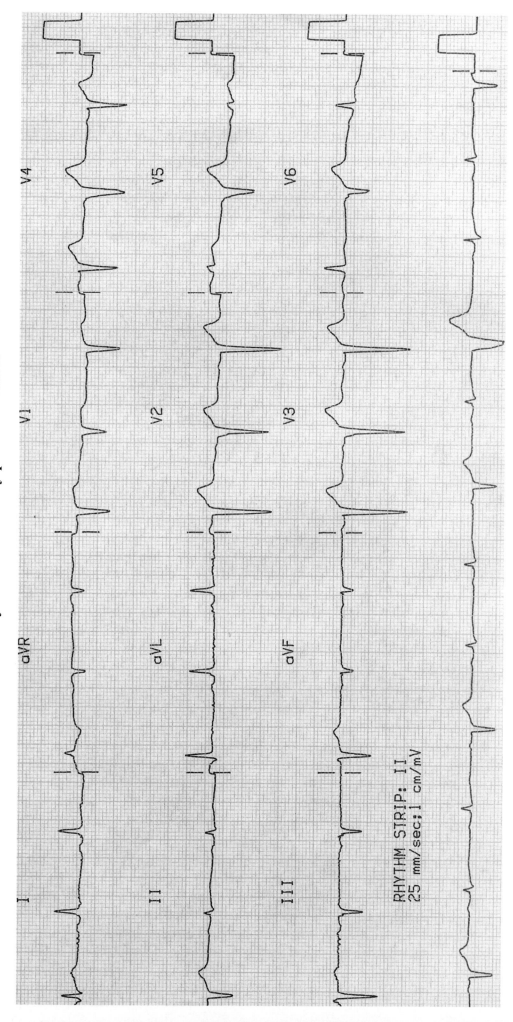

A-17

NARRATIVE INTERPRETATION

Rhythm:	**Sinus**
Rate:	**68**
Intervals:	**PR 0.14, QRS 0.08, QT 0.38**
Axis:	**+15 degrees**

Abnormalities
R wave greater than S wave leads V1 and V2. Flat T wave leads I, aVL, V6.

Synthesis
Sinus rhythm. Posterior wall MI of indeterminate age. Nonspecific T abnormalities.

TEST ANSWERS: 1, 94, 106.

Comment: This tracing demonstrates an isolated posterior wall MI. Tall R waves in the right precordial leads may also be seen in persons with RVH. An upright T wave in lead V1 or concomitant evidence of inferior wall MI supports the former diagnosis. This patient had a confirmed posterior wall MI secondary to occlusion of the left circumflex coronary artery.

FURTHER READING

Chaitman BR: Posterior myocardial infarction revisited. *J Am Coll Cardiol* 12:1167–1168, 1988.

Eisenstein I, Sammarco ME, Madrid WL, Selvester RH: Electrocardiographic and vectorcardiographic diagnosis of posterior wall myocardial infarction. *Chest* 88:409–416, 1985.

Huey BL, Beller GA, Kaiser DL, Gibson RS: A comprehensive analysis of myocardial infarction due to left circumflex artery occlusion: Comparison with infarction due to right coronary artery and left anterior descending artery occlusion. *J Am Coll Cardiol* 12:1156–1166, 1988.

A-17

Clinical History

A 55-year-old man with a history of a myocardial infarction.

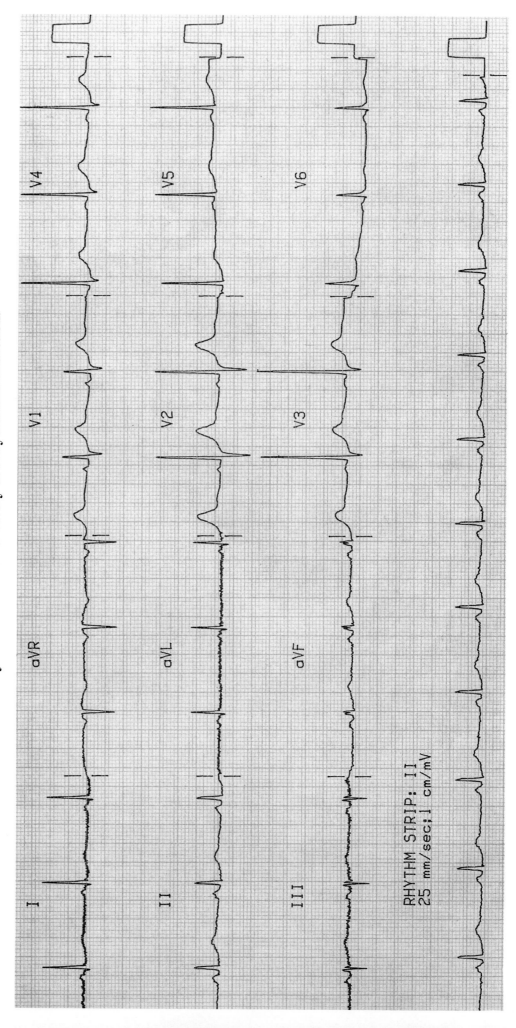

43

A-18

NARRATIVE INTERPRETATION

Rhythm:	**Wide complex tachycardia suggestive of ventricular tachycardia**
Rate:	**140**
Intervals:	**PR −, QRS 0.16, QT 0.36**
Axis:	**+210 degrees**

Abnormalities
No P waves evident. Wide complex rhythm. Axis rightward of +90 degrees.

Synthesis
Ventricular tachycardia. Right-axis deviation.

TEST ANSWERS: 30, 65.

Comment: Remember that wide complex rhythms must be regarded as ventricular in origin until proven otherwise. This is especially true in patients with a history of coronary heart disease or left ventricular dysfunction. The fact that this patient was hemodynamically stable should not dissuade one from first considering ventricular tachycardia, rather than supraventricular tachycardia with aberrant conduction. Electrocardiographic clues to ventricular tachycardia include the markedly prolonged QRS duration and the RS pattern in lead V1.

FURTHER READING
Akhtar M, Shenasa M, Jazayeri M, et al: Wide QRS complex tachycardia. *Ann Intern Med* 109:905–912, 1988.

Brugada P, Brugada J, Mont L, et al: A new approach to the differential diagnosis of a regular tachycardia with a wide QRS complex. *Circulation* 83:1649–1659, 1991.

Tchou P, Young P, Mahmud R, et al: Useful clinical criteria for the diagnosis of ventricular tachycardia. *Am J Med* 84:53–56, 1988

Wellens HJJ, Barr FWHM, Lie KI: The value of the electrocardiogram in the differential diagnosis of a tachycardia with a widened QRS complex. *Am J Med* 84:27–33, 1978.

A-18

Clinical History

A 64-year-old man who walks into the emergency room complaining of lightheadedness. He has a history of a myocardial infarction.

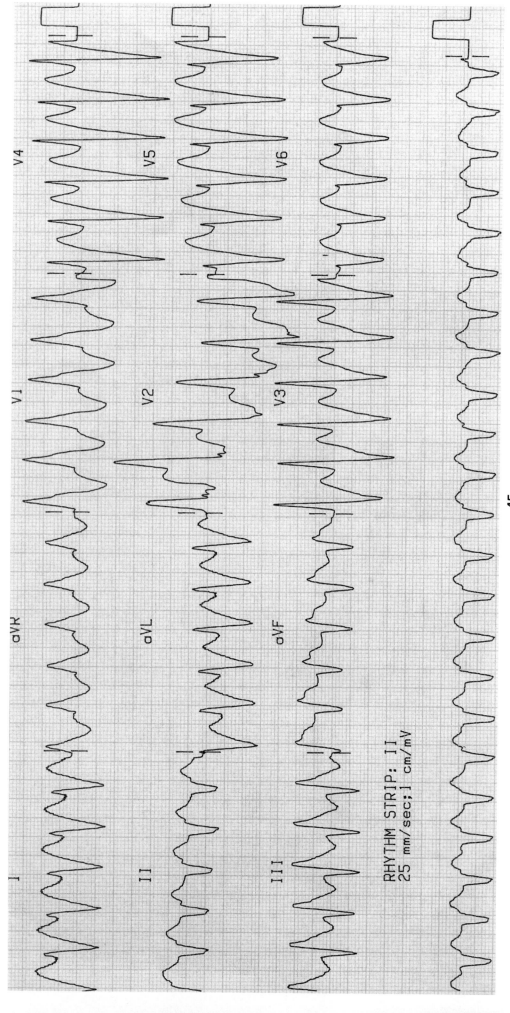

A-19

NARRATIVE INTERPRETATION

Rhythm:	**Sinus**
Rate:	**85**
Intervals:	**PR 0.14, QRS 0.08, QT 0.32**
Axis:	**+60 degrees**

Abnormalities

ST elevation leads I, aVL, V2–V6. Biphasic T waves leads I, aVL, V2–V3, V6. Inverted T waves leads V4–V5.

Synthesis

Sinus rhythm. ST-T-wave abnormalities suggestive of acute or recent myocardial injury.

TEST ANSWERS: 1, 100.

Comment: Note that these T-wave changes involve the entire precordium as well as leads I and aVL. They suggest myocardial injury and should not be identified as juvenile T-wave changes, a normal variant. The ST segments in leads I and aVL as well as the entire precordium are slightly elevated and show abnormal downward concavity. Such findings suggest early MI. This patient had further ischemic changes and subsequently developed a non-Q-wave MI. On coronary angiography, he had a subtotal occlusion of the proximal left anterior descending artery.

The ST abnormalities of pericarditis are sometimes difficult to distinguish from those of myocardial injury. In pericarditis, the ST-segment elevation is usually concave upward. The presence of PR depression is another clue for pericarditis.

A-19

Clinical History

A 36-year-old man with atypical chest pain and mild dyspnea.

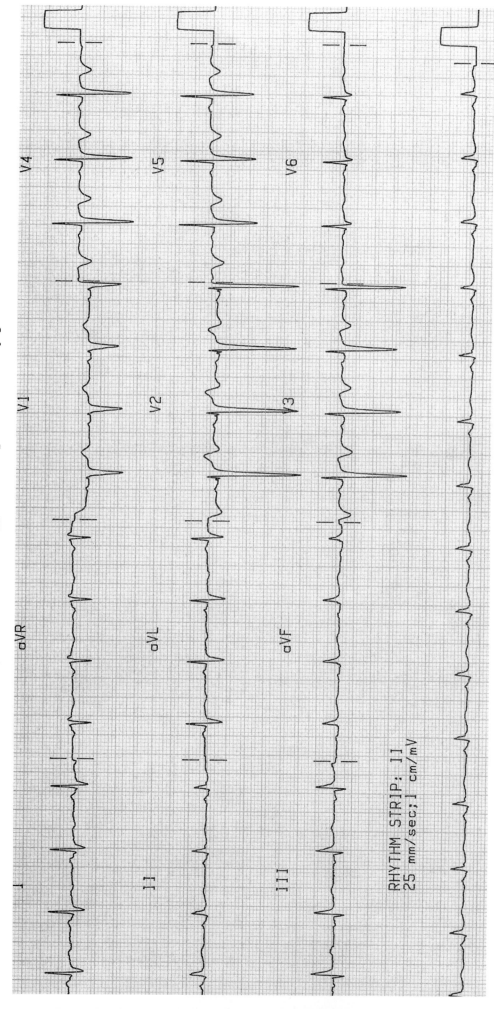

A-20

NARRATIVE INTERPRETATION

Rhythm:	**Atrial fibrillation with controlled ventricular response**
Rate:	**82 (average)**
Intervals:	**PR – , QRS 0.08, QT 0.38**
Axis:	**0 degrees**

Abnormalities

Ventricular pacemaker complexes on demand with capture. Pacemaker fusion complex. Q waves leads II, III, aVF, V5. R waves less than 3 mm leads V1–V4. ST elevation leads II, III, aVF, V3–V6. ST depression leads I, aVL. T-wave inversion leads II, III, aVF, V3–V6. R wave lead aVL + S wave lead V3 greater than 28 mm in a male.

Synthesis

Atrial fibrillation with controlled ventricular response. Ventricular pacemaker functioning on demand, rate 75 with appropriate capture. Pacemaker fusion complex. Left ventricular hypertrophy by voltage criteria. Inferior wall MI of indeterminate age. Anteroseptal (extensive anterior) wall MI of indeterminate age. Probable ventricular aneurysm. Clinical correlation or serial tracings required to exclude acute transmural ischemia/infarction.

TEST ANSWERS: 20, 35, 51, 56, 78, 84, (88), 92, 95.

Comment: This tracing points out the importance of serial tracings to confirm the diagnosis of acute injury. The ST-T-wave findings are compatible with an evolving acute MI. However, this asymptomatic patient had no new changes on his electrocardiogram, indicating that the persistent ST elevation was likely due to a ventricular aneurysm.

Reverse or poor R-wave progression is generally used as an indicator of anteroseptal MI. The presence of a deep Q wave in lead V5 suggests more extensive necrosis of the anterior wall.

Note that the fourth complex on the rhythm strip is a fusion beat that combines depolarization from both atrial conduction and the pacemaker. Also note that the first complex of the 12 lead has a pacemaker spike that occurs just after the initiation of the QRS. There is no apparent deformity of the QRS from pacemaker activation, therefore these complexes have been referred to as *pseudofusion* complexes.

A-20

A 69-year-old asymptomatic man with a history of multiple myocardial infarctions, most recently 1 year ago.

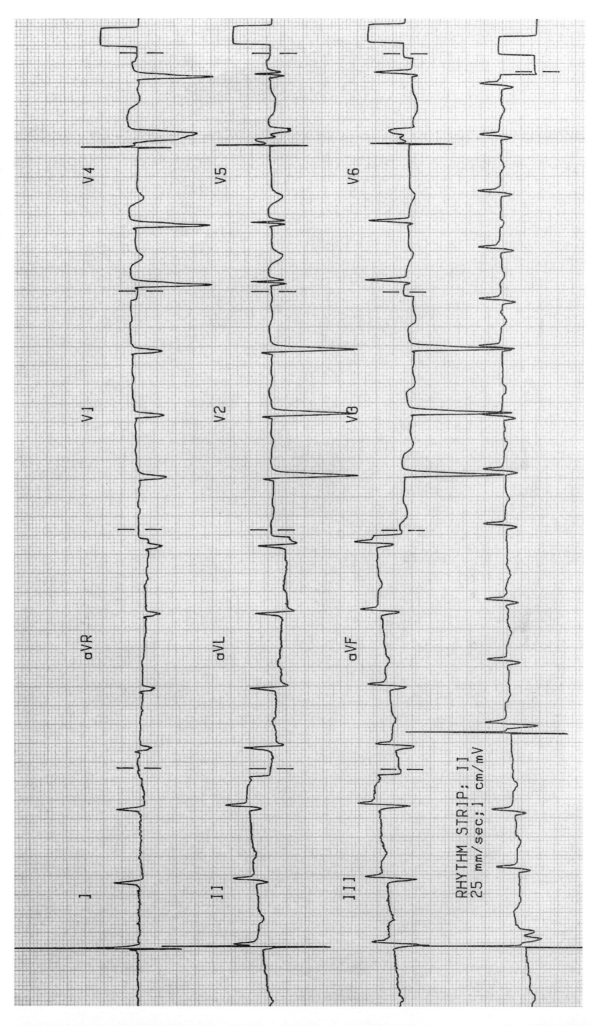

A-21

NARRATIVE INTERPRETATION

Rhythm:	**Sinus bradycardia with first-degree AV block**
Rate:	**53**
Intervals:	**PR 0.21, QRS 0.08, QT 0.40**
Axis:	**+15 degrees**

Abnormalities
Heart rate less than 60 bpm. Prolonged PR interval. RSr' pattern leads V1–V2.

Synthesis
Sinus bradycardia. First-degree AV block. RSr' pattern, normal variant.

TEST ANSWERS: 3, 42, 98.

Comment: The RSR' pattern in lead V1 without any additional evidence of conduction abnormality is reported in up to 2.4 percent of normal individuals. The secondary R wave has been attributed to activation of the right ventricular outflow tract. Criteria defining this pattern as normal include a primary R wave less than 8 mm, a secondary R wave less than 6 mm, and an R' amplitude less than the R wave. The normal variant demonstrated in this tracing should not be confused with incomplete RBBB. The diagnosis of incomplete RBBB includes characteristic secondary ST-T-wave abnormalities and is likely to have a more prominent terminal R wave.

The borderline first-degree AV block is not obvious in all leads but may be identified in the lead II rhythm strip.

FURTHER READING
Tapia FA, Proudfit WL: Secondary R waves in right precordial leads in normal persons and in patients with cardiac disease. *Circulation* 21:28–37, 1960.

A-21

Clinical History
A 44-year-old asymptomatic man.

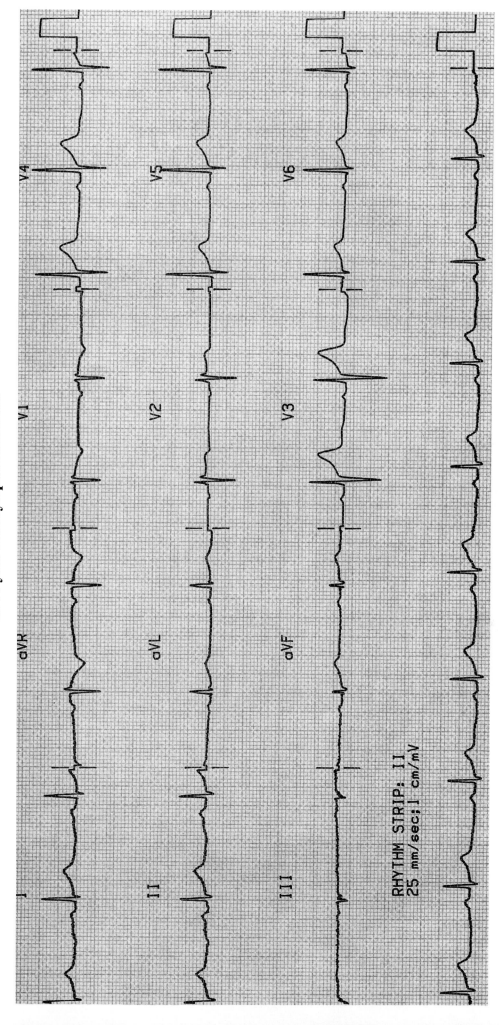

A-22

NARRATIVE INTERPRETATION

Rhythm:	**Sinus**
Rate:	**80**
Intervals:	**PR 0.16, QRS 0.10, QT 0.36**
Axis:	**−30 degrees**

Abnormalities
R wave lead aVL greater than 11 mm. S wave lead V2 + R wave lead V5 greater than 35 mm. R wave lead aVL + S wave lead V3 greater than 28 mm in a male. R wave V1–V3 less than 3 mm. T-wave inversion lead aVL. VPC.

Synthesis
Sinus rhythm. VPC. LVH by voltage criteria and associated ST-T-wave abnormalities. Poor R-wave progression.

TEST ANSWERS: 1, 26, 66, 78, 103.

Comment: This patient exhibits multiple voltage criteria for LVH. Both the precordial and limb lead voltage easily exceed normal limits. Poor R-wave progression is noted secondary to a leftward shift of the transitional zone from the hypertrophied left ventricle. The T-wave inversion in lead aVL is likely secondary to LVH. The Q wave in aVL should not be interpreted as indicative of a lateral wall MI.

A-22

Clinical History
A 68-year-old man with hypertension.

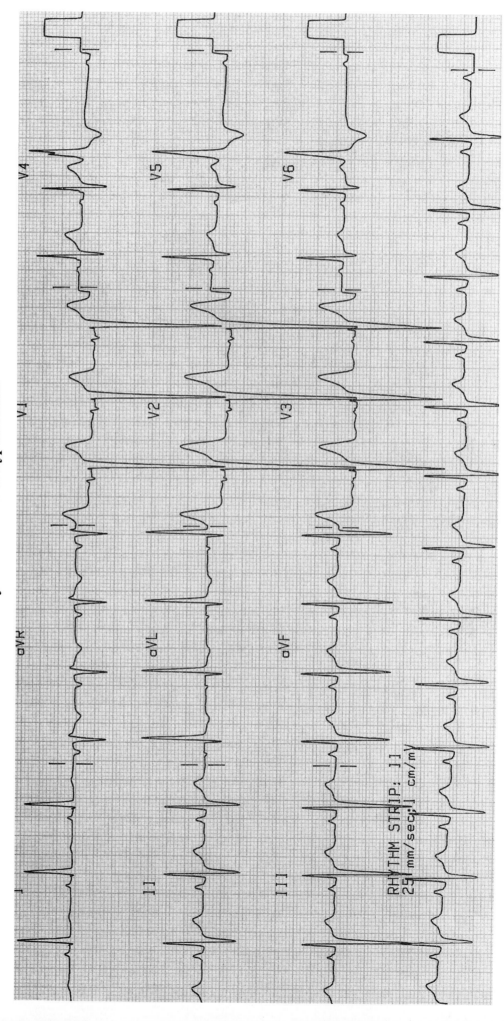

A-23

NARRATIVE INTERPRETATION

Rhythm:	**Sinus bradycardia**
Rate:	**58**
Intervals:	**PR 0.16, QRS 0.12, QT 0.34**
Axis:	**+60 degrees**

Abnormalities
Heart rate less than 60 bpm. Broad, notched QRS with rsR' pattern lead V1 accompanied by T-wave inversion in leads V1–V3.

Synthesis
Sinus bradycardia. RBBB with associated ST-T-wave abnormalities.

TEST ANSWERS: 3, 70, 104.

Comment: *New* RBBB is most often seen in individuals who either already have or will develop clinical cardiovascular disease. The Framingham study found the 10-year incidence of cardiovascular mortality to be threefold higher in persons with newly acquired RBBB compared with age-matched controls without RBBB. In contrast, a subset of healthy persons younger than 40 years of age with new RBBB remained free of cardiovascular disease.

FURTHER READING
Schneider JF, Thomas HE, Kreger BE, et al: Newly acquired right bundle branch block. *Ann Intern Med* 92:37–44, 1980.

A-23

Clinical History

A 50-year-old woman with hypertension. A year ago her electrocardiogram was normal.

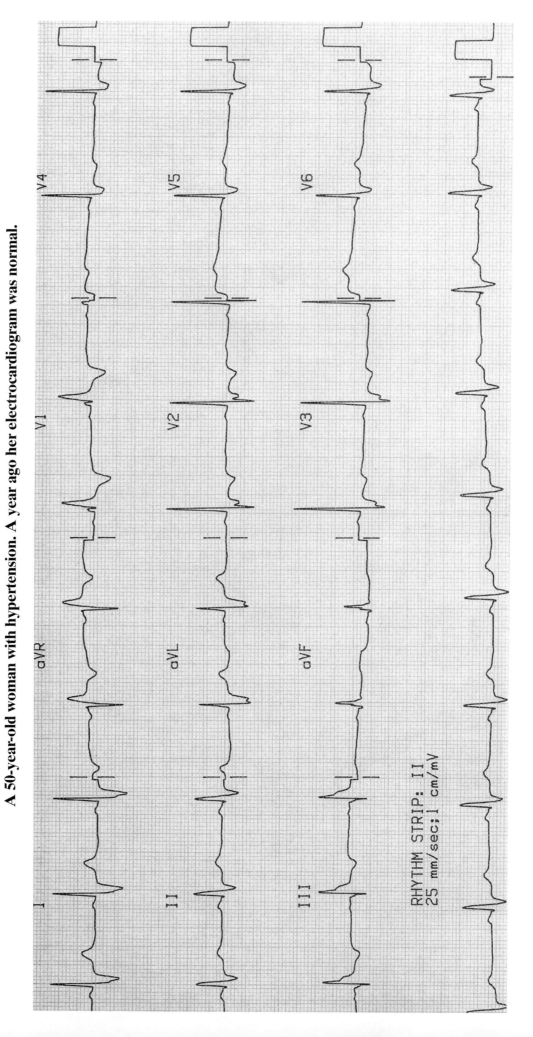

A-24

NARRATIVE INTERPRETATION

Rhythm:	**Sinus**
Rate:	**88**
Intervals:	**PR 0.16, QRS 0.08, QT 0.32**
Axis:	**+45 degrees**

Abnormalities
VPCs. Paired VPCs. Slight ST elevation leads I, II, III, aVF, V1–V6.

Synthesis
Sinus rhythm. VPCs, multiform. Paired VPCs on rhythm strip. Nonspecific ST abnormalities.

TEST ANSWERS: 1, 27, 28, 106.

Comment: This patient demonstrates frequent ventricular ectopy and nonspecific ST abnormalities after cardiac surgery. The diffuse ST changes are likely secondary to postoperative pericardial inflammation. A definitive diagnosis of pericarditis cannot be made on this tracing.

The presence of complex ventricular ectopy after coronary artery bypass surgery does not carry an adverse prognosis. In one study of 92 postoperative patients, complex ventricular arrhythmias were seen in 57 patients. These patients were no more likely to develop sudden death, syncope, or other complications than patients without ventricular ectopy.

FURTHER READING
Rubin DA, Nieminski RN, Monteferrante JC, et al: Ventricular arrhythmias after coronary artery bypass graft surgery: Incidence, risk factors, and long-term prognosis. *J Am Coll Cardiol* 6:307–310, 1985.

A-24

Clinical History

A 55-year-old man who is 8 days status postcoronary artery bypass surgery. He complains of mild palpitations.

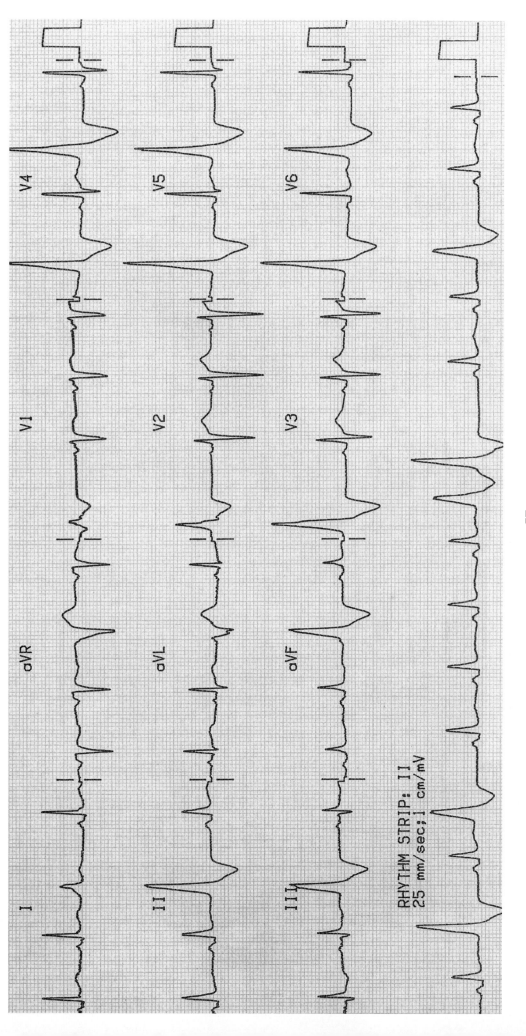

A-25

NARRATIVE INTERPRETATION

Rhythm:	**Sinus with first-degree AV block**
Rate:	**80**
Intervals:	**PR 0.36, QRS 0.08, QT 0.36**
Axis:	**−15 degrees**

Abnormalities
Prolonged PR interval. Q waves leads II, III, aVF, V5, V6. QS leads V1–V4. ST elevation leads V1–V5. Slight ST elevation leads I, aVL, V6.

Synthesis
Sinus rhythm with first-degree AV block. Inferior wall MI of indeterminate age. Extensive anterior wall MI of indeterminate age. Probable ventricular aneurysm.

TEST ANSWERS: 1, 42, 88, 92, 95.

Comment: ST elevation lasting more than 2 weeks following an acute MI is indicative of the likely formation of a left ventricular aneurysm. The diagnosis however, cannot be made definitively by electrocardiography and imaging techniques should be used for confirmation. The patient in this example had suffered multiple MIs. Echocardiography confirmed that the persistent ST-segment elevation in the prior anterior and lateral wall infarction zones was indicative of a large ventricular aneurysm.

A-25

Clinical History

A 79-year-old asymptomatic man with a history of coronary heart disease.

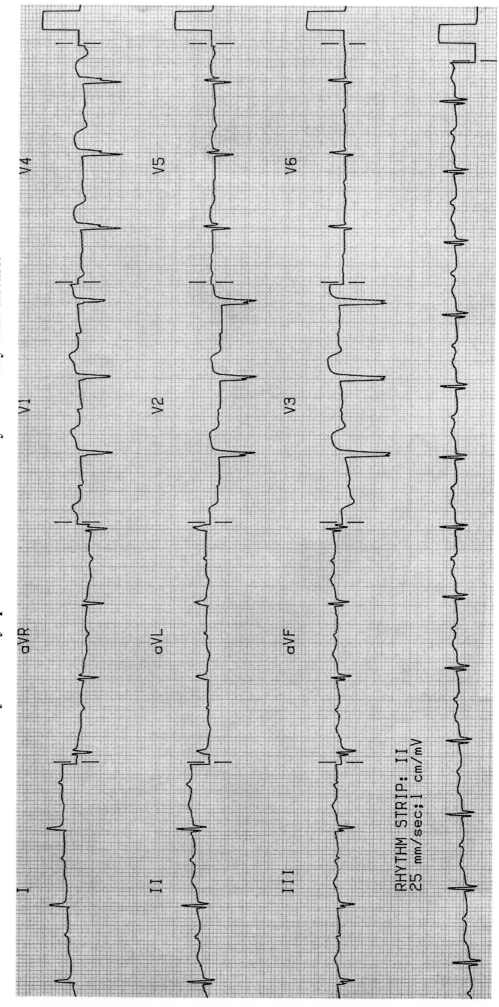

RHYTHM STRIP: II
25 mm/sec; 1 cm/mV

A-26

NARRATIVE INTERPRETATION

Rhythm:	**Sinus**
Rate:	**65**
Intervals:	**PR 0.18, QRS 0.08, QT 0.36**
Axis:	**+75 degrees**

Abnormalities

Abnormal P terminal force V1. Broad, notched P wave lead II. S wave lead V2 + R wave lead V5 greater than 40 mm (patient age 30–40 years).

Synthesis

Sinus rhythm. Left atrial abnormality. LVH by voltage criteria.

TEST ANSWERS: 1, 60, 78.

Comment: This patient had echocardiographically demonstrated left atrial dilatation. The abnormal P-terminal force in lead V1 is easily noted. On careful examination, a second criterion for left atrial enlargement is present, namely a broad, notched P wave in lead II with a peak-to-peak interval of the notches of 40 ms. Note that increased voltage for LVH is present in this young man as precordial voltage exceeds age-adjusted limits for LVH (>40 mm for age 30–40 years). This patient had left ventricular and left atrial enlargement on the basis of aortic insufficiency.

FURTHER READING

Alpert MA, Mususwamy K: Electrocardiographic diagnosis of left atrial enlargement. *Arch Intern Med* 149:1161–1165, 1989.

Hazen MS, Marwick TH, Underwood DA: Diagnostic accuracy of the resting electrocardiogram in detection and estimation of left atrial enlargement: An echocardiographic correlation in 551 patients. *Am Heart J* 122:823–828, 1991.

Manning GW, Smiley JR: QRS voltage criteria for left ventricular hypertrophy in a normal male population. *Circulation* 29:224–230, 1964.

Walker CHM, Rose RL: Importance of age, sex, and body habitus in the diagnosis of left ventricular hypertrophy from the precordial electrocardiogram in childhood and adolescence. *Pediatrics* 28:705–711, 1961.

A-26

Clinical History

A 34-year-old man with dyspnea and diastolic heart murmur.

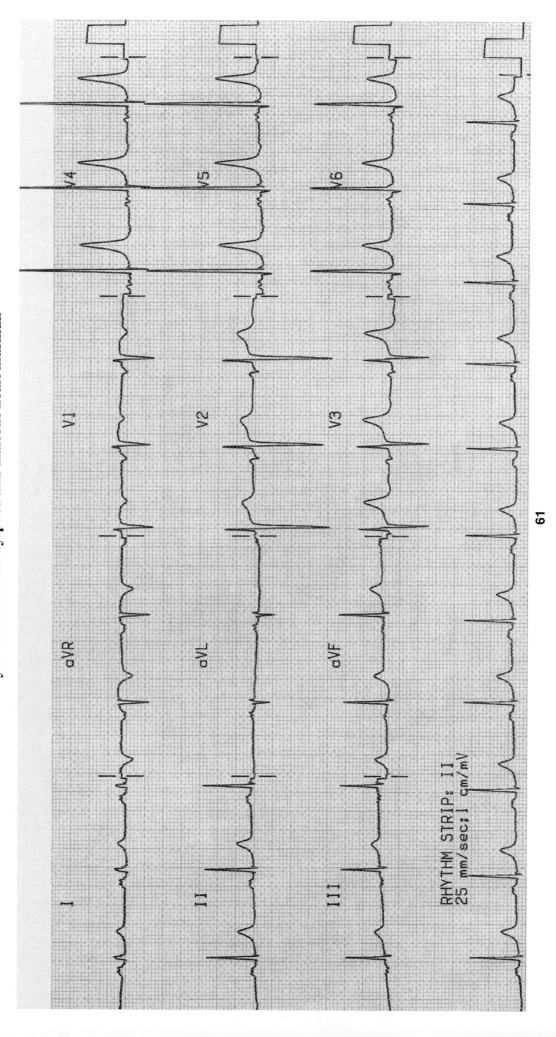

A-27

NARRATIVE INTERPRETATION

Rhythm:	**Atrial flutter with 4:1 AV conduction**
Rate:	**Atrial rate 240, ventricular rate 60**
Intervals:	**PR –, QRS 0.10, QT 0.42**
Axis:	**–15 degrees**

Abnormalities
RSR' leads V1–V2. Low T wave voltage limb leads. Biphasic T waves leads V5–V6.

Synthesis
Atrial flutter with 4:1 AV conduction. Incomplete RBBB. Nonspecific T-wave abnormalities.

TEST ANSWERS: 19, 51, 71, 106.

Comment: Under normal circumstances, patients with atrial flutter will have a physiologic conduction delay at the AV node that results in 2:1 AV conduction. This should not be interpreted as AV *block.* Higher conduction ratios usually imply either conduction disease or the effects of medications such as digitalis, beta blockers, diltiazem, verapamil, and others that may impair AV conduction. It is reasonable to assume that this elderly man had conduction system disease to explain the 4:1 conduction. Although the T waves in the limb leads are at least partially obscured by the flutter waves, there appears to be virtually no T-wave voltage and it is appropriate to comment on this feature of the electrocardiogram.

A-27

Clinical History
A 90-year-old asymptomatic man. He takes no medications.

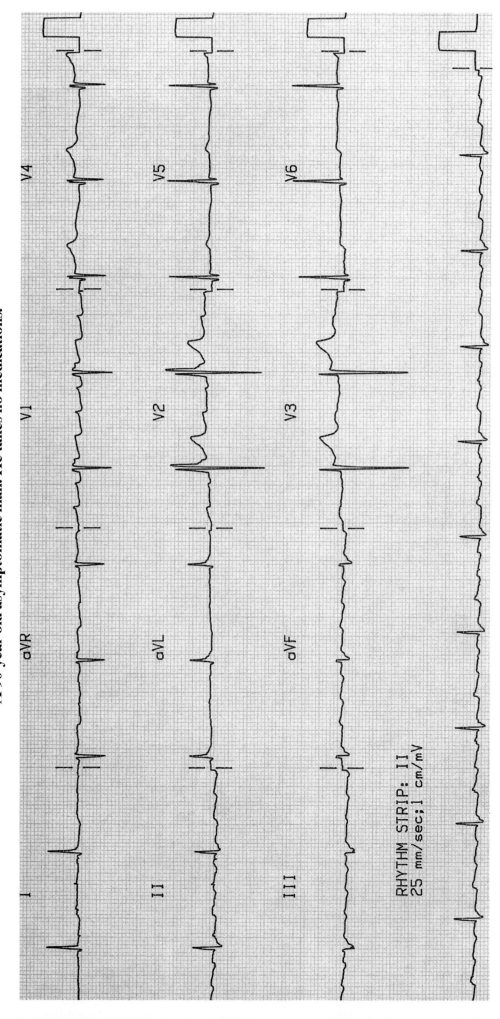

A-28

NARRATIVE INTERPRETATION

Rhythm:	**Sinus tachycardia**
Rate:	**105**
Intervals:	**PR 0.16, QRS 0.08 QT 0.32**
Axis:	**+75 degrees**

Abnormalities

Heart rate greater than 100 bpm. ST elevation leads II, III, aVF, V4–V6. ST depression leads I, aVL, V1–V2.

Synthesis

Sinus tachycardia. Inferior and anterolateral wall MI with ST abnormalities of acute MI. Reciprocal changes versus anterior myocardial ischemia. (Possible acute posterior MI.)

TEST ANSWERS: 4, 85, 91, (93), 100, 101.

Comment: This patient demonstrates acute ST-segment abnormalities consistent with acute MI involving the inferior and anterolateral walls. Early posterior wall infarction is also possible on the basis of ST depression in the anterior precordial leads. A single electrocardiogram is insufficient to distinguish this from reciprocal changes. Serial tracings or subsequent wall motion studies are routinely required for definitive diagnosis. Most studies indicate that patients with inferior wall MI who also demonstrate precordial ST depression have more extensive myocardial damage and an adverse prognosis.

FURTHER READING

Mirvis DM: Physiologic basis for anterior ST-segment depression in patients with acute inferior wall myocardial infarction. *Am Heart J* 116:1308–1322, 1988.

Schweitzer P: The electrocardiographic diagnosis of acute myocardial infarction in the thrombolytic era. *Am Heart J* 119:642–654, 1990.

A-28

Clinical History

A 59-year-old man with 45 min of chest discomfort.

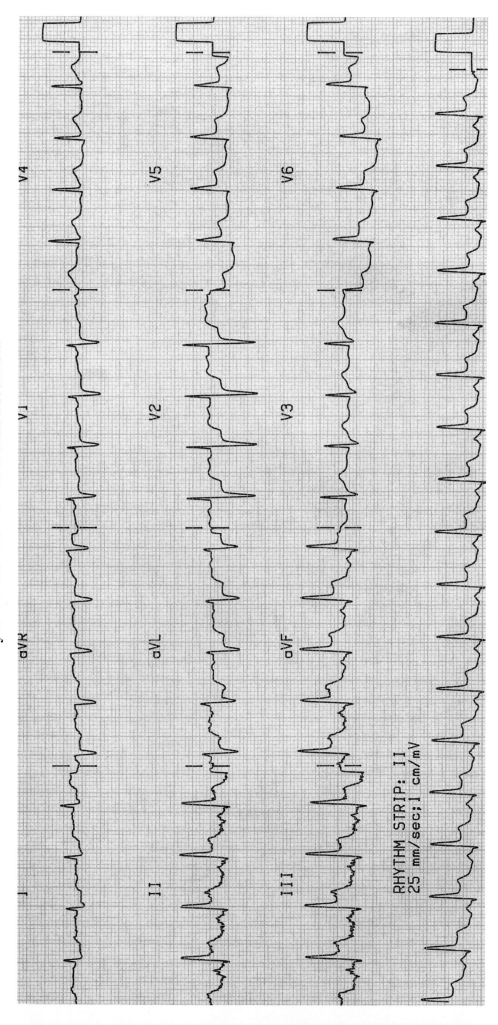

A-29

NARRATIVE INTERPRETATION

Rhythm:	**Atrial fibrillation**
Rate:	**145 (average)**
Intervals:	**PR —, QRS 0.08, QT 0.30**
Axis:	**+15 degrees**

Abnormalities
Rapid, irregular heart rate.

Synthesis
Atrial fibrillation with a rapid ventricular response.

TEST ANSWERS: 20, 50.

Comment: On first glance, the reader might misinterpret this rhythm as supraventricular tachycardia because it appears quite regular. On closer inspection, there is slight variation of the RR intervals and no organized P-wave activity, indicative of atrial fibrillation. The rapid ventricular response is physiologic in the absence of intrinsic conduction disease or AV blocking agents.

66

A-29

Clinical History

A 66-year-old woman with palpitations.

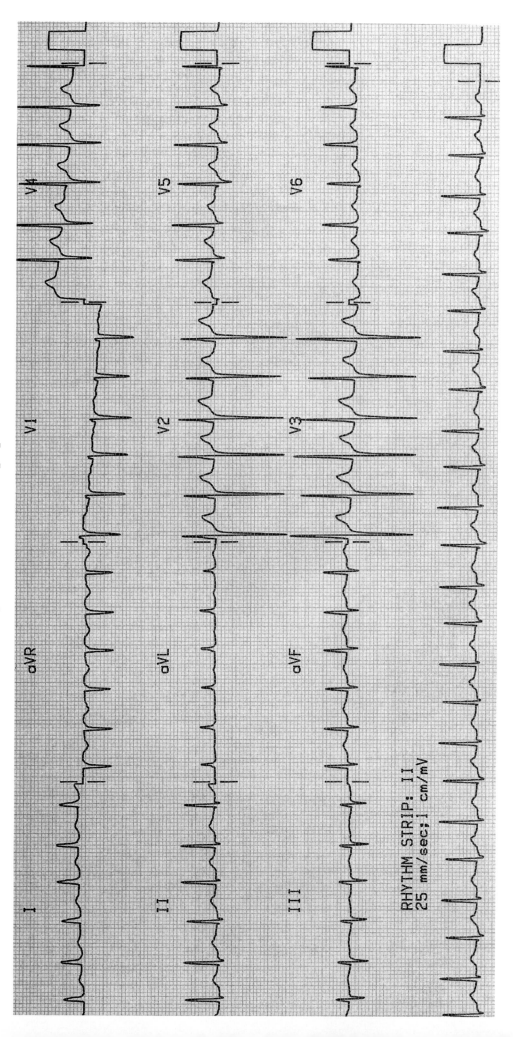

A-30

NARRATIVE INTERPRETATION

Rhythm:	**Sinus**
Rate:	**80**
Intervals:	**PR 0.18, QRS 0.11, QT 0.40**
Axis:	**+60 degrees**

Abnormalities
S wave lead V2 + R wave lead V5 greater than 35 mm. R wave lead aVL + S wave lead V3 greater than 28 mm in a male. T-wave inversion leads I, II, V5–V6. Prolonged QRS duration.

Synthesis
Sinus rhythm. LVH by voltage criteria with associated ST-T-wave abnormalities and intraventricular conduction delay.

TEST ANSWERS: 1, 76, 78, 103.

Comment: Remember to check the standardization of each electrocardiogram. This tracing is recorded at one-half standard and the complexes are half the usual size. After correcting for the standardization, this patient has obvious LVH with increased precordial voltage and associated ST-T-wave abnormalities. Cardiac catheterization demonstrated severe aortic stenosis and insufficiency.

A-30

Clinical History

**A 66-year-old man admitted for elective cardiac catheterization.
He has a loud systolic murmur.**

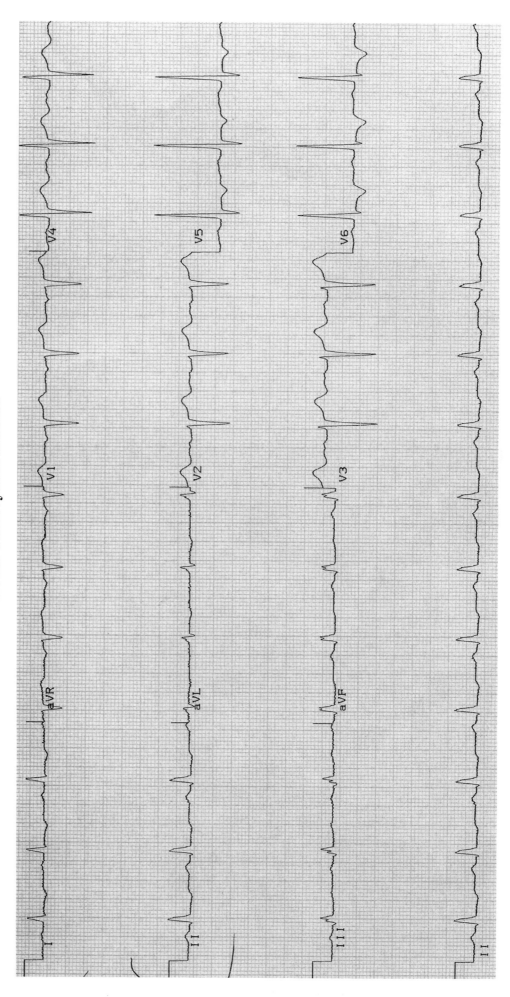

A-31

NARRATIVE INTERPRETATION

Rhythm:	Sinus
Rate:	65
Intervals:	PR 0.24, QRS 0.12, QT 0.36
Axis:	+105 degrees

Abnormalities
Axis rightward of +90 degrees. Prolonged PR interval. Broad QRS with rSR' and T-wave inversion leads V1–V2.

Synthesis
Sinus rhythm. First-degree AV block. RBBB with associated ST-T-wave abnormalities. Right-axis deviation. Left posterior fascicular block.

TEST ANSWERS: 1, 42, 65, 70, 73, 104.

Comment: In patients with RBBB, the QRS axis should be interpreted using the first 0.06 s. In this example, the axis is abnormally rightward and is consistent with left posterior fascicular block. Additional diagnostic criteria of LPFB include a small initial R wave in aVL and narrow Q waves in the inferior limb leads. This patient has trifascicular block based on the presence of RBBB, LPFB, and first-degree AV block.

One might be suspicious that the ST configuration in leads V2–V5 represent the first manifestations of acute MI. Here, old tracings are invaluable and this patient's initial electrocardiogram was found to be unchanged from prior tracings. Interestingly, changes indicative of MI became quite evident on the second hospital day (see next example).

A-31

Clinical History

A 74-year-old man admitted to the coronary care unit (CCU).

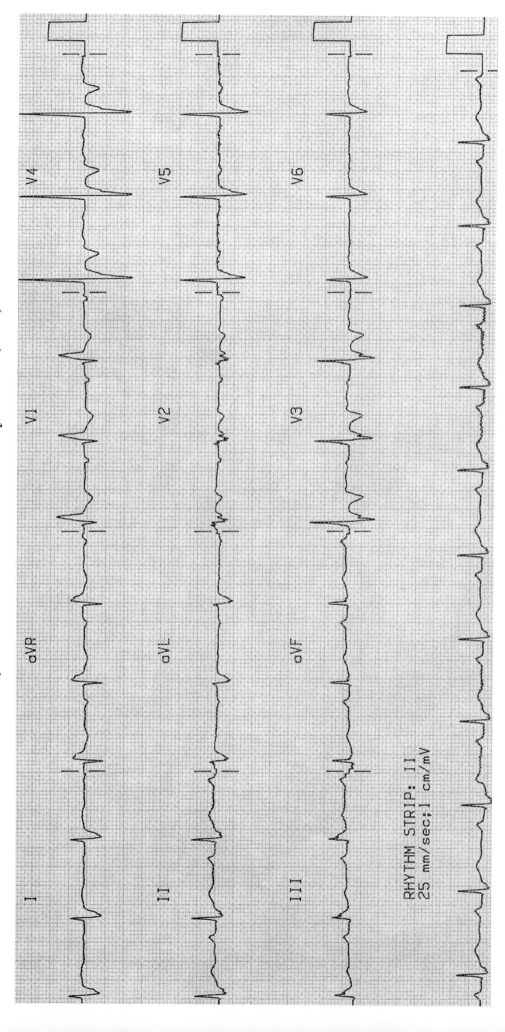

A-32

NARRATIVE INTERPRETATION

Rhythm:	**Sinus bradycardia with first-degree AV block**
Rate:	**48**
Intervals:	**PR 0.24, QRS 0.14, QT 0.52**
Axis:	**+ 105 degrees**

Abnormalities
Heart rate less than 60 bpm. Prolonged PR interval. Axis rightward of +90 degrees. Broad QRS with rSR' lead V1. Deep T-wave inversion leads I, aVL, V2–V6. T-wave upright lead V1. Straight ST segment leads I, aVL, V1–V6 with slight ST elevation leads V1–V3.

Synthesis
Sinus bradycardia. First-degree AV block. RBBB. Right axis deviation. Left posterior fascicular block. ST-T-wave abnormalities suggesting myocardial injury.

TEST ANSWERS: 3, 42, 65, 70, 73, 100.

Comment: This tracing demonstrates extensive anterior and lateral wall changes suggesting early injury in the presence of a RBBB and left posterior fascicular block. The significant findings are the markedly inverted T waves with a straight ST segment in the lateral leads and across the precordium. There is slight ST elevation in leads V1–V3 suggesting acute or recent myocardial injury. Also note the upright T wave in lead V1, where inversion would be expected in uncomplicated RBBB. Here the ST-T-wave findings are no longer secondary to the conduction abnormality and reflect an acute coronary syndrome. Compare this tracing with the previous example.

A-32

Clinical History

A 74-year-old man admitted to the CCU who has developed chest discomfort.

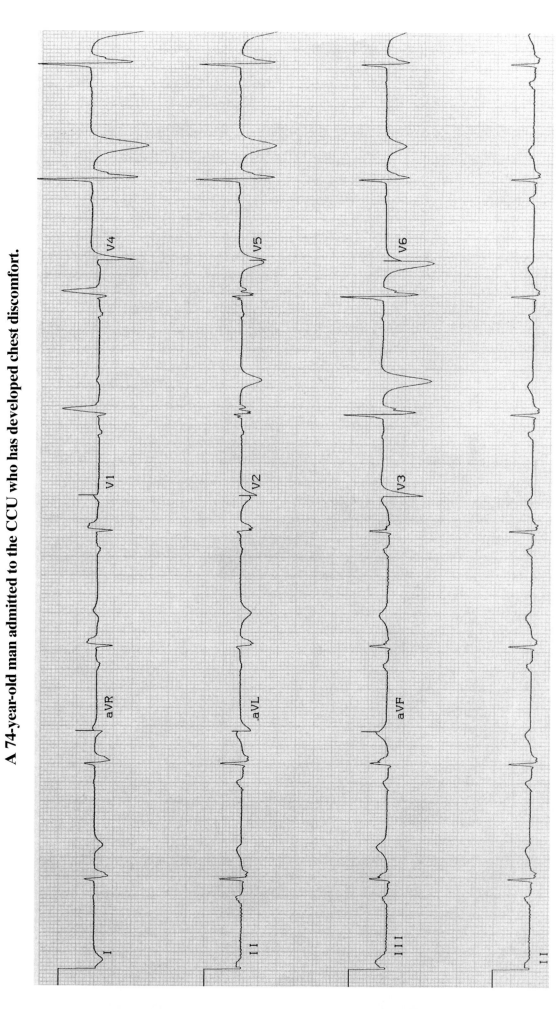

A-33

NARRATIVE INTERPRETATION

Rhythm:	**Sinus**
Rate:	**75**
Intervals:	**PR 0.16, QRS 0.08, QT 0.36**
Axis:	**−45 degrees**

Abnormalities
Axis leftward of −30 degrees.

Synthesis
Sinus rhythm. Left axis deviation. Left anterior fascicular block.

TEST ANSWERS: 1, 64, 72.

Comment: This patient has left anterior fascicular block (LAFB) as her only electrocardiographic abnormality. In population studies, the prevalence of LAFB has ranged from 1 to 14 percent. The prognosis of patients with LAFB is not different from that of individuals without this abnormality. It is important to realize that not everyone with left axis deviation has LAFB. Other conditions causing left axis deviation include inferior wall MI, chronic pulmonary disease (pseudo left axis deviation), LVH, and a variety of congenital cardiac anomalies.

FURTHER READING
Barrett PA, Peter CT, Swan HJC, et al: The frequency and prognostic significance of electrocardiographic abnormalities in clinically normal individuals. *Prog Cardiovasc Dis* 23:299–319, 1981.

Perloff JK, Roberts NK, Cabeen WR Jr: Left axis deviation: A reassessment. *Circulation* 60:12–21, 1979.

A-33

Clinical History

A 49-year-old asymptomatic woman.

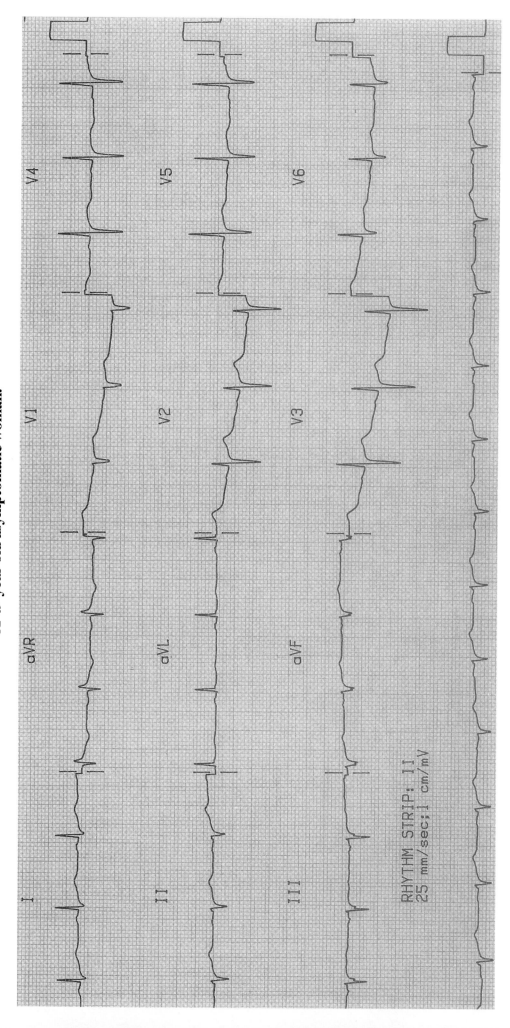

RHYTHM STRIP: II
25 mm/sec; 1 cm/mV

A-34

NARRATIVE INTERPRETATION

Rhythm:	**Sinus with first-degree AV block**
Rate:	**85**
Intervals:	**PR 0.22, QRS 0.08, QT 0.40**
Axis:	**+120 degrees**

Abnormalities
Prolonged PR interval. qR lead V1. Prominent R wave lead V2. Axis rightward of +90 degrees.

Synthesis
Sinus rhythm. First-degree AV block. Right axis deviation. RVH.

TEST ANSWERS: 1, 42, 65, 79.

Comment: This patient had severe primary pulmonary hypertension with RVH. Marked right axis deviation is evident with prominent R forces in the right precordial leads. Other causes of rightward axis besides RVH include left posterior hemiblock and lateral wall MI.

FURTHER READING
Surawicz B: Electrocardiographic diagnosis of chamber enlargement. *J Am Coll Cardiol* 8:711–724, 1986.

A-34

Clinical History
A 49-year-old woman with severe dyspnea.

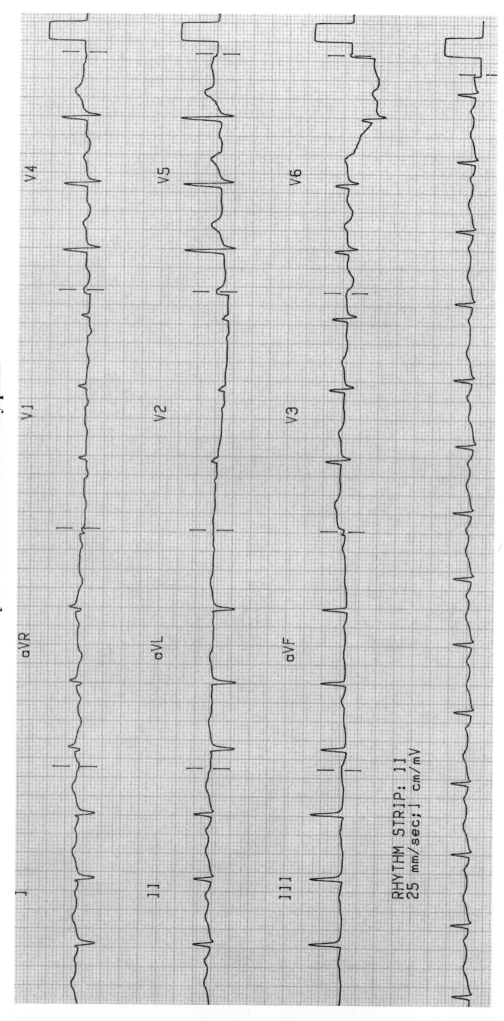

RHYTHM STRIP: II
25 mm/sec; 1 cm/mV

A-35

NARRATIVE INTERPRETATION

Rhythm:	**Accelerated AV junctional rhythm**
Rate:	**95**
Intervals:	**PR –, QRS 0.08, QT 0.34**
Axis:	**–45 degrees**

Abnormalities
Inverted P wave leads II, III, aVF. Axis leftward of –30 degrees. Slight ST depression leads V3–V6.

Synthesis
Accelerated AV junctional rhythm. Left axis deviation. Left anterior fascicular block. Nonspecific ST-segment abnormalities.

TEST ANSWERS: 23, 64, 72, 106.

Comment: The inverted P waves that occur after the QRS are indicative of a junctional focus. The rhythm is an *accelerated* junctional rhythm because of the elevated heart rate. Normally, the AV junction functions as a subsidiary escape pacemaker at a rate of 35 to 50 bpm. The increased rate seen in this example is the result of increased automaticity at the AV junction. Accelerated AV junctional rhythm is usually seen in patients with underlying cardiac disease such as acute MI, myocarditis, COPD, or after cardiac surgery. It may also reflect digitalis toxicity. Another term for this rhythm is *nonparoxysmal junctional tachycardia.*

A-35

Clinical History

A 65-year-old man with lightheadedness.

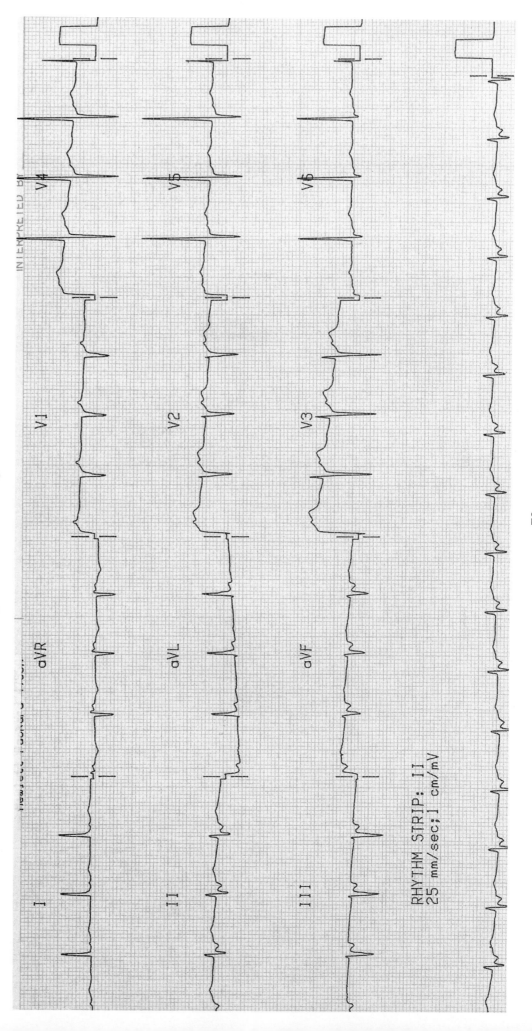

A-36

NARRATIVE INTERPRETATION

Rhythm:	**Atrial flutter**
Rate:	**Atrial rate 380, ventricular rate 190**
Intervals:	**PR –, QRS 0.08, QT –**
Axis:	**–30 degrees**

Abnormalities

R wave lead aVL greater than 11 mm. R wave lead I + S wave lead V3 greater than 28 mm in a male. ST depression leads I, aVL, V2–V6. T wave flat leads I, aVL, V6.

Synthesis

Atrial flutter with 2:1 AV conduction. LVH by voltage criteria and associated ST-T-wave abnormalities.

TEST ANSWERS: 19, 50, 78, 103.

Comment: This patient has developed atrial flutter following cardiac surgery. The rapid atrial rate is indicative of type II atrial flutter. Type I and type II flutter are characterized by atrial rates of 240 to 340 and 340 to 433 bpm, respectively. Type I flutter may be converted to sinus rhythm with electrical cardioversion, antiarrhythmic agents, or rapid atrial pacing. In contrast, type II atrial flutter cannot be affected by pacing. Remember that with atrial rates in this range, 2:1 AV conduction is a physiologic response of the AV node and does not represent AV nodal disease. The electrical axis in the lead II rhythm strip is seen to vary from normal to slightly leftward. This is probably secondary to respiratory variation.

A-36

Clinical History

A 70-year-old man following cardiac surgery.

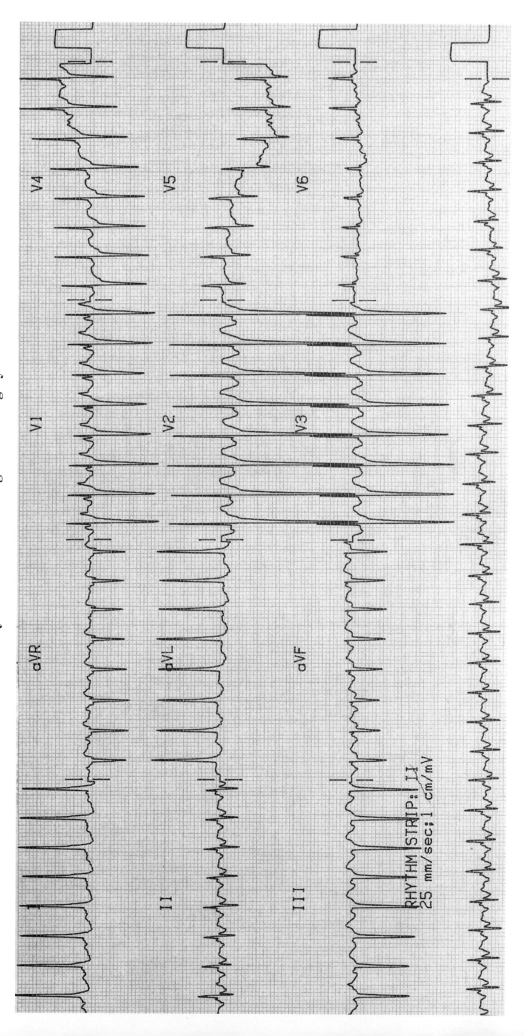

A-37

NARRATIVE INTERPRETATION

Rhythm:	**Sinus bradycardia with second-degree AV block, Mobitz type I**
Rate:	**55**
Intervals:	**PR variable, QRS 0.12, QT 0.44**
Axis:	**+30 degrees**

Abnormalities

Sinus rate less than 60 bpm. Gradual prolongation of the PR interval with eventual failure to conduct P wave. Q wave leads II, III, aVF. Prolonged QRS duration. ST depression leads V4–V6. S wave lead V2 + R wave lead V5 greater than 35 mm. R wave lead aVL + S wave lead V3 greater than 28 mm in a male. T-wave inversion leads II, III, aVF.

Synthesis

Sinus bradycardia. Second-degree AV block, Mobitz type I (Wenckebach). Inferior wall MI of indeterminate age. LVH. Intraventricular conduction delay (IVCD). ST-T-wave abnormalities associated with LVH or IVCD or both.

TEST ANSWERS: 3, 43, 76, 78, 92, 103.

Comment: This tracing demonstrates a number of electrocardiographic abnormalities. There is progressive prolongation of the PR interval with eventual failure to conduct one P wave to the ventricles, a manifestation of Mobitz type I, second-degree AV block. In classic Wenckebach, there is progressive shortening of the RR interval, and the RR interval containing the blocked P wave is less than twice the sum of two PP intervals. Note in this example that the PR interval following the blocked P wave is greater than 0.20 s, but first-degree AV block is generally not diagnosed in the presence of higher degrees of AV block. The ST-T-wave abnormalities in this example are most likely related to LVH.

A-37

Clinical History

A 66-year-old man in the coronary care unit (CCU).

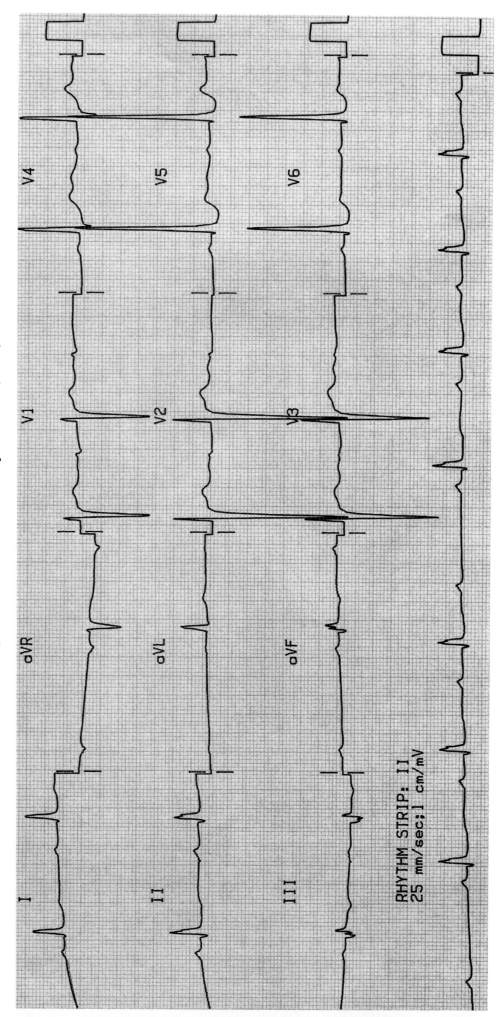

RHYTHM STRIP: II
25 mm/sec; 1 cm/mV

A-38

NARRATIVE INTERPRETATION

Rhythm:	**Supraventricular tachycardia**
Rate:	**160**
Intervals:	**PR –, QRS 0.08, QT 0.28**
Axis:	**–15 degrees**

Abnormalities
Rapid heart rate. ST depression leads I, II, aVL, aVF, V3–V6. Alternating heights of R wave, most prominent in lead V3.

Synthesis
Supraventricular tachycardia. Electrical alternans. Nonspecific ST-segment abnormalities.

TEST ANSWERS: 18, 69, 106.

Comment: This patient has paroxysmal supraventricular tachycardia. This is a "catch-all" term for a number of arrhythmias. The characterization of this rhythm as atrial tachycardia is deferred because P waves are not clearly evident. The most common cause of PSVT in adults is AV nodal reentrant tachycardia, representing at least 50 percent of patients. This rhythm is characterized by reentry within the AV node and results in a narrow complex arrhythmia of about 140 to 200 bpm. Characteristically, the P wave is buried in the QRS complex.

A subtle finding in this example is electrical alternans, seen best in lead V3. Some authors suggest that this finding indicates that a concealed AV nodal bypass tract is involved in the generation of the arrhythmia.

FURTHER READING
Ganz LI, Friedman PL: Supraventricular tachycardia. *N Engl J Med* 332:162–173, 1995.
Kalbfleisch SJ, El-Atassi R, Calkins H, et al: Differentiation of paroxysmal narrow QRS complex tachycardias using the 12-lead electrocardiogram. *J Am Coll Cardiol* 21:85–89, 1993.

Clinical History

A 45-year-old man with sudden onset of palpitations.

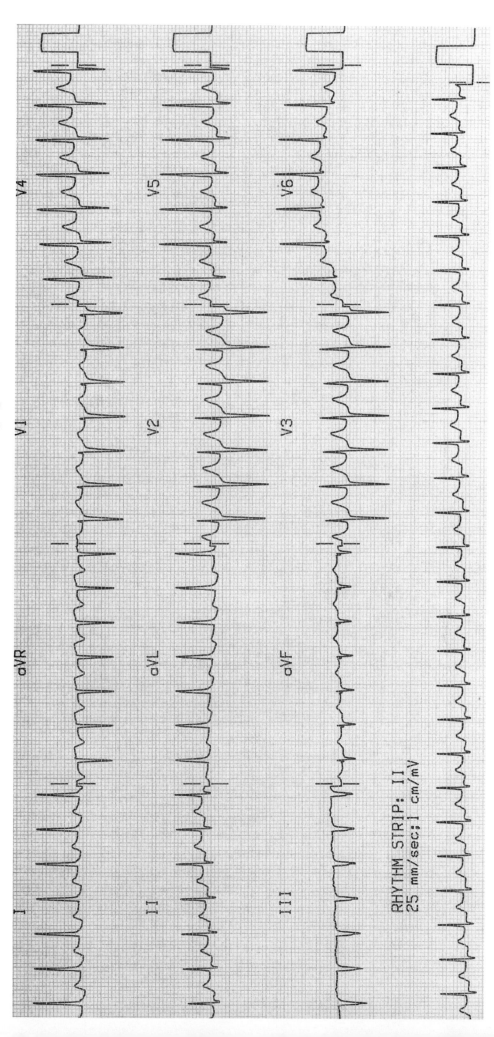

A-39

NARRATIVE INTERPRETATION

Rhythm:	**Sinus**
Rate:	**92**
Intervals:	**PR 0.16, QRS 0.08, QT 0.40**
Axis:	**−15 degrees**

Abnormalities

VPCs in a bigeminal pattern. Abnormal P terminal force lead V1. R wave lead aVL + S wave lead V3 greater than 20 mm in a female. T wave flat in lead I, inverted in lead aVL. Prolonged QTc interval.

Synthesis

Sinus rhythm with ventricular bigeminy. Left atrial abnormality. LVH by voltage criterion with associated ST-T-wave abnormalities. Prolonged QTc.

TEST ANSWERS: 1, 26, 60, 78, 103, 109.

Comment: The rhythm is sinus with ventricular bigeminy. Remember that every other P wave is "buried" within the VPC and the sinus rate is actually twice that of the visualized P waves. Patients with ventricular bigeminy may complain of palpitations or may be asymptomatic. More serious symptoms may arise if the ectopic beats fail to perfuse with a resulting fall in effective cardiac output or blood pressure.

A-39

Clinical History

A 62-year-old asymptomatic woman seen 2 days after gallbladder surgery.

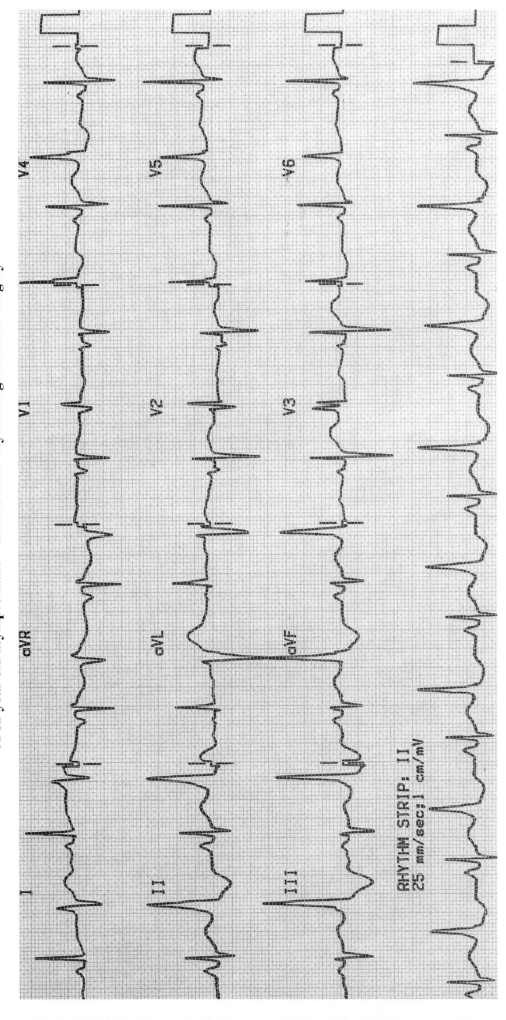

A-40

NARRATIVE INTERPRETATION

Rhythm:	**Sinus**
Rate:	**62**
Intervals:	**PR 0.16, QRS 0.08, QT 0.36**
Axis:	**+90 degrees**

Abnormalities

R wave leads V1–V3 less than 3 mm. ST elevation leads V2–V4. T-wave inversion leads V2–V5. T-wave biphasic lead V5.

Synthesis

Sinus rhythm. Poor R-wave progression. Anteroseptal (anterior) wall MI with ST-T-wave abnormalities suggesting recent myocardial injury.

TEST ANSWERS: 1, 66, 81, (83), 100.

Comment: This patient suffered an acute anteroseptal wall MI. Technically, the poor R-wave progression best localizes the injury to the anteroseptal wall, although the ST-T-wave abnormalities extend a bit further to the anterior wall. He had a history of radiation therapy to the mediastinum for Hodgkin's disease. This has been reported to induce focal coronary obstruction in patients otherwise without coronary atherosclerosis. The Q wave in aVL does not support the diagnosis of lateral wall MI, as there are no additional Q waves either in lead I or leads V5–V6. Patients with a vertical axis will often demonstrate a QS wave in lead aVL. The negative to biphasic P wave and inverted T wave in aVL also suggest that the Q wave in this lead is a normal variant.

FURTHER READING

Chinnasami, BR, Schwartz RC, Pink SB, et al: Isolated left main coronary stenosis and mediastinal irradiation. *Clin Cardiol* 15:459–461, 1992.

Dunsmore LD, LoPointe MA, Dunsmore RA: Radiation-induced coronary artery disease. *J Am Coll Cardiol* 8:239–244, 1986.

A-40

Clinical History

**A 37-year-old man admitted to the coronary care unit with 2 days of chest discomfort.
He has a history of treatment for Hodgkin's disease.**

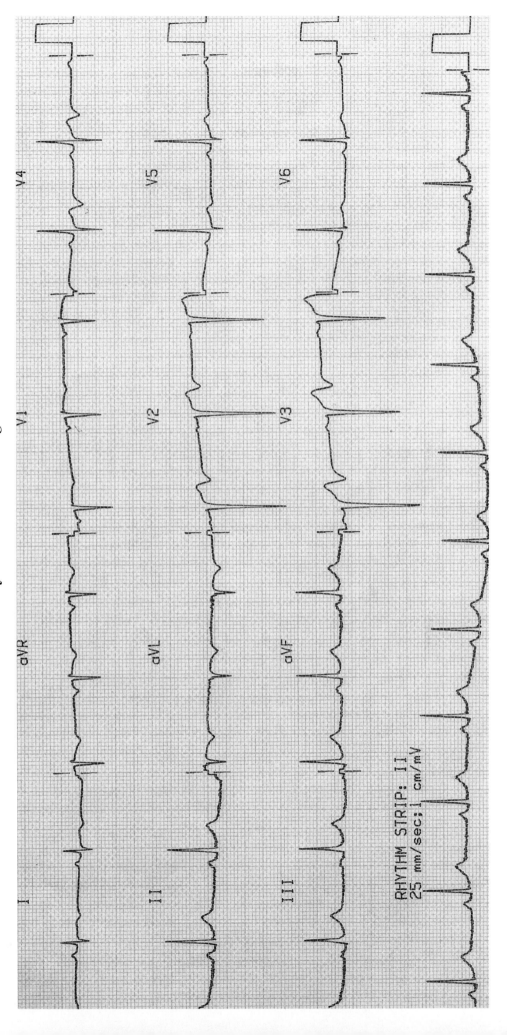

TEST B

B-1

NARRATIVE INTERPRETATION

Rhythm:	**Sinus bradycardia with second-degree AV block, Mobitz type I**
Rate:	**58**
Intervals:	**PR variable, QRS 0.14, QT 0.40**
Axis:	**−45 degrees**

Abnormalities
Heart rate less than 60 bpm. VPC. Incremental prolongation of PR interval with eventual failure to conduct P wave. Broad, notched QRS in leads I, aVL, V6, with associated T-wave inversion. Axis leftward of −30 degrees.

Synthesis
Sinus bradycardia with second-degree AV block, Mobitz type I. VPC. LBBB with associated ST-T-wave changes. Left-axis deviation.

TEST ANSWERS: 3, 26, 43, 64, 74, 104.

Comment: Note in this example that the shortest PR interval of the Wenckebach sequence is prolonged beyond 0.2 s. However, first-degree AV block should not be diagnosed in the presence of a higher degree of AV block.

This patient also has complete LBBB. A major diagnostic criterion of LBBB is absence of the normal septal activation from left to right. In LBBB, the initial forces depolarize the septum from right to left, instead of the usual left to right. Accordingly, there cannot be *septal* Q waves in leftward leads. A Q wave may occasionally be seen in lead aVL, but should not appear in either lead I or leads V5–V6. In this example, one might initially consider a Q wave present in lead I, but on closer inspection, a small R wave is evident.

FURTHER READING
Willems JL, Robles de Medina EO, Bernard R, et al: Criteria for intraventricular conduction disturbances and preexcitation. *J Am Coll Cardiol* 5:1261–1275, 1985.

B-1

Clinical History

A 73-year-old asymptomatic man with a history of hypertension.

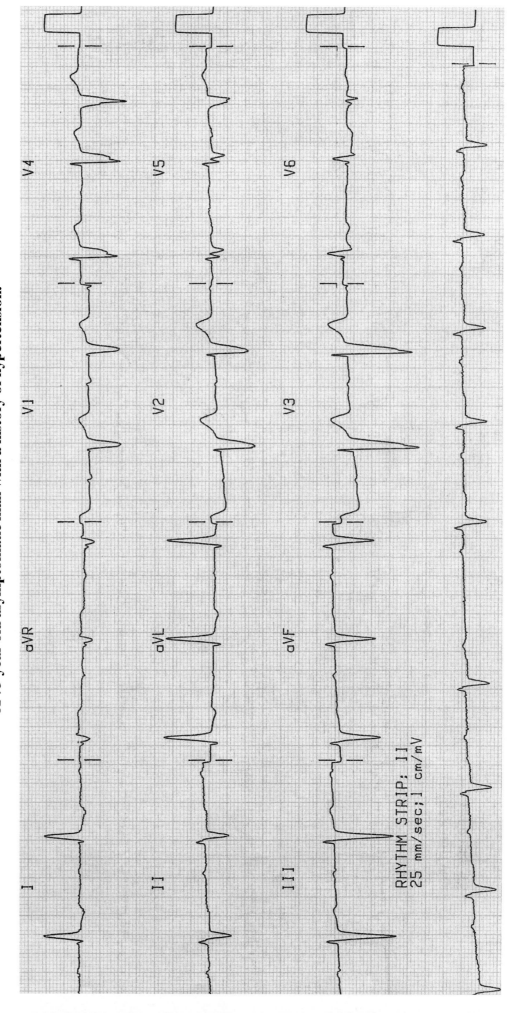

B-2

NARRATIVE INTERPRETATION

Rhythm:	**Sinus**
Rate:	**72**
Intervals:	**PR 0.16, QRS 0.08, QT 0.38**
Axis:	**+45 degrees**

Abnormalities
High J point with concave upward ST elevation leads I, II, aVL, aVF, V2–V6.

Synthesis
Sinus rhythm. Normal variant, isolated J-point elevation.

TEST ANSWERS: 1, 96.

Comment: This tracing represents the normal variant of early repolarization seen in some healthy individuals. A large study of nearly 50,000 healthy Air Force personnel found that 2 percent had benign ST elevation similar to the type shown in this example. Normally, the ST segment is isoelectric with the T-P segment. ST elevation to a greater degree may represent early repolarization or acute pericarditis. Interestingly, 1 year later, this patient with early repolarization developed acute pericarditis with more profound ST-segment abnormalities (see next tracing).

FURTHER READING
Klatsky AL, Oehm R, Cooper RA, et al: The early repolarization normal variant electrocardiogram: Correlates and consequences. *Am J Med* 115:171–177, 2003.

Haydar ZR, Brantley DA, Gittings NS, et al: Early repolarization: An electrocardiographic predictor of enhanced aerobic fitness. *Am J Cardiol* 85:264–266, 2000.

Parisi AF, Beckmann CH, Lancaster MC: The spectrum of ST segment elevation in the electrocardiograms of healthy adult men. *J Electrocardiol* 4:137–144, 1971.

B-2

Clinical History

A 22-year-old military recruit on routine examination.

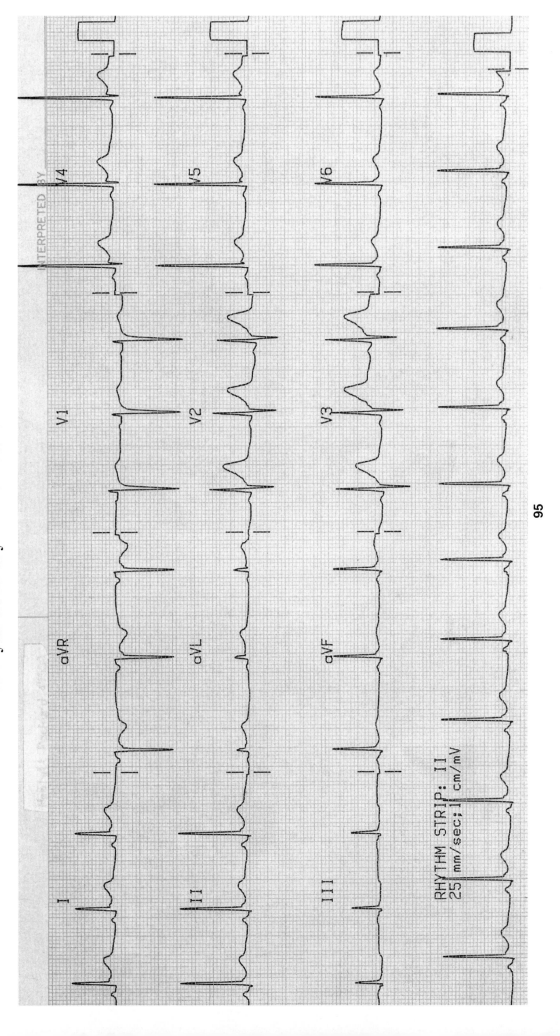

B-3

NARRATIVE INTERPRETATION

Rhythm:	**Sinus**
Rate:	**85**
Intervals:	**PR 0.18, QRS 0.08, QT 0.28**
Axis:	**+45 degrees**

Abnormalities
PR depression (most pronounced in) leads II, aVF. J-point elevation throughout. Diffuse ST elevation.

Synthesis
Sinus rhythm. PR depression, J-point elevation, and ST elevation consistent with early, acute pericarditis.

TEST ANSWERS: 1, 63, 105.

Comment: This is an interesting tracing in that this patient had resting ST abnormalities characteristic of early repolarization and subsequently developed acute pericarditis (see previous example). It is often difficult to differentiate these two entities. PR depression, if evident, suggests pericarditis; however, this is not a universal finding. Some authors suggest that if the ratio of the amplitudes of the ST segment and T wave (ST/T ratio) measured in lead V6 is greater than 0.25, acute pericarditis is present. In this example, the diffuse ST elevation that involves every lead except aVR is characteristic of pericarditis and should not be confused with acute myocardial injury. The ST elevation of acute myocardial injury is usually localized to leads representing a specific region of the myocardium and characteristically has a concave downward (coved) configuration.

FURTHER READING

Gintzon LE, Laks MM: The differential diagnosis of acute pericarditis from the normal variant: New electrocardiographic criteria. *Circulation* 65:1004–1009, 1982.

Spodick DH: Differential characteristics of the electrocardiogram in early repolarization and acute pericarditis. *N Engl J Med* 295:523–526, 1976.

Wanner WR, Schaal SF, Bashore TM, et al: Repolarization variant versus acute pericarditis. *Chest* 83:180–184, 1983.

B-3

Clinical History

A 23-year-old man with pleuritic chest pain.

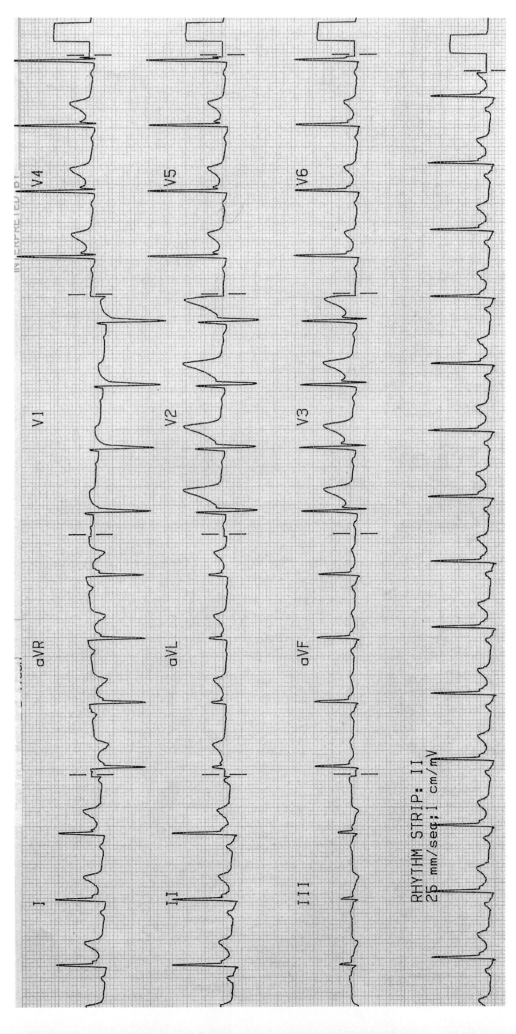

B-4

NARRATIVE INTERPRETATION

Rhythm:	**Sinus**
Rate:	**99**
Intervals:	**PR 0.16, QRS 0.12, QT 0.28**
Axis:	**0 degrees**

Abnormalities
Broad, slurred QRS leads I, aVL, V5–V6, with ST depression and T-wave inversion. (S wave lead V2 + R wave lead V5 equals 50 mm.)

Synthesis
Sinus rhythm. LBBB with associated ST-T-wave changes (consider LVH).

TEST ANSWERS: 1, 74, (78), 104

Comment: It is controversial to make a diagnosis of LVH in the presence of LBBB. However, LVH and LBBB commonly coexist. Standard electrocardiographic criteria for LVH cannot be used in the presence of LBBB because of voltage changes related to the conduction abnormality. A number of modifications of criteria for LVH in the presence of LBBB have been proposed. One report found that the criterion of SV2 + RV5 greater than 45 mm had a specificity of 100 percent and a sensitivity of 86 percent in patients with LBBB and echocardiographic evidence of LVH. Despite this, the diagnosis of LVH in the presence of LBBB must be made with caution. Therefore, the author has added "consider LVH" in this example.

FURTHER READING

Flowers NC: Left bundle branch block: A continuously evolving concept. *J Am Coll Cardiol* 9:684–697, 1987.

Kafka H, Burggraf GW, Milliken JA: Electrocardiographic diagnosis of left ventricular hypertrophy in the presence of left bundle branch block: An echocardiographic study. *Am J Cardiol* 55:103–106, 1985.

Klein RC, Vera Z, DeMaria JA, Mason DT: Electrocardiographic diagnosis of left ventricular hypertrophy in the presence of left bundle branch block. *Am Heart J* 108:502–506, 1984.

Vandenberg BF, Romhilt DW: Electrocardiographic diagnosis of left ventricular hypertrophy in the presence of bundle branch block. *Am Heart J* 122:818–822, 1991.

B-4

Clinical History

A 78-year-old woman with cardiomegaly and bilateral pleural effusions.

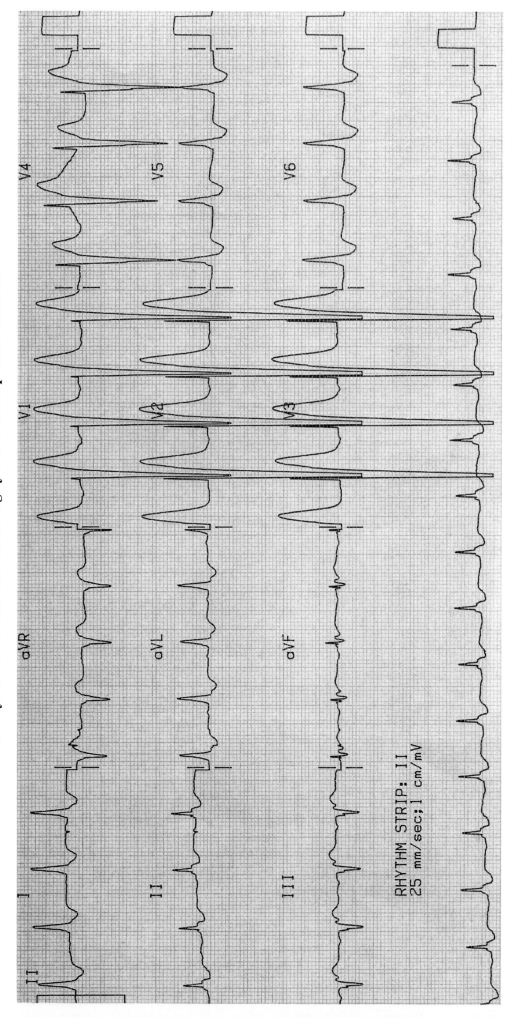

B-5

NARRATIVE INTERPRETATION

> **Rhythm:** **Wide complex tachycardia consistent with ventricular tachycardia**
> **Rate:** **185**
> **Intervals:** **PR –, QRS 0.12, QT –**
> **Axis:** **–60 degrees**

Abnormalities
Rapid heart rate with wide QRS complex. Axis leftward of –30 degrees.

Synthesis
Ventricular tachycardia. Left-axis deviation.

TEST ANSWERS: 30, 64.

Comment: The clinical stability of this patient should not dissuade the clinician from a diagnosis of ventricular tachycardia. A number of clues suggest the origin of this rhythm as ventricular rather than supraventricular with aberrancy. The configuration of the QRS complex both in V1 and V6 suggests ventricular tachycardia, as does the leftward axis. Despite the attending physician's recollection of an abnormal baseline electrocardiogram, the underlying diagnosis of a cardiomyopathy should always lead the clinician to consider ventricular tachycardia first. It is generally wise to treat any wide complex arrhythmia in a patient with structural heart disease as ventricular tachycardia until proven otherwise. This patient's baseline electrocardiogram may be seen in the previous example.

FURTHER READING

Akhtar M, Shenasa M, Jazayeri M, et al: Wide QRS complex tachycardia. *Ann Intern Med* 109:905–912, 1988.
Brugada P, Brugada J, Mont L, et al: A new approach to the differential diagnosis of a regular tachycardia with a wide QRS complex. *Circulation* 83:1649–1659, 1991.
Tchou P, Young P, Mahmud R, et al: Useful clinical criteria for the diagnosis of ventricular tachycardia. *Am J Med* 84:53–56, 1988.
Wellens HJJ, Barr FWHM, Lie KI: The value of the electrocardiogram in the differential diagnosis of a tachycardia with a widened QRS complex. *Am J Med* 84:27–33, 1978.

B-5

Clinical History

A 78-year-old woman who presents to the emergency department with mild lightheadedness and dyspnea. Her physician reports she has a history of a cardiomyopathy and an abnormal electrocardiogram.

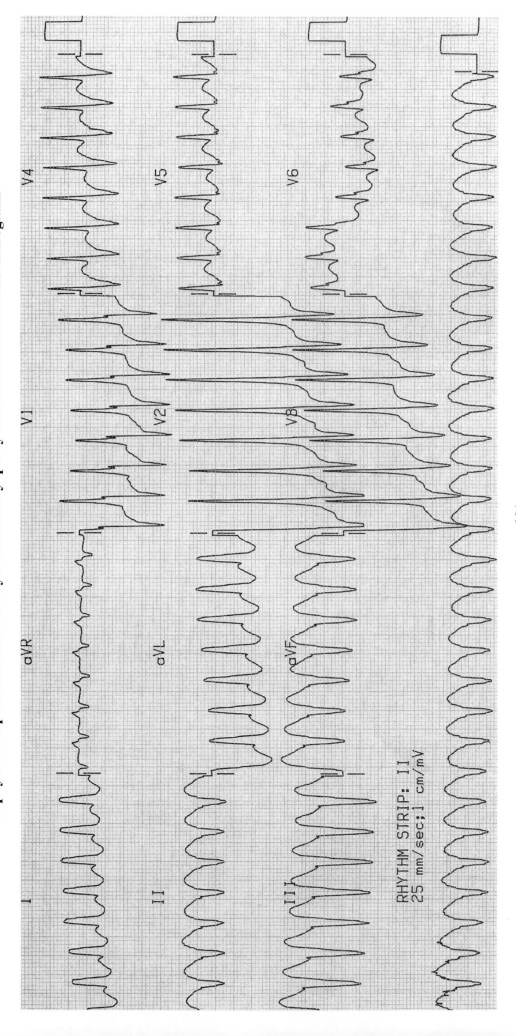

B-6

NARRATIVE INTERPRETATION

Rhythm:	**Sinus**
Rate:	**88**
Intervals:	**PR 0.16, QRS 0.08, QT 0.38**
Axis:	**+60 degrees**

Abnormalities
Abnormal P terminal force V1. R wave V1–V3 less than 3 mm. S wave lead V2 + R wave lead V5 greater than 35 mm.

Synthesis
Sinus rhythm. Left atrial abnormality. Poor R-wave progression. LVH by voltage criteria.

TEST ANSWERS: 1, 60, 66, 78.

Comment: This patient had mitral stenosis with left atrial enlargement confirmed by echocardiography. A deep and wide P terminal force in lead V1 is easily appreciated. A notched P wave is also seen in left atrial abnormality; however, in this example, the peak-to-peak duration of the two notches in lead II is not greater than 40 ms.

LVH is not expected from mitral stenosis and was a reflection of this patient's concomitant hypertension. Poor R-wave progression was also likely secondary to LVH.

FURTHER READING
Hazen MS, Marwick TH, Underwood DA: Diagnostic accuracy of the resting electrocardiogram in detection and estimation of left atrial enlargement: An echocardiographic correlation in 551 patients. *Am Heart J* 122:823–828, 1991.

B-6

Clinical History

A 56-year-old woman with a history of rheumatic fever.

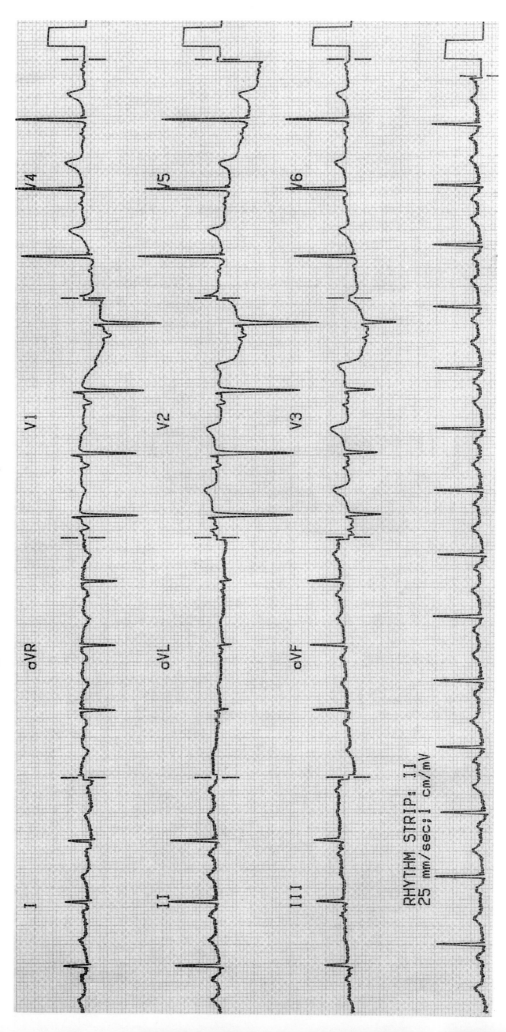

B-7

NARRATIVE INTERPRETATION

Rhythm:	**Atrial fibrillation with complete AV block;**
	AV junctional rhythm
Rate:	**54**
Intervals:	**PR –, QRS 0.12, QT 0.44**
Axis:	**–75 degrees**

Abnormalities

Slow, regular complexes in the presence of atrial fibrillation. Broad, notched QRS with RsR' pattern lead V1–V2 with T-wave inversion leads V1–V3. T-wave inversion leads I, aVL, V4–V6. Axis leftward of –30 degrees (rS waves leads II, III, aVF with broad, initial R wave lead V1).

Synthesis

Atrial fibrillation with complete AV block. AV junctional escape rhythm. RBBB with associated ST-T-wave abnormalities. Left-axis deviation. LAFB (cannot exclude inferior and posterior wall MI of indeterminate age).

TEST ANSWERS: 20, 22, 47, 64, 70, 72, (92), (94), 104.

Comment: The underlying rhythm is atrial fibrillation. The expected irregular conduction to the ventricles is absent because of complete AV block from digitalis toxicity. A subsidiary pacemaker in the AV junction has responded with an escape rhythm. Without prior tracings, one cannot be certain that the complexes were not of ventricular origin. However, the rate of a ventricular escape focus would most likely be slower.

It is difficult to exclude an inferior wall MI in this tracing, but note the small R waves in leads II, III, and aVF, making inferior MI unlikely. A confounding factor is that, LAFB can mask a previous Q wave by directing the initial vector inferiorly. Also note the broad initial R wave in lead V1, which suggests a possible posterior wall MI. Again, this diagnosis is made tenuous in the presence of a conduction abnormality and without an obvious inferior wall MI. Despite the suspicion of prior MI, this patient had normal coronary arteries on catheterization. Therefore, the rS complexes in the inferior leads and the broad R wave in lead V1 were due to the LAFB and RBBB, respectively.

FURTHER READING

Kastor JA, Yurchak PM: Recognition of digitalis intoxication in the presence of atrial fibrillation. *Ann Intern Med* 67:1045–1054, 1967.

B-7

Clinical History

A 73-year-old man 2 days following aortic valve surgery. He has been receiving digoxin.

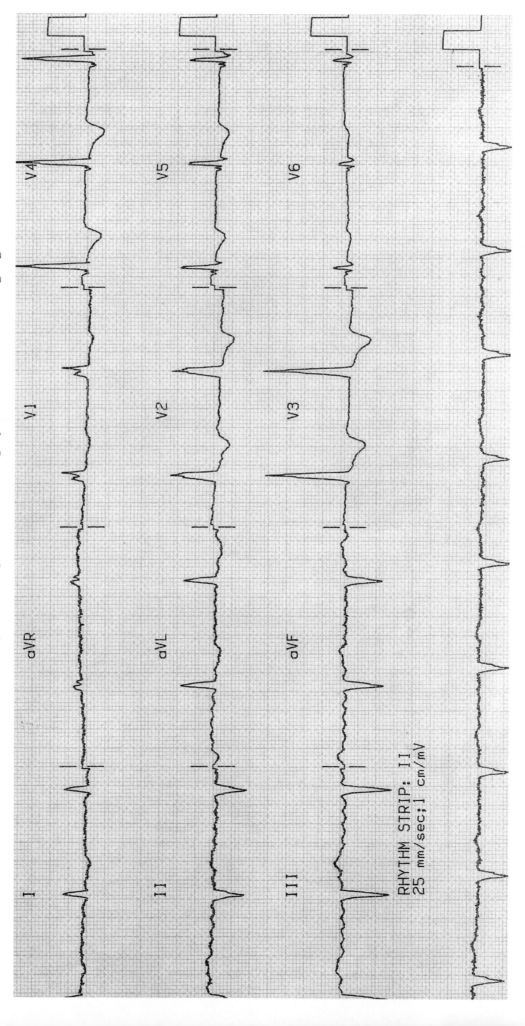

B-8

NARRATIVE INTERPRETATION

Rhythm:	**Sinus bradycardia**
Rate:	**57**
Intervals:	**PR 0.11, QRS 0.10, QT 0.44**
Axis:	**+110 degrees**

Abnormalities

Heart rate less than 60 bpm. Short PR interval. Delta waves negative in leads II, III, aVF, V1–V6. Prolonged QRS with generalized ST-T-wave abnormalities.

Synthesis

Sinus bradycardia. Ventricular preexcitation pattern (WPW).

TEST ANSWERS: 3, 49.

Comment: On first glance, the reader might mistakenly interpret this tracing as a lateral and posterior wall MI. On closer examination, the delta wave becomes evident, particularly in lead III, indicating preexcitation. The delta wave is negative in leads I and aVL and positive in the anterior precordial leads, which creates a pseudoinfarction pattern. This pattern is helpful in localizing the bypass tract to a left lateral location.

FURTHER READING

Goldberger AL: ECG simulators of myocardial infarction. Part I. Pathophysiology and differential diagnosis of pseudoinfarct Q wave patterns. *PACE* 5:106–119, 1982.

Goldberger AL: ECG simulators of myocardial infarction. Part II. Pathophysiology and differential diagnosis of pseudoinfarct ST-T-wave patterns. *PACE* 5:414–430, 1982.

Horowitz LN: Electrophysiologic evaluation of patients with preexcitation syndromes. *Cardiol Clin* 4:447–457, 1986.

Reddy GV, Schamroth L: The localization of bypass tracts in the Wolff-Parkinson-White syndrome from the surface electrocardiogram. *Am Heart J* 113:984–993, 1987.

B-8

Clinical History
A 33-year-old asymptomatic man.

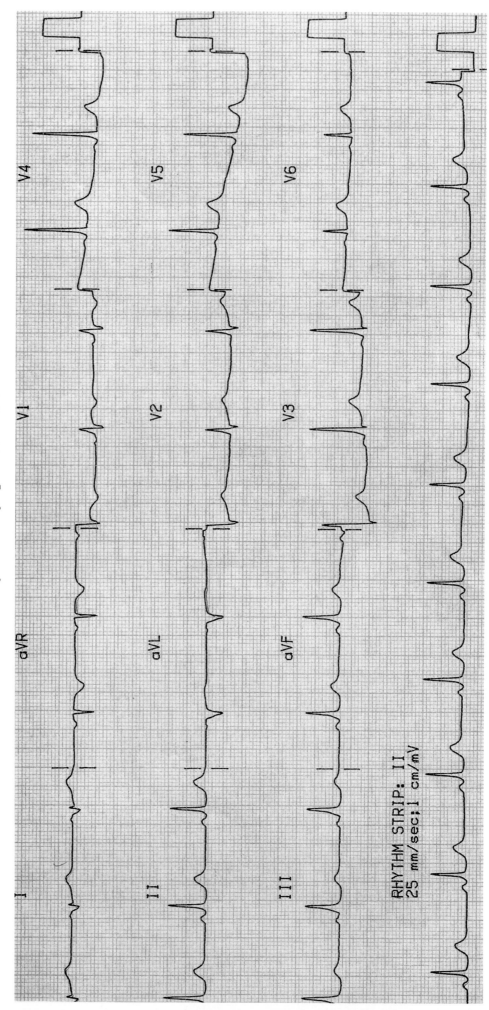

RHYTHM STRIP: II
25 mm/sec; 1 cm/mV

B-9

NARRATIVE INTERPRETATION

Rhythm:	**Sinus tachycardia**
Rate:	**110**
Intervals:	**PR 0.16, QRS 0.08, QT 0.32**
Axis:	**+45 degrees**

Abnormalities
Heart rate greater than 100 bpm.

Synthesis
Sinus tachycardia. Otherwise normal electrocardiogram.

TEST ANSWER: 4.

Comment: It is important for the reader to remember that standard voltage criteria for LVH do not apply to persons ≤30 years of age. One large series that compared voltage criteria for LVH according to age found that the upper limit of normal for SV1 + RV5 (or V6) was 53 mm in patients 16 to 25 years of age compared with 37 mm in patients 31 to 50 years of age (see criteria section for recommendations to diagnose LVH in younger patients).

FURTHER READING
Berk WA: ECG findings in nonpenetrating trauma: A review. *J Emerg Med* 5:209–215, 1987.

Manning GW, Smiley JR: QRS voltage criteria for left ventricular hypertrophy in a normal male population. *Circulation* 29:224–230, 1964.

Tenzer ML: The spectrum of myocardial contusion: A review. *J Trauma* 25:620–627, 1985.

Walker CHM, Rose RL: Importance of age, sex and body habitus in the diagnosis of left ventricular hypertrophy from the precordial electrocardiogram in childhood and adolescence. *Pediatrics* 28:705–711, 1961.

B-9

Clinical History

A 17-year-old male seen in the emergency department following a football injury.

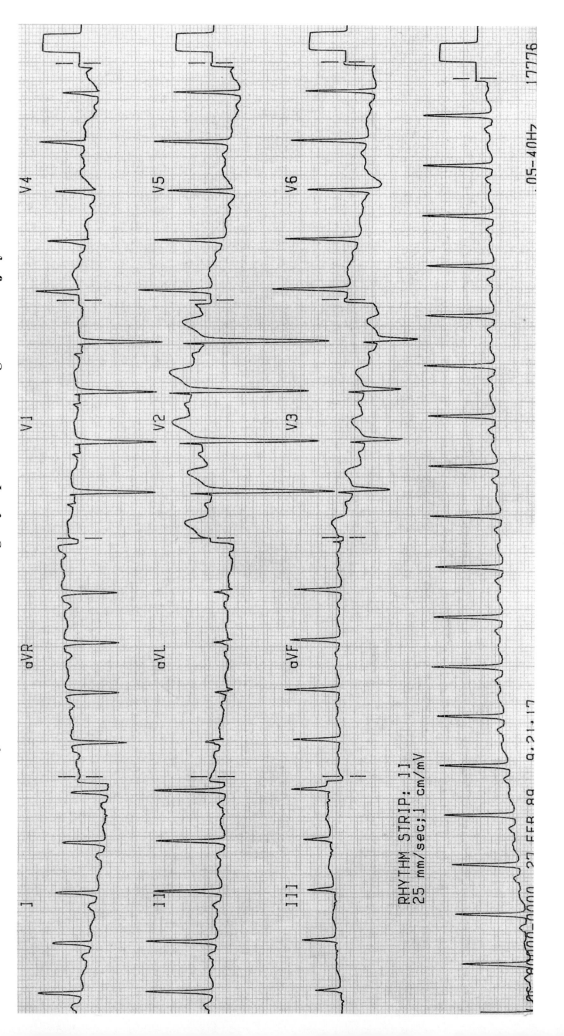

B-10

NARRATIVE INTERPRETATION

Rhythm:	**Sinus**
Rate:	**78**
Intervals:	**PR 0.16, QRS 0.16, QT 0.40**
Axis:	**−60 degrees**

Abnormalities

Axis leftward of − 30 degrees. Q waves leads II, III, aVF. Broad QRS with rsR′ with T-wave inversion lead V1. T-wave inversion leads II, III, aVF.

Synthesis

Sinus rhythm. Inferior wall MI of indeterminate age. Left-axis deviation. RBBB with associated ST-T-wave abnormalities.

TEST ANSWERS: 1, 64, 70, 92, 104, (106).

Comment: This is an interesting tracing because it illustrates the combined presence of inferior wall MI, left-axis deviation, and RBBB. In RBBB, the first portion of the QRS complex (first 0.06 s) may be interpreted normally. Accordingly, the deep inferior Q waves are diagnostic of this patient's prior inferior wall MI. The left-axis deviation is a result of the inferior wall MI and is not secondary to a left anterior fascicular block. Note that there are late R waves present in leads III and aVF, a finding that indicates inferiorly directed terminal forces. In LAFB these forces should remain in a superior direction and would demonstrate an S wave in these leads. The T-wave inversions in the inferior limb leads are likely secondary to the prior MI but may also be classified as nonspecific.

FURTHER READING

Fisher ML, Mugmon MA, Carliner NH, et al: Left anterior fascicular block: Electrocardiographic criteria for its recognition in the presence of inferior myocardial infarction. *Am J Cardiol* 44:845–849, 1979.

Milliken JA: Isolated and complicated left anterior fascicular block: A review of suggested electrocardiographic criteria. *J Electrocardiol* 16:199–212, 1983.

Warner RA, Hill NE, Mookherjee S, Smulyan H: Electrocardiographic criteria for the diagnosis of combined inferior myocardial infarction and left anterior hemiblock. *Am Heart J* 51:718–722, 1983.

B-10

Clinical History

A 54-year-old man admitted for elective cholecystectomy.

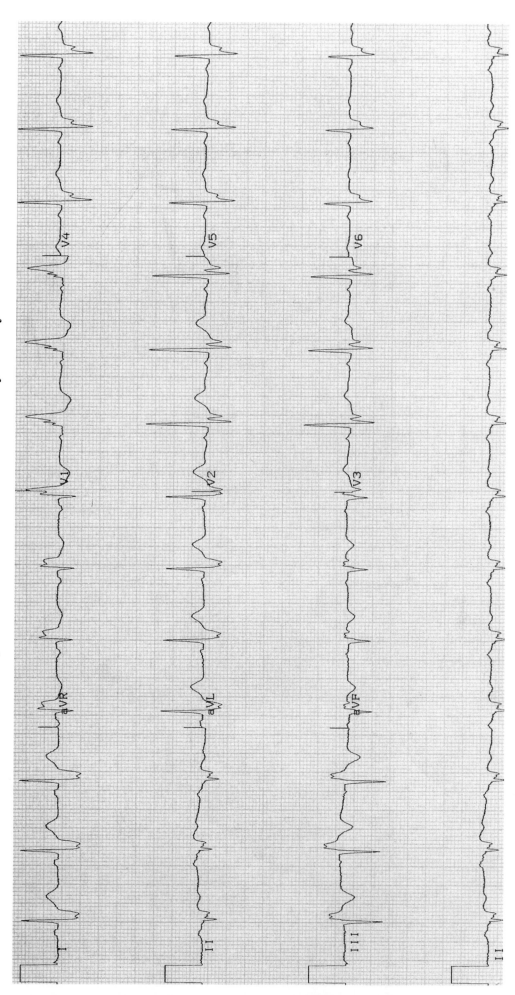

B-11

NARRATIVE INTERPRETATION

Rhythm:	**Supraventricular tachyarrhythmia, probably atrial flutter with 2:1 AV conduction**
Rate:	**Ventricular rate 140, atrial rate 280 (probable)**
Intervals:	**PR –, QRS 0.08, QT 0.26**
Axis:	**+15 degrees**

Abnormalities
Rapid heart rate. ST depression leads I, II, III, aVF, V4–V6. T-wave inversion leads II, III, aVF, V4–V6. S wave lead V2 + R wave lead V5 greater than 35 mm.

Synthesis
Supraventricular tachyarrhythmia, probably atrial flutter with 2:1 AV conduction. LVH by voltage criteria. Associated ST-T-wave abnormalities.

TEST ANSWERS: (18), 19, (50), 78, 103.

Comment: The differentiation of sinus tachycardia, supraventricular tachycardia, and atrial flutter with 2:1 AV conduction can often be quite difficult based on a single electrocardiogram. The reader should suspect atrial flutter whenever the heart rate is approximately 150 bpm, even if only a single abnormal P wave is evident. The second P wave of atrial flutter may be "buried" in the QRS complex. In this example, there is no unequivocal P wave, although it is suspected to be superimposed on the T wave of the preceding complex.

The clinician can often determine the actual rhythm at the bedside by using vagal maneuvers such as carotid sinus pressure. Patients with sinus tachycardia characteristically show only slight slowing of the heart rate with this maneuver, whereas those with supraventricular tachycardia may convert to regular sinus rhythm. Carotid pressure will not convert atrial flutter to sinus, but it may may diminish AV conduction enough to uncover flutter waves (see next tracing).

B-11

Clinical History

A 56-year-old man in the emergency department with *unexplained* tachycardia.

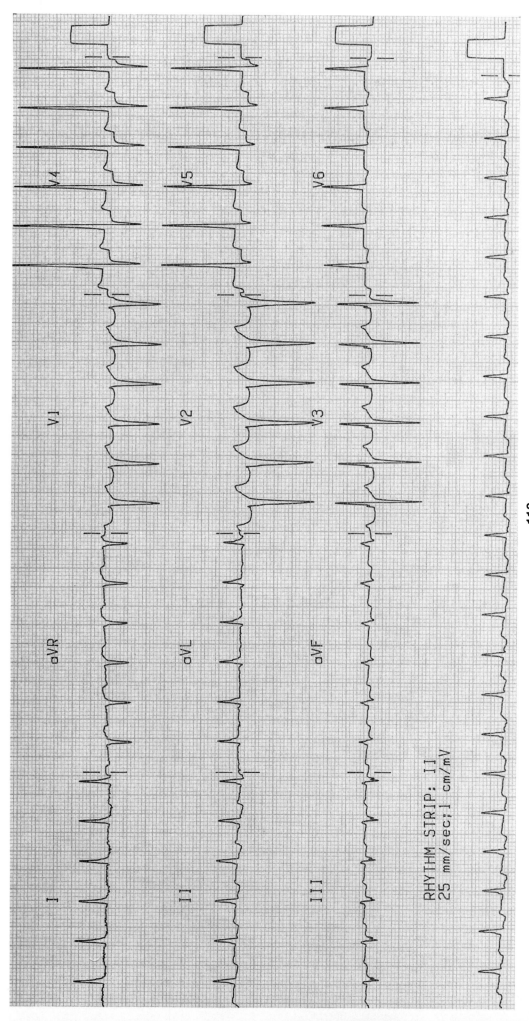

B-12

NARRATIVE INTERPRETATION

Rhythm:	**Atrial flutter with 4:1 AV conduction**
Rate:	**Atrial rate 296, ventricular rate 74**
Intervals:	**PR −, QRS 0.08, QT 0.34**
Axis:	**+15 degrees**

Abnormalities
ST depression leads I, II, aVF, V4–V6. T-wave inversion leads V4–V6. R wave less than 3 mm leads V1–V3. S wave lead V2 + R wave lead V5 greater than 35 mm.

Synthesis
Atrial flutter with 4:1 AV conduction. LVH. Associated ST-T-wave abnormalities. Poor R-wave progression.

TEST ANSWERS: 19, 51, 66, 78, 103.

Comment: The patient in the previous tracing has been given adenosine, increasing the degree of AV block and "uncovering" atrial flutter waves. The physiologic 2:1 AV conduction of the previous tracing is now nonphysiologic 4:1 AV conduction due to the medication. Adenosine has multiple cardiac effects in addition to its inhibition of AV conduction. These include slowing of the SA node, decreasing atrial contractility, and coronary vasodilation.

Other intravenous medications that have proven useful in the acute care setting to assist with rhythm determination include verapamil, diltiazem, and short-acting beta-blockers such as esmolol.

FURTHER READING
Belardinelli L, Linden JH, Berne RM: The cardiac effects of adenosine. *Prog Cardiovasc Dis* 32:73–97, 1989.

B-12

Clinical History

A 56-year-old man in the emergency department with unexplained tachycardia. He has been administered adenosine.

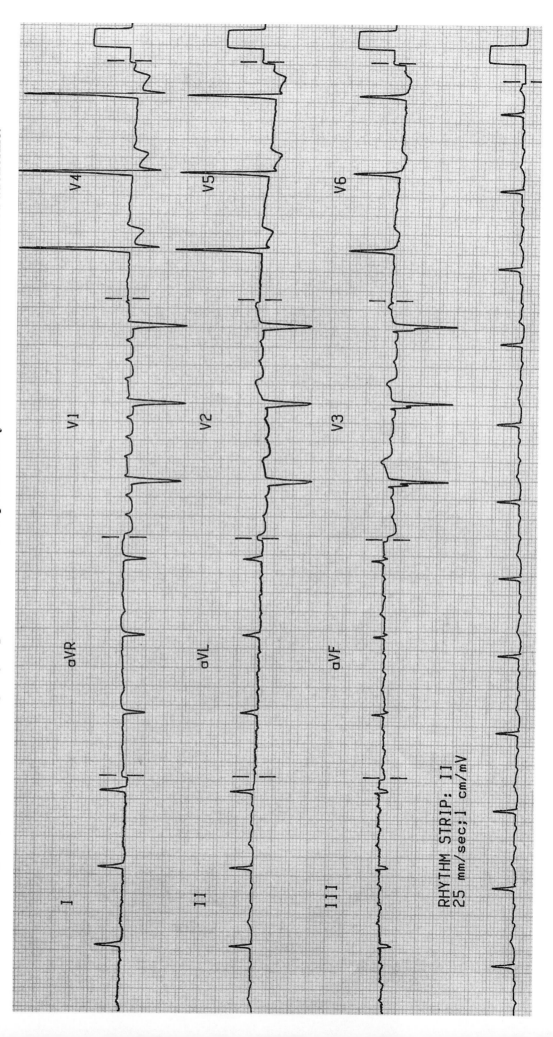

B-13

NARRATIVE INTERPRETATION

Rhythm:	**Multifocal atrial rhythm (MAR); multifocal atrial tachycardia (MAT)**
Rate:	**95 (MAR), 140 (MAT)**
Intervals:	**PR −, QRS 0.08, QT 0.36**
Axis:	**+120 degrees**

Abnormalities

Frequent, multifocal APCs. Period of MAT on rhythm strip. Axis rightward of + 90 degrees. ST depression leads II, III, aVF, V1–V3. Tall R wave lead V1. Deep S waves leads V5–V6.

Synthesis

Multifocal atrial rhythm with period of multifocal atrial tachycardia. Right axis deviation. RVH. Associated (or nonspecific) ST abnormalities.

TEST ANSWERS: 13, 14, 65, 79, 103, (106).

Comment: This tracing demonstrates both the rhythm disturbances and QRS morphology seen in patients with severe COPD and cor pulmonale. Right ventricular hypertrophy is suggested by right axis deviation, tall R waves in the right precordial leads, and deep S waves in the left precordial leads. The ST-T abnormalities in the right precordial leads are most likely also related to RVH.

Multifocal atrial rhythm and multifocal atrial tachycardia are rhythm disturbances associated with COPD. By definition, multifocal atrial rhythm describes a rhythm of less than 100 bpm where there is no dominant atrial mechanism. This distinguishes it from sinus rhythm with frequent APCs where there is a clear sinus focus. Multifocal atrial tachycardia is diagnosed when there are multiple atrial foci at a rate greater than 100 bpm. Both rhythms appear in this example.

FURTHER READING

Kastor JA: Multifocal atrial tachycardia. *N Engl J Med* 322:1713–1717, 1990.

B-13

Clinical History
A 60-year-old heavy smoker.

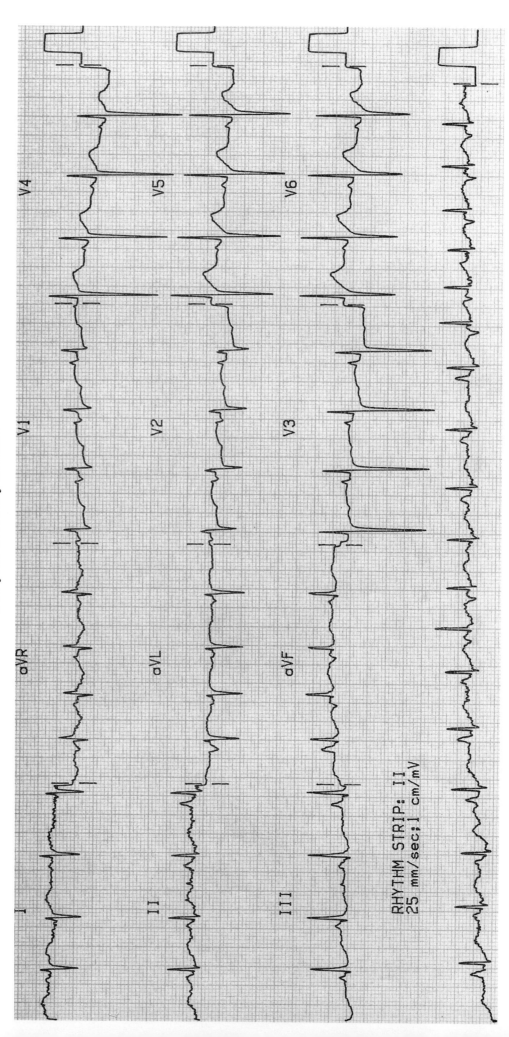

RHYTHM STRIP: II
25 mm/sec; 1 cm/mV

B-14

NARRATIVE INTERPRETATION

Rhythm:	**Sinus**
Rate:	**95**
Intervals:	**PR 0.16, QRS 0.08, QT 0.36**
Axis:	**0 degrees**

Abnormalities
Limb lead voltage less than 5 mm. VPC. APC.

Synthesis
Sinus rhythm. VPC. APC. Low-voltage limb leads.

TEST ANSWERS: 1, 10, 26, 67.

Comment: Low limb-lead voltage is present in this patient. Causes of low voltage include COPD, pericardial effusion, multiple MIs with loss of viable myocardium, myxedema, amyloidosis, and marked obesity.

The first complex of the tracing is most likely a VPC, although this cannot be confirmed without visualization of the prior complex. On careful inspection, APCs are also evident. Note that the eighth complex is premature and shows an altered P-wave configuration.

B-14

Clinical History
A 75-year-old man with sepsis.

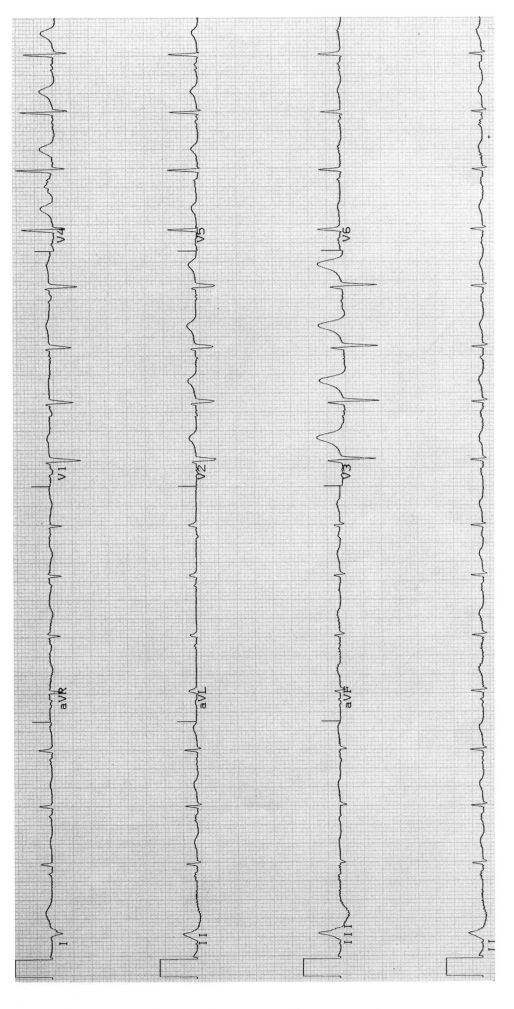

B-15

NARRATIVE INTERPRETATION

Rhythm:	**Sinus, with sinus arrhythmia**
Rate:	**65**
Intervals:	**PR 0.16, QRS 0.08, QT 0.38**
Axis:	**+60 degrees**

Abnormalities
Variation in PP interval of more than 0.16 s.

Synthesis
Sinus rhythm with sinus arrhythmia; otherwise normal electrocardiogram.

TEST ANSWERS: 1, 2.

Comment: Sinus arrhythmia is defined when the basic rhythm is sinus, but the P-to-P interval varies by at least 0.16 s. It is usually seen when the intrinsic sinus rate is slow. A gradual lengthening and shortening of the P-to-P intervals differentiate this rhythm from sinoatrial block.

Sinus arrhythmia may be divided into respiratory and nonrespiratory forms. Respiratory sinus arrhythmia is a result of alterations in vagal tone induced by the respiratory cycle. Inspiration raises the heart rate and expiration slows it. Respiratory sinus arrhythmia is most common in younger persons and does not reflect cardiac pathology. Nonrespiratory sinus arrhythmia is unrelated to the respiratory cycle and may result from drugs such as opiates and digitalis. Elderly persons with slow intrinsic heart rates may also show marked nonrespiratory sinus arrhythmia.

B-15

Clinical History
An asymptomatic 18-year-old man.

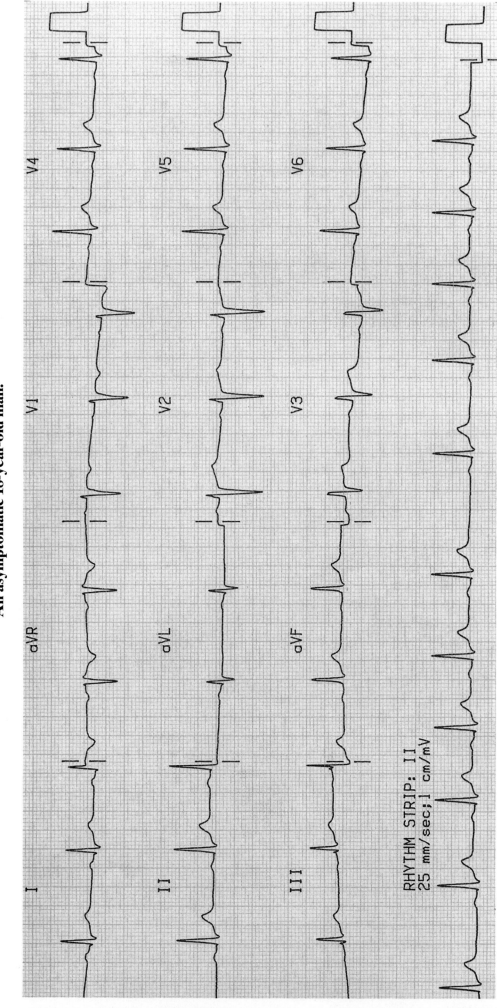

RHYTHM STRIP: II
25 mm/sec; 1 cm/mV

B-16

NARRATIVE INTERPRETATION

Rhythm:	**Sinus**
Rate:	**46**
Intervals:	**PR 0.16, QRS 0.08, QT 0.32**
Axis:	**+30 degrees**

Abnormalities

Slow heart rate. VPCs, interpolated with postextrasystolic PR prolongation. Q wave leads II, III, aVF. ST-segment elevation (coved) leads III, aVF. T-wave inverted leads III, aVF. T-wave biphasic lead II. T-wave greater than S wave lead V2.

Synthesis

Sinus bradycardia with frequent, uniform, interpolated VPCs. Inferior wall MI with ST-T-wave abnormalities suggesting recent injury. Possible posterior wall MI of indeterminate age.

TEST ANSWERS: 3, 26, 58, 91, (94), 100.

Comment: This is an excellent example of the concealed retrograde conduction characteristic of interpolated VPCs. Interpolated VPCs most often occur when the sinus mechanism is slow. The ventricular depolarization conducts retrograde into the AV junction and renders it partially refractory to the next supraventricular impulse. When the next sinus beat occurs, the impulse is slowed and conducts to the ventricles with a prolonged PR interval. The retrograde conduction of the VPC is *concealed* in that it is not actually seen electrocardiographically, but may be inferred by its PR prolonging effect on the next impulse.

A probable recent, evolving inferior wall MI is present, although the true duration cannot be determined from a single tracing. The reader should also consider a posterior MI in view of the tall R wave in lead V2.

B-16

Clinical History

A 59-year-old man in the coronary care unit (CCU).

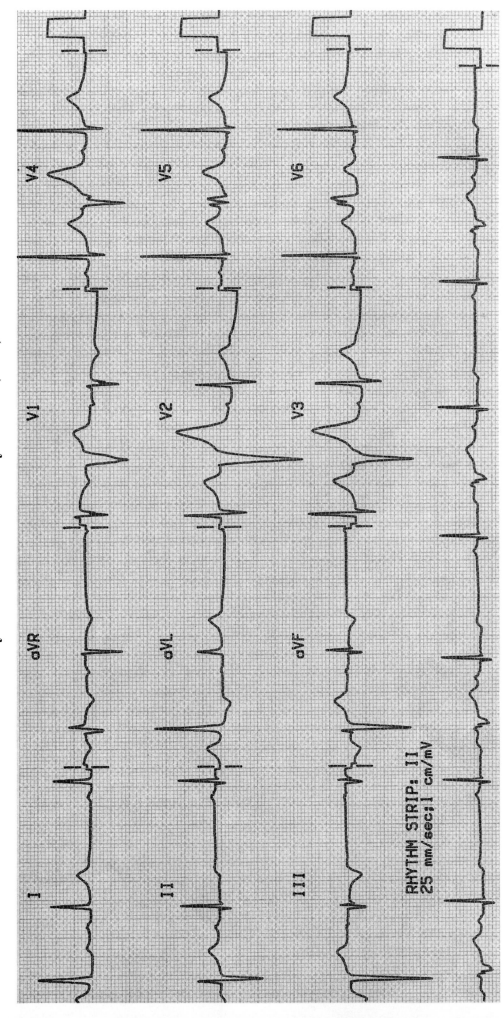

B-17

NARRATIVE INTERPRETATION

Rhythm:	**Sinus bradycardia**
Rate:	**47**
Intervals:	**PR 0.18, QRS 0.16, QT 0.52**
Axis:	**−45 degrees**

Abnormalities
Slow heart rate. Broad notched QRS leads I, aVL, V6 with associated ST depression and T-wave inversion leads I, aVL, V6. Axis leftward of −30 degrees.

Synthesis
Sinus bradycardia. LBBB with associated ST-T-wave abnormalities. Left axis deviation.

TEST ANSWERS: 3, 64, 74, 104.

Comment: The development of a *new* LBBB is an important marker for significant underlying heart disease. The Framingham study found that newly acquired LBBB identified a high-risk population with advanced hypertensive or atherosclerotic heart disease. Within 10 years of follow-up, 50 percent of those with new onset LBBB were dead from cardiovascular disease. Importantly, progression to complete heart block is infrequent, and permanent pacemaker insertion is not indicated.

FURTHER READING
Schneider JF, Thomas HE, Kreger BE, et al: Newly acquired left bundle branch block. *Ann Intern Med* 90:303–310, 1979.

B-17

Clinical History

An 83-year-old woman who is being treated for hypertension. A year ago her electrocardiogram demonstrated LVH.

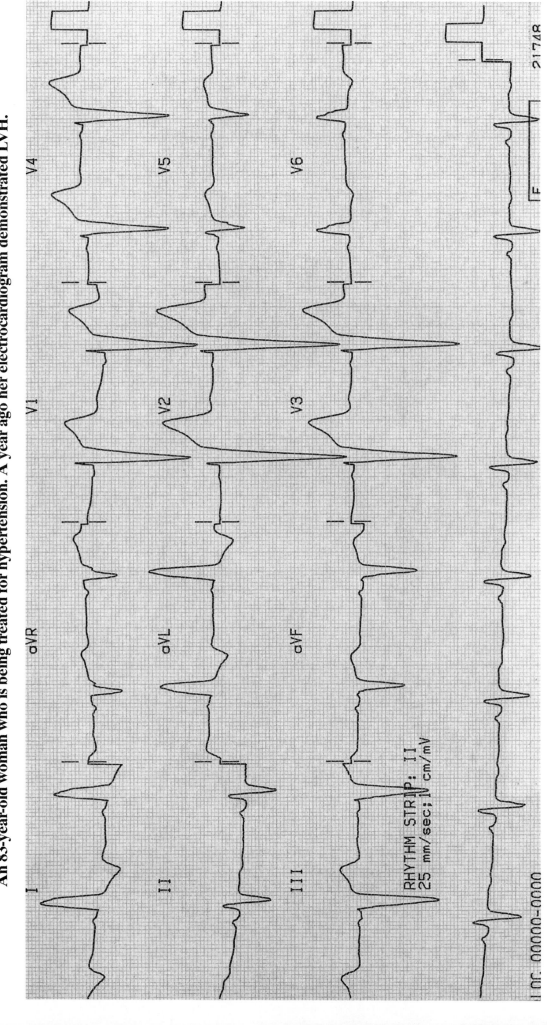

B-18

NARRATIVE INTERPRETATION

Rhythm:	**Sinus**
Rate:	**70**
Intervals:	**PR 0.18, QRS 0.08, QT 0.40**
Axis:	**−45 degrees**

Abnormalities

Axis leftward of −30 degrees. Q wave leads II, III, aVF. R wave greater than S wave with upright T wave leads V1–V2.

Synthesis

Sinus rhythm. Inferior and posterior wall MI of indeterminate age. Left axis deviation. Left anterior fascicular block.

TEST ANSWERS: 1, 64, 72, 92, 94.

Comment: Interpretation of this electrocardiogram is not as easy as it might initially seem. There is an old inferior wall MI. There is also evidence of a posterior wall infarction on the basis of a broad, tall R wave in lead V1 (and V2), with an upright T wave in lead V1. This is a very reliable finding in the presence of an inferior wall MI.

This tracing also illustrates the difficulty in determining whether left anterior fascicular block (LAFB) coexists with inferior wall MI. These entities may induce left axis deviation alone or together. Note, however, that there is a terminal conduction delay in aVR that occurs after the R wave in aVL, which is indicative of a counterclockwise vector loop in the frontal plane. This is characteristic of LAFB. The "notch" in lead II and aVF also suggests a concomitant LAFB and inferior wall MI.

FURTHER READING

Fisher ML, Mugmon MA, Carliner NH, et al: Left anterior fascicular block: Electrocardiographic criteria for its recognition in the presence of inferior myocardial infarction. *Am J Cardiol* 44:845–849, 1979.

Warner RA, Hill NE, Mookherjee S, Smulyan H: Electrocardiographic criteria for the diagnosis of combined inferior myocardial infarction and left anterior hemiblock. *Am Heart J* 51:718–722, 1983.

126

B-18

Clinical History

A 52-year-old asymptomatic man seen after a recent hospitalization.

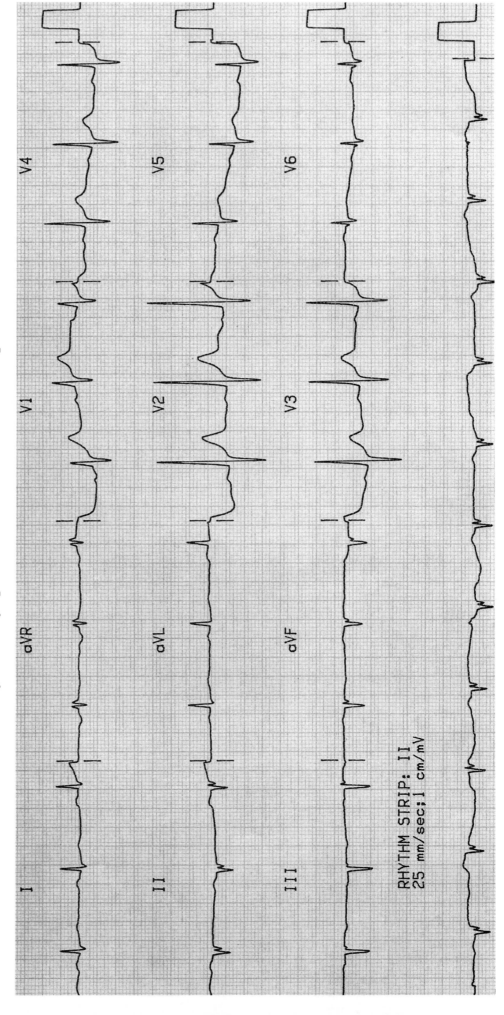

B-19

NARRATIVE INTERPRETATION

Rhythm:	**Sinus bradycardia**
Rate:	**54**
Intervals:	**PR 0.14, QRS 0.08, QT 0.40**
Axis:	**+60 degrees**

Abnormalities

Heart rate less than 60 bpm. ST elevation leads II, III, aVF, V2–V6. Biphasic T waves leads II, III, aVF, V2. T-wave inversion leads V3–V6. S wave lead V2 + R wave lead V5 greater than 35 mm.

Synthesis

Sinus bradycardia. ST-T-segment changes suggesting acute myocardial injury. LVH by voltage criteria.

TEST ANSWERS: 3, 78, 100.

Comment: Diffuse ST elevation is present in the inferior leads and across the precordium. There are no diagnostic Q waves to allow further characterization, so it is proper to simply indicate acute myocardial injury without further localization. This ST-T-wave pattern suggests the presence of a high-grade stenosis of the left anterior descending coronary artery.

This patient sustained an anterior, apical, non-Q-wave MI. He underwent cardiac catheterization and subsequent angioplasty of a 95 percent stenosis of the proximal left anterior descending coronary artery.

FURTHER READING

de Zwaan C, Bar FWHM, Wellens HJJ: Characteristic electrocardiographic pattern indicating a critical stenosis high in left anterior descending coronary artery in patients admitted because of impending myocardial infarction. *Am Heart J* 103:730–737, 1982.

B-19

Clinical History

A 63-year-old hypertensive man with chest pressure for 2 h.

I aVR V1 V4

II aVL V2 V5

III aVF V3 V6

RHYTHM STRIP: II
25 mm/sec; 1 cm/mV

INTERPRETED B

B-20

NARRATIVE INTERPRETATION

Rhythm: Sinus
Rate: 82
Intervals: PR 0.16, QRS 0.14, QT 0.38
Axis: +105 degrees

Abnormalities
Axis rightward of +90 degrees. Broad notched QRS with rSR' pattern and T-wave inversion lead V1.

Synthesis
Sinus rhythm. RBBB. Associated ST-T-wave abnormalities. Right axis deviation. Left posterior fascicular block.

TEST ANSWERS: 1, 65, 70, 73, 104.

Comment: Remember that in patients with RBBB the initial portion of the QRS complex may still be interpreted in the usual fashion. A rightward axis is clearly evident in this example and suggests a left posterior fascicular block. Also note that in LPFB, the initial forces are directed leftward and superior via the left anterior fascicle, which produces small Q waves in the inferior leads. The narrow Q waves in this example are the result of the LPFB and not from an inferior wall MI. The ST findings in the inferior leads may raise suspicion of acute myocardial injury, but they are still consistent with the RBBB alone. The clinical history supports this interpretation.

B-20

Clinical History
An 89-year-old asymptomatic man.

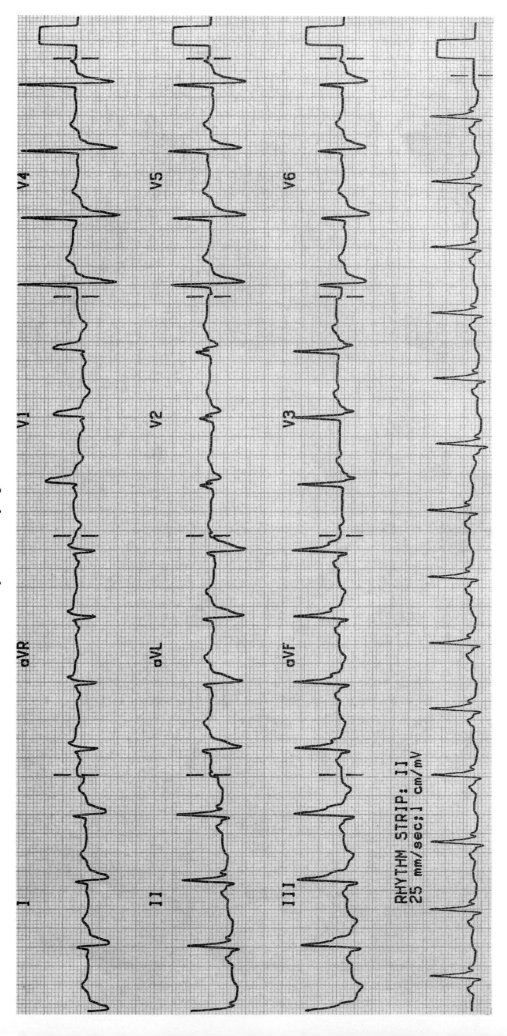

B-21

NARRATIVE INTERPRETATION

Rhythm:	**Sinus**
Rate:	**75**
Intervals:	**PR –, QRS –, QT –**
Axis:	**–**

Abnormalities

Dual-chamber pacemaker with appropriate atrial sensing and pacing and appropriate ventricular sensing and pacing. DDD mode. VPC.

Synthesis

Sinus rhythm. VPC. Dual-chamber pacemaker functioning in DDD mode with appropriate atrial and ventricular sensing, and capture.

TEST ANSWERS: 1, 26, 38.

Comment: This tracing illustrates all the functions of a dual-chamber pacemaker programmed to the DDD mode. The first three letters of the pacemaker code indicate which chamber is paced, which chamber is sensed, and the mode of response to sensing. A DDD pacemaker operates in an AV sequential manner; it paces the ventricle as required after either sensing an atrial depolarization or following a paced atrial beat. Note that until the intrinsic P waves appeared in the eighth complex on the rhythm strip, one could not confirm the presence of atrial sensing. Appropriate ventricular sensing is confirmed by the response following the VPC.

When analyzing pacemaker electrocardiograms, one should first analyze the underlying rhythm. Then determine which chambers are paced, which are sensed, and the relationship of these factors to each other. Remember, that not all dual-chamber pacemakers are programmed to DDD.

FURTHER READING

Garson A Jr: Stepwise approach to the unknown pacemaker ECG. Am *Heart J* 119:924–941 1990.

B-21

Clinical History

A 78-year-old woman seen on routine examination.

B-22

NARRATIVE INTERPRETATION

Rhythm:	**Atrial fibrillation**
Rate:	**60 (average)**
Intervals:	**PR −, QRS 0.11, QT 0.42**
Axis:	**−45 degrees**

Abnormalities

Axis leftward of −30 degrees. ST depression leads I, aVL. T-wave inversion leads I, aVL. S wave lead V2 + R wave lead V5 greater than 35 mm. R wave lead I + S wave lead III greater than 25 mm. R wave lead aVL + S wave lead V3 greater than 28 mm in a man. R wave V1–V3 less than 3 mm. Prolonged QRS duration.

Synthesis

Atrial fibrillation with a controlled ventricular response. Left-axis deviation. Left anterior fascicular block. Intraventricular conduction delay. Left ventricular hypertrophy. ST-T-wave abnormalities associated with ventricular hypertrophy. Poor R-wave progression.

TEST ANSWERS: 20, 51, 64, 66, 72, 76, 78, 103.

Comment: This tracing illustrates a number of abnormalities. Atrial fibrillation is present, however the ventricular response is slower than would be expected and suggests either intrinsic conduction disease or medications that block AV node conduction.

Multiple criteria for left ventricular hypertrophy are present. The intraventricular conduction delay, ST-T-wave abnormalities, and poor R wave progression are all likely to be related to ventricular hypertrophy or enlargement. This patient demonstrated four chamber enlargement secondary to an ischemic cardiomyopathy (see next two tracings).

B-22

Clinical History
A 70-year-old man admitted to the CCU.

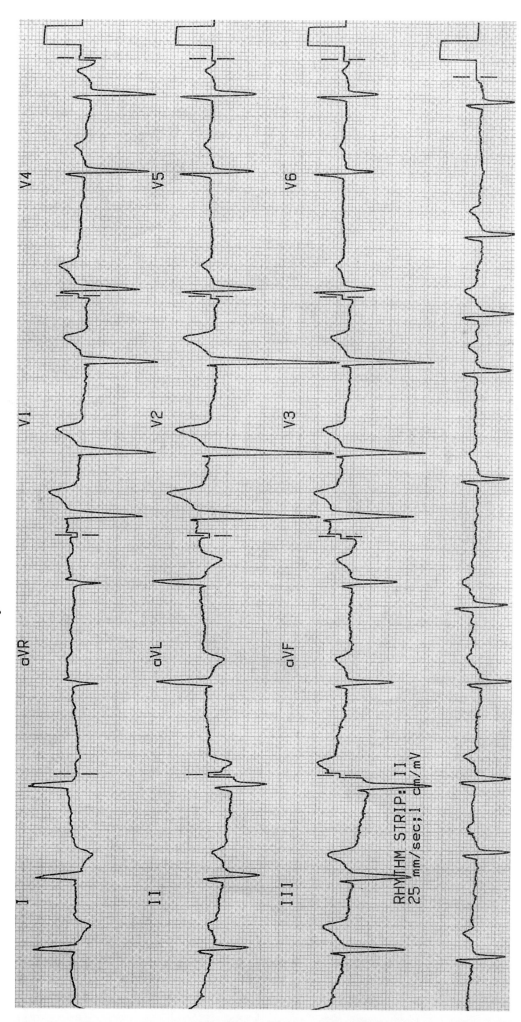

B-23

NARRATIVE INTERPRETATION

Rhythm:	**Atrial fibrillation**
Rate:	**118 (average)**
Intervals:	**PR −, QRS 0.11, QT 0.36**
Axis:	**−45 degrees**

Abnormalities

Rapid heart rate. Prolonged QRS duration. Wide complex beats on rhythm strip. Axis leftward of −30 degrees. ST depression leads I, II, aVL, aVF, V4–V6. T-wave inversion leads I, aVL. S wave lead V2 + R wave lead V6 greater than 35 mm. R wave lead aVL + S wave lead V3 greater than 28 mm in a man. R wave V1–V3 less than 3 mm.

Synthesis

Atrial fibrillation with a rapid ventricular response. VPCs. Left-axis deviation. Left anterior fascicular block. Left ventricular hypertrophy. ST-T-wave abnormalities suggestive of myocardial ischemia. Poor R-wave progression. Intraventricular conduction delay.

TEST ANSWERS: 20, 26, 50, 64, 66, 72, 76, 78, 102, (103).

Comment: This is a follow-up to the previous tracing. Compared with the earlier example, there are additional ST abnormalities that reflect myocardial ischemia. The ST depression is more prominent in leads I and aVL and is now much more characteristic of myocardial ischemia than of LVH in leads II and V4–V6.

The increase in the heart rate allows the interpreter to characterize the AV response as *physiologic* (see next tracing).

136

B-23

Clinical History
A 70-year-old man admitted to the CCU.

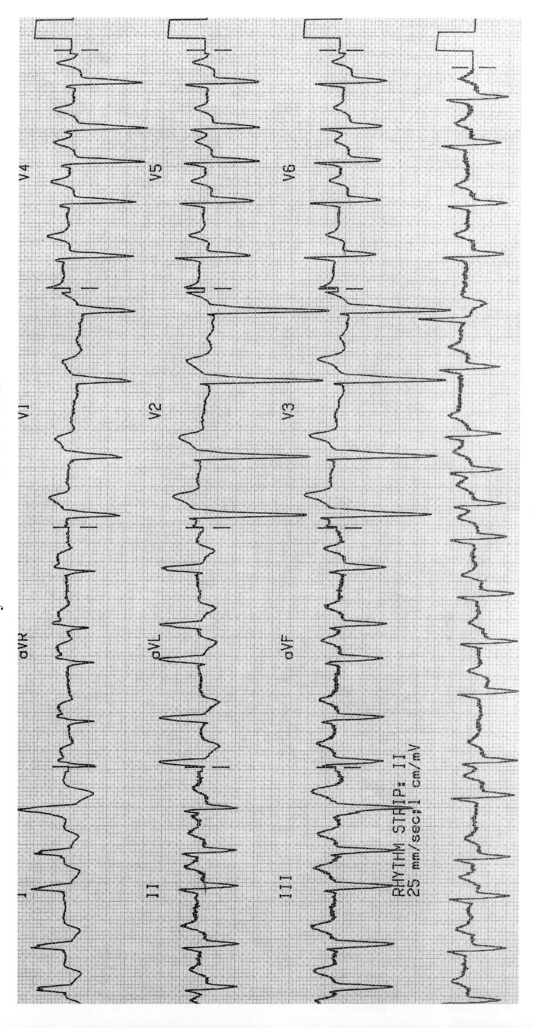

B-24

NARRATIVE INTERPRETATION

Rhythm:	**Atrial fibrillation with high-grade AV block;**
	AV junctional escape rhythm
Rate:	**40**
Intervals:	**PR –, QRS 0.11, QT 0.46**
Axis:	**–45 degrees**

Abnormalities

Slow heart rate. ST depression leads I, aVL. T-wave inversion leads I, aVL, V6. Axis leftward of –30 degrees. R-wave voltage V1–V3 less than 3 mm. R wave lead aVL + S wave lead V3 greater than 28 mm in a man. Prolonged QRS duration. VPC.

Synthesis

Atrial fibrillation with high-degree AV block. AV junctional escape rhythm. VPC. Left-axis deviation. Left anterior fascicular block. Left ventricular hypertrophy. Poor R-wave progression. Intraventricular conduction delay. ST-T wave abnormalities associated with ventricular hypertrophy.

TEST ANSWERS: 20, 22, 26, 46, (51), 64, 66, 72, 76, 78, 103, (106).

Comment: This example is the third tracing in this series. This patient required treatment with both beta blockers and diltiazem to control myocardial ischemia. The result on the cardiac conduction system was high-grade AV block with an AV junctional escape rhythm. The majority of the complexes have the identical RR interval and indicate a junctional escape focus. Complete AV block is not evident because the fifth and seventh complexes on the rhythm strip occur earlier than expected, reflecting AV conduction of the atrial impulses. Remember that this rhythm disturbance, often characteristic of digitalis toxicity, may occur from other medications.

138

B-24

Clinical History

A 70-year-old man admitted to the CCU. He has been administered anti-ischemic agents.

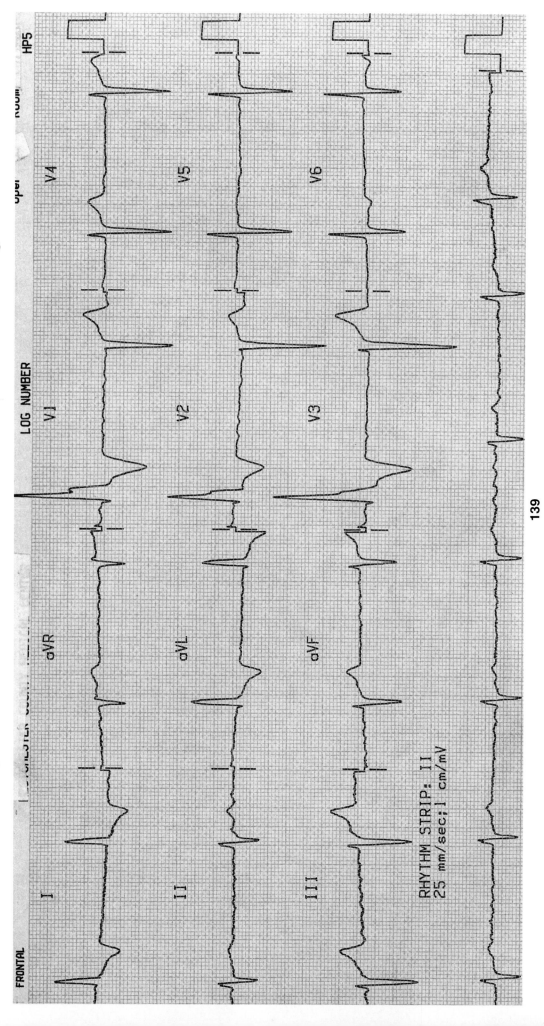

B-25

NARRATIVE INTERPRETATION

Rhythm:	**Sinus bradycardia with first-degree AV block**
Rate:	**55**
Intervals:	**PR 0.26, QRS 0.10, QT 0.44**
Axis:	**+30 degrees**

Abnormalities

Slow heart rate. Prolonged PR interval. P-wave duration greater than 0.12 s. Slightly prolonged QRS interval with absent septal Q waves and slurred initial upstroke in leads V4–V6. ST depression leads I, II, aVL, aVF, V4–V6. S wave lead V2 + R wave lead V5 greater than 35 mm.

Synthesis

Sinus bradycardia. First-degree AV block. Nonspecific atrial abnormality. Incomplete LBBB. LVH by voltage criteria. ST-T-wave abnormalities associated with ventricular hypertrophy and/or conduction abnormality.

TEST ANSWERS: 3, 42, 62, 75, 78, 103, 104, (106).

Comment: This patient demonstrates the frequent association of LVH and incomplete LBBB. Standard voltage criteria for LVH may be used in the presence of incomplete LBBB. The concomitant conduction abnormality is suggested by absent septal Q waves and a slurred upstroke in the left precordial leads. Both incomplete LBBB and LVH may result in prolongation of the QRS complex and ST-T-wave abnormalities (see next tracing).

An additional finding in this tracing is nonspecific atrial abnormality. This may be diagnosed when there is a prolongation of the P wave without specific criteria for left or right atrial abnormality.

FURTHER READING

Barold SS, Linhart JW, Hildner FJ, et al: Incomplete left bundle branch block. *Circulation* 38:702–710 1968.
Schamroth L, Bradlow BA: Incomplete left bundle branch block. *Br Heart J* 26:285–288, 1964.

Clinical History
A 76-year-old man with valvular heart disease.

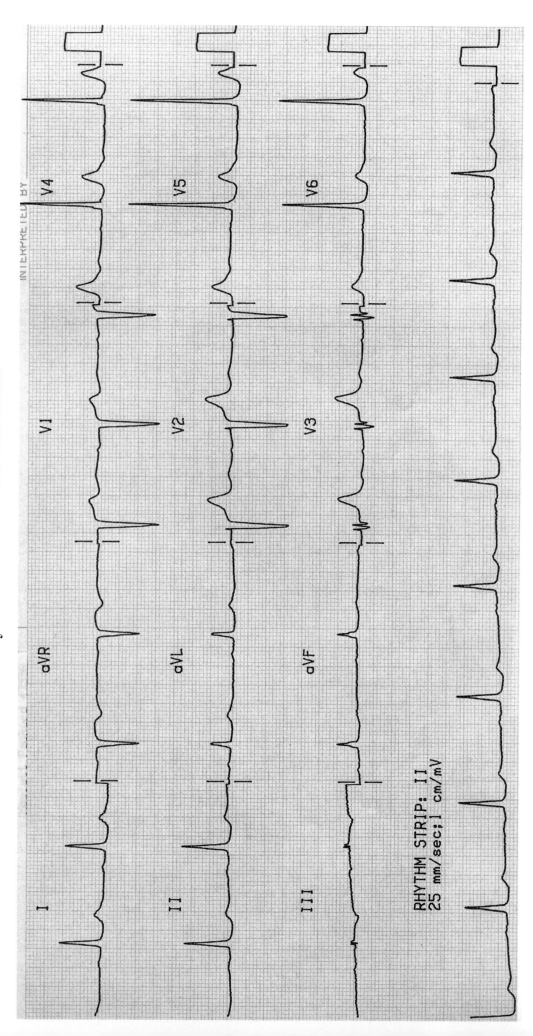

B-26

NARRATIVE INTERPRETATION

> **Rhythm:** Sinus with first-degree AV block
> **Rate:** 72
> **Intervals:** PR 0.26, QRS 0.14, QT 0.36
> **Axis:** +30 degrees

Abnormalities
Prolonged PR interval. P-wave duration greater than 0.12 s. Broad, notched QRS with ST depression and T-wave inversion leads I, aVL, V5–V6.

Synthesis
Sinus rhythm. First-degree AV block. Nonspecific atrial abnormality. LBBB with associated ST-T-wave abnormalities.

TEST ANSWERS: 1, 42, 62, 74, 104.

Comment: This tracing may be compared with the previous example from the same patient. The incomplete LBBB has now become complete. Standard voltage criteria for LVH, which may be used with incomplete LBBB, are now invalid. Some authors have suggested that LVH may still be diagnosed with complete LBBB if the sum of the voltage of the S wave in lead V2 and the R wave in lead V5 is greater than 45 mm. In this example, the precordial voltage actually decreases when complete LBBB develops.

FURTHER READING

Kafka H, Burggraf GW, Milliken JA: Electrocardiographic diagnosis of left ventricular hypertrophy in the presence of left bundle branch block: An echocardiographic study. *Am J Cardiol* 55:103–106, 1985.

Klein RC, Vera Z, DeMaria JA, Mason DT: Electrocardiographic diagnosis of left ventricular hypertrophy in the presence of left bundle branch block. *Am Heart J* 108:502–506, 1984.

Vandenberg BF, Romhilt DW: Electrocardiographic diagnosis of left ventricular hypertrophy in the presence of bundle branch block. *Am Heart J* 122:818–822, 1991.

B-26

Clinical History
A 76-year-old man with valvular heart disease.

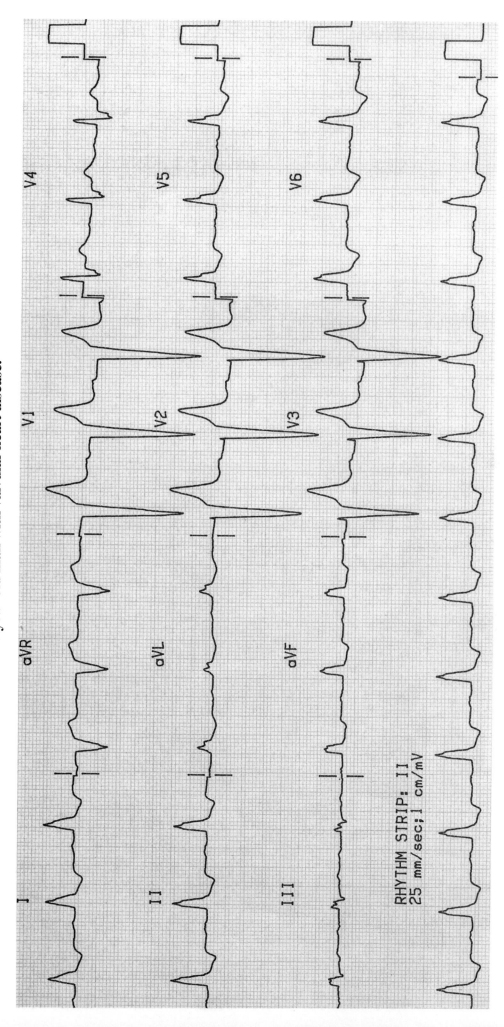

B-27

NARRATIVE INTERPRETATION

Rhythm:	**Accelerated AV junctional rhythm**
Rate:	**130**
Intervals:	**PR 0.12, QRS 0.08, QT 0.28**
Axis:	**+45 degrees**

Abnormalities

Rapid heart rate with inverted P waves II, III, aVF, and PR interval at lower limit of normal. VPC. QRS voltage in limb leads less than 5 mm. ST elevation leads I, II, III, aVF, V6. R-wave voltage less than 3 mm leads V1–V3.

Synthesis

Atrial tachycardia (cannot exclude accelerated AV junctional rhythm). VPC. Low-voltage limb leads. Poor R-wave progression. ST abnormalities suggest acute or recent myocardial injury.

TEST ANSWERS: 15, (23), 26, 66, 67, 100.

Comment: This is a difficult rhythm to characterize on the surface ECG. The differential diagnosis includes atrial tachycardia, the uncommon form of AV nodal reentrant tachycardia and accelerated AV junctional rhythm, otherwise known as *nonparoxysmal junctional tachycardia.*

The ST-segment abnormalities suggest early myocardial injury of the inferior and lateral walls, but are not diagnostic of acute Q-wave MI.

Low voltage in the limb leads and poor R-wave progression present in this example was likely due to this patient's marked obesity and COPD.

FURTHER READING

Alpert MA, Boyd TE, Cohen MV, et al: The electrocardiogram in morbid obestiy. *Am J Cardiol* 85:908–907, 2000.

B-27

Clinical History

A 61-year-old obese man with dyspnea.

RHYTHM STRIP: II
25 mm/sec; 1 cm/mV

B-28

NARRATIVE INTERPRETATION

Rhythm:	**Sinus bradycardia with wandering atrial pacemaker within the SA node**
Rate:	**47**
Intervals:	**PR 0.16, QRS 0.08, QT 0.40**
Axis:	**+75 degrees**

Abnormalities
Slow heart rate. Changing P-wave morphology. T-wave inversion leads V2–V6. Prominent U wave lead V3.

Synthesis
Sinus bradycardia with wandering atrial pacemaker within the SA node. Nonspecific T-wave abnormalities. Prominent U waves.

TEST ANSWERS: 3, 5, 106, 110.

Comment: Wandering atrial pacemaker within the SA node refers to a change in the origin of conduction with maintenance of a sinus mechanism. This rhythm is characterized by differing P-wave morphologies and minimal, if any, change in the PR interval. The pacemaker may also "wander" to the AV junction, which would produce inverted P waves in leads II, III, and aVF with a shortening of the PR interval. It is important to exclude an artifactual change in the P wave caused by respiratory variation. In this example, the abrupt change in P-wave morphology in the fourth through sixth beats on the rhythm strip indicate the true presence of a wandering atrial pacemaker.

146

B-28

Clinical History

A 68-year-old asymptomatic man.

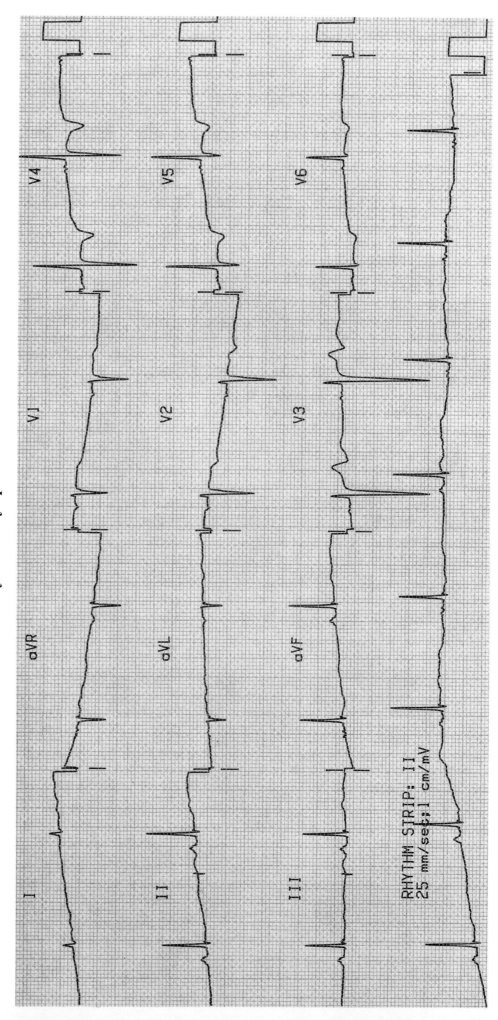

B-29

NARRATIVE INTERPRETATION

Rhythm:	**Sinus**
Rate:	**64**
Intervals:	**PR 0.16, QRS 0.09, QT 0.40**
Axis:	**−45 degrees**

Abnormalities
APCs. Axis leftward of −30 degrees.

Synthesis
Sinus rhythm. APCs. Left-axis deviation. Left anterior fascicular block.

TEST ANSWERS: 1, 10, 64, 72.

Comment: Atrial premature complexes (APCs) are frequently observed in normal persons. Studies of healthy airmen found that 0.7 to 3 percent had APCs on routine 12-lead electrocardiograms. One study using 24 h Holter monitoring of 50 male medical students found that 56 percent had APCs. The frequency of atrial extrasystoles may increase due to excessive fatigue, alcohol, or caffeine. Atrial ectopy is common in patients with COPD, valvular heart disease, or thyrotoxicosis.

FURTHER READING
Barrett PA, Peter CT, Swan HJC, et al: The frequency and prognostic significance of electrocardiographic abnormalities in clinically normal individuals. *Prog Cardiovasc Dis* 23:299–319, 1981.

B-29

Clinical History
A 44-year-old man with palpitations.

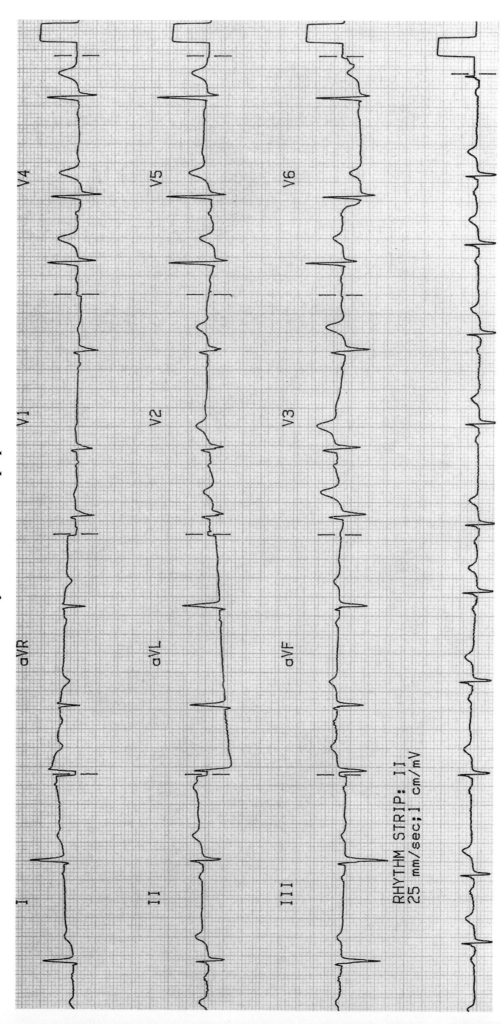

B-30

NARRATIVE INTERPRETATION

Rhythm:	**Sinus with 2:1 AV block**
Rate	Atrial rate 72, ventricular rate 36
Intervals:	PR 0.20 (in conducted beats), QRS 0.08, QT 0.52
Axis:	+15 degrees

Abnormalities
2:1 AV conduction.

Synthesis
Sinus rhythm with second-degree AV block, 2:1. Otherwise within normal limits.

TEST ANSWERS: 1, 45.

Comment: With 2:1 AV block, it is not possible from the surface electrocardiogram to distinguish between Mobitz type I (Wenckebach) and Mobitz type II. In order to confirm a Wenckebach sequence, at least two cycles of PR prolongation are required to demonstrate the progressively prolonged PR interval before the dropped beat occurs. When every other beat is nonconducted, as in the current example, the opportunity to observe gradual prolongation of the PR interval simply does not exist. Type I block is most often located in the AV node, whereas type II block with a narrow QRS complex is most likely to be in the His bundle.

A number of clues can help the clinician to distinguish between these two entities. In type I (intra-nodal) block, atropine will generally improve and carotid sinus pressure worsen conduction. In type II (intra-His) block, the opposite effects will generally occur.

FURTHER READING
Langendorf R, Cohen H, Gozo EG Jr: Observations on second-degree atrioventricular block, including new criteria for the differential diagnosis between type I and type 11 block. *Am J Cardiol* 29:111–119, 1972.
Mangiardi LM, Bonamini R, Conte M, et al: Bedside evaluation of atrioventricular block with narrow QRS complexes: Usefulness of carotid sinus massage and atropine administration. *Am J Cardiol* 49:1136–1145, 1982.
Zipes DP: Second-degree atrioventricular block. *Circulation* 60:465–472, 1979.

B-30

Clinical History
A 62-year-old man with lightheadedness.

I

aVR

V1

V4

II

aVL

V2

V5

III

aVF

V3

V6

RHYTHM STRIP: II
25 mm/sec; 1 cm/mV

B-31

NARRATIVE INTERPRETATION

Rhythm:	**Sinus bradycardia**
Rate:	**57**
Intervals:	**PR 0.16, QRS 0.08, QT 0.40**
Axis:	**+45 degrees (corrected)**

Abnormalities

Slow heart rate. Right-left arm electrode reversal. Slight ST depression lead II (actual lead III). T-wave inversion lead II (actual lead III). T biphasic lead aVF.

Synthesis

Incorrect electrode placement (right-left arm reversal). Sinus bradycardia. Nonspecific ST-T-wave abnormalities.

TEST ANSWERS: 3, 106, 112.

Comment: This tracing demonstrates a common misplacement of the recording electrodes with reversal of the right and left arm electrodes. Lead I appears as lead III normally would and vice versa. Similarly, the configuration of leads aVL and aVR is reversed. Lead aVF is unaffected and may be interpreted normally. The precordial leads are unaltered, a feature that helps to distinguish arm electrode reversal from dextrocardia. Patients with dextrocardia will demonstrate a reversed configuration in both the limb and chest leads.

152

B-31

Clinical History

A 50-year-old man with chest discomfort.

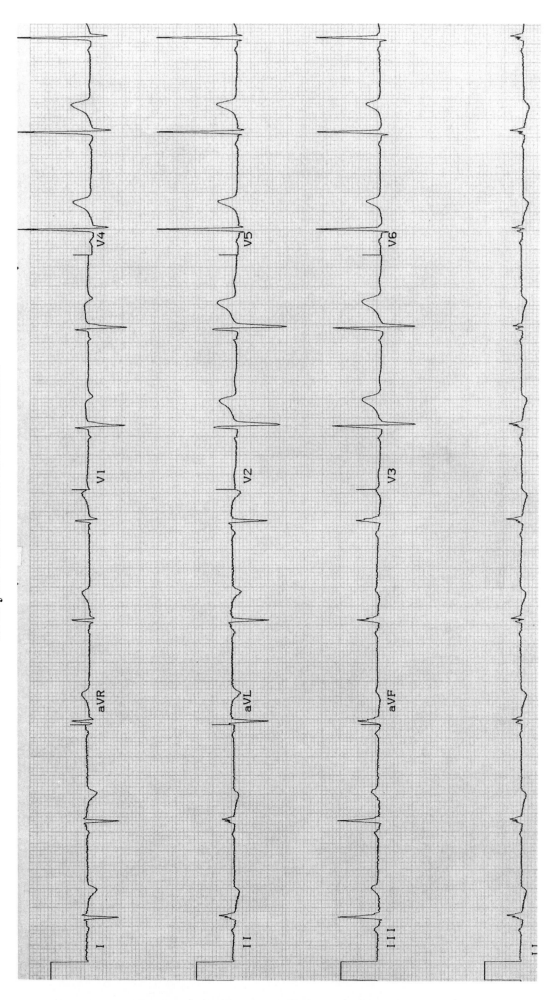

B-32

NARRATIVE INTERPRETATION

Rhythm:	**Atrial fibrillation**
Rate:	**86 (average)**
Intervals:	**PR −, QRS 0.08, QT 0.38**
Axis:	**+45 degrees**

Abnormalities

Multiform VPCs. ST depression leads I, II, aVL, aVF, V4–V6. S wave lead V2 + R wave lead V5 greater than 35 mm.

Synthesis

Atrial fibrillation with a controlled ventricular response. Multiform VPCs. LVH by voltage criteria. Associated, diffuse ST-T-wave abnormalities.

TEST ANSWERS: 20, 27, 51, 78, 103.

Comment: Patients with atrial fibrillation frequently have wide complex beats. It is often challenging to differentiate ventricular complexes from supraventricular complexes with aberrant conduction. A number of criteria have been proposed, but most have been found lacking in sensitivity and specificity.

This patient had an underlying rhythm of atrial fibrillation with frequent wide complex beats. The fixed coupling of the complexes favor ventricular ectopy, whereas variable coupling would have supported aberrancy.

Examination of the morphology of the wide complexes may also provide additional clues. The complexes seen here demonstrate a right bundle branch pattern with an rR' configuration in lead V1. Unfortunately, this particular pattern does not allow for a firm prediction of their origin.

Interestingly, this patient eventually converted to sinus rhythm with VPCs having the identical morphology to the wide complex beats seen here.

FURTHER READING

Gulamhusein S, Yee R, Ko PT, Klein GJ: Electrocardiographic criteria for differentiating aberrancy and ventricular extrasystole in chronic atrial fibrillation: Validation by intracardiac recordings. *J Electrocardiol* 18:41–50, 1985.

Marriott HJL, Sandler IA: Criteria, old and new, for differentiating between ectopic ventricular beats and aberrant ventricular conduction in the presence of atrial fibrillation. *Prog Cardiovasc Dis* 9:18–28, 1966.

Wellens HJJ, Barr FWHM, Lie KI: The value of the electrocardiogram in the differential diagnosis of a tachycardia with a widened QRS complex. *Am J Med* 84:27–33, 1978.

B-32

Clinical History

An 88-year-old woman in the CCU. Medications include digoxin.

RHYTHM STRIP: II
25 mm/sec; 1 cm/mV

B-33

NARRATIVE INTERPRETATION

Rhythm:	**Sinus**
Rate:	**84**
Intervals:	**PR 0.20, QRS 0.08, QT 0.50**
Axis:	**+45 degrees**

Abnormalities

ST depression leads I, II, aVL, aVF, V2–V6. T-wave inversion leads V1–V6. S wave lead V2 + R wave lead V5 greater than 35 mm. Prolonged QT interval for heart rate.

Synthesis

Sinus rhythm. Prolonged QTc. LVH by voltage criteria. Diffuse, nonspecific ST-T-wave abnormalities.

TEST ANSWERS: 1, 78, (103), 106, 109.

Comment: The patient from the previous example has converted to sinus rhythm after treatment with digoxin and quinidine. There is evidence of quinidine toxicity by virtue of marked prolongation of the QT interval. It is possible that some of the QT interval prolongation is due to incorporation of the U wave in the measurement. Nevertheless, the clinician must be alerted to quinidine toxicity and the potential for proarrhythmia in patients treated with drugs that prolong the QT interval.

FURTHER READING

Schweitzer P: The values and limitations of the QT interval in clinical practice. *Am Heart J* 124: 1121–1126, 1992.

Woosley RL, Sale M: QT interval: A measure of drug action. *Am J Cardiol* 72:36B–43B, 1993.

B-33

Clinical History

An 88-year-old woman in the CCU. Medications include digoxin and quinidine sulfate.

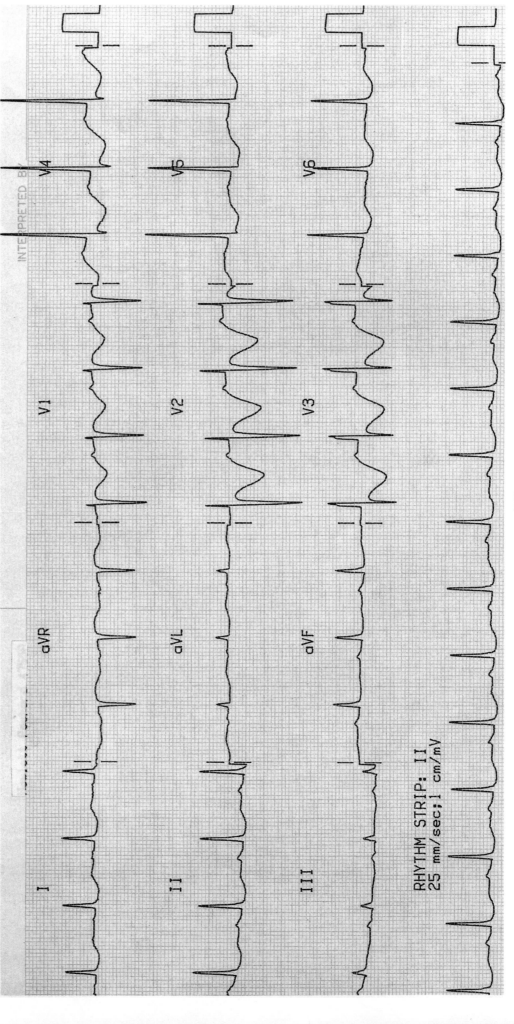

B-34

NARRATIVE INTERPRETATION

Rhythm:	**Sinus with multifocal atrial rhythm**
Rate:	70
Intervals:	**PR 0.16, QRS 0.08, QT 0.36**
Axis:	**+30 degrees**

Abnormalities
Frequent APCs, normally conducted. Nonconducted APC. ST depression leads I, II, aVL, aVF, V4–V6. S wave lead V2 + R wave lead V5 greater than 35 mm.

Synthesis
Sinus rhythm with multifocal atrial rhythm. LVH by voltage criteria. Associated ST-T-wave abnormalities.

TEST ANSWERS: 1, (10), 12, 13, 78, 103.

Comment: This tracing demonstrates sinus rhythm in only the last four complexes (the fourth complex from the end is obscured but is likely to be a sinus beat). In the remainder of the tracing, and the entire rhythm strip, there is no discernible sinus mechanism. Multiple atrial foci are evident, with varying P wave morphologies and PR intervals. Accordingly, the rhythm is properly classified as a multifocal, or chaotic, atrial rhythm. Sinus rhythm with frequent APCs is an alternative.

The fifth complex of the 12-lead is a premature, nonconducted, atrial beat. The origin of the complexes with inverted P waves in leads II, III, and aVF are most likely *low* atrial rather than junctional because the PR interval is at least 0.12 s or more. One cannot completely exclude the possibility that these beats are junctional with antegrade block.

158

B-34

Clinical History

A 64-year-old man seen in preoperative evaluation.

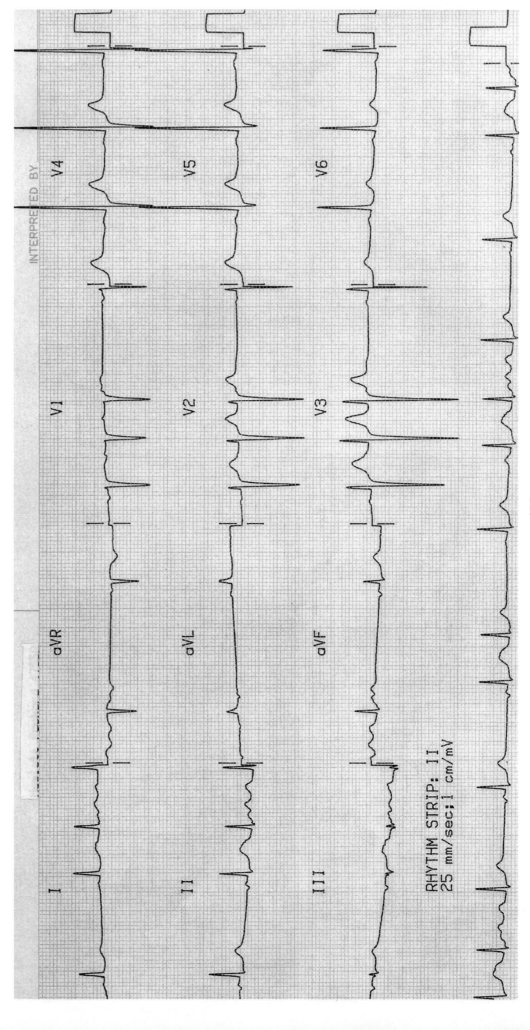

B-35

NARRATIVE INTERPRETATION

Rhythm:	**Sinus with third-degree AV block; AV junctional** escape rhythm
Rate:	**Sinus rate 100; AV junctional rate 53**
Intervals:	**PR −, QRS 0.08, QT 0.38**
Axis:	**+60 degrees**

Abnormalities
P waves fail to conduct to ventricles. VPCs. ST elevation leads II, III, aVF. ST depression leads I, aVL, V2. T-wave inversion leads I, aVL.

Synthesis
Sinus rhythm with complete (third-degree) AV block. AV junctional escape rhythm. VPCs. Acute inferior wall MI with ST-T-wave abnormalities of acute myocardial injury. Nonspecific ST-T-wave abnormalities consistent with MI or reciprocal change.

TEST ANSWERS: 1, 22, 26, 47, 91, 100, 101.

Comment: Various degrees of AV block may accompany acute inferior wall MI. Complete AV block is seen in 3 to 7 percent of patients who have not been treated with thrombolytic therapy. In patients with inferior wall MI, the conduction abnormality is a result of profound vagal influences. If the escape rhythm is satisfactory and there is no hemodynamic compromise, most patients will not require temporary pacemaker therapy. The rhythm disturbance generally resolves within a number of days, although an occasional patient may require 2 weeks to regain normal conduction.

FURTHER READING
Nicod P, Gilpin E, Dittrich H, et al: Long-term outcome in patients with inferior myocardial infarction and complete atrioventricular block. *J Am Coll Cardiol* 12:589–594, 1988.

B-35

Clinical History
A 71-year-old woman in the CCU.

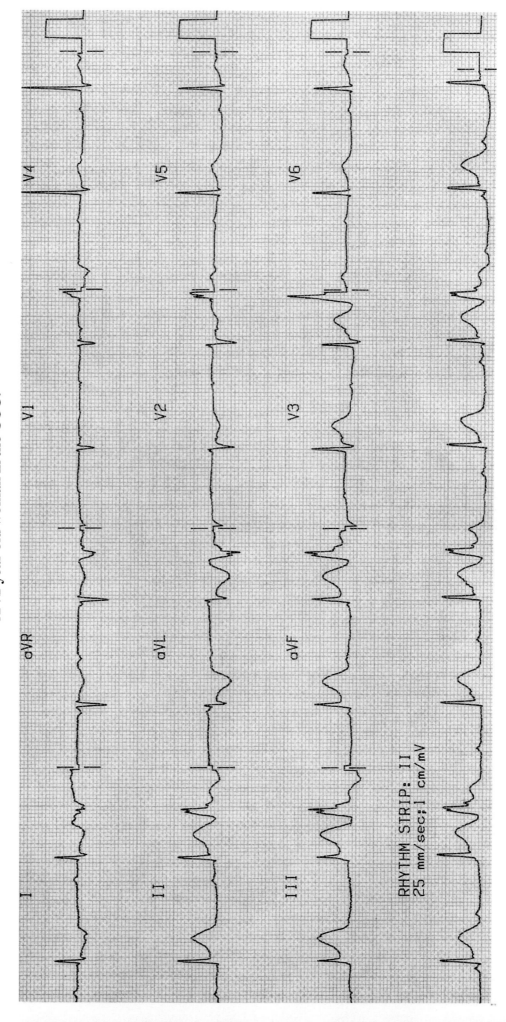

B-36

NARRATIVE INTERPRETATION

Rhythm:	**Sinus**
Rate:	**66**
Intervals:	**PR 0.18, QRS 0.10, QT 0.40**
Axis:	**+60 degrees**

Abnormalities
ST depression leads II, III, aVF, V5–V6. S wave lead V2 + R wave lead V5 greater than 35 mm.

Synthesis
Sinus rhythm. LVH by voltage criteria. Nonspecific ST abnormalities.

TEST ANSWERS: 1, 78, (103), 106.

Comment: This tracing reminds the interpreter to always check the standardization. One could mistakenly overlook the increased voltage for LVH if failing to notice that the chest leads are recorded at half-standard.

An isolated, broad, notched Q wave is present in lead aVL; however, the absence of a Q wave in lead I precludes the diagnosis of a lateral wall MI.

The minor ST abnormalities are not characteristic of those usually associated with LVH and are best considered nonspecific.

162

B-36

Clinical History

A 70-year-old man admitted with chest pain.

** CHEST LEADS AT 1/2 STD. **

B-37

NARRATIVE INTERPRETATION

Rhythm:	**Sinus bradycardia**
Rate:	**44**
Intervals:	**PR 0.14, QRS 0.08, QT 0.52**
Axis:	**+60 degrees**

Abnormalities
Slow heart rate. Somatic tremor artifact. ST depression leads I, II, V5–V6. T-wave inversion leads II, II, aVF. S wave lead V2 + R wave lead V5 greater than 35 mm. Prominent U waves. Inverted U wave leads V4–V6.

Synthesis
Sinus bradycardia. LVH by voltage criteria. Associated ST-T-wave abnormalities. Prominent U waves. Inverted U waves. Somatic tremor with baseline artifact.

TEST ANSWERS: 3, 78, 103, 110, 111, 113.

Comment: On first inspection, the reader might misinterpret this electrocardiogram as atrial fibrillation because of the irregular baseline. Moreover, the slow regular rhythm might suggest atrial fibrillation with complete AV block and an AV junctional escape rhythm. On closer review, note the discrete P waves in the right precordial leads, particularly in lead V3. This slow, regular rhythm is sinus bradycardia with a somatic tremor caused by Parkinson's disease.

LVH is present in this electrocardiogram with increased precordial voltage and ST-T-wave abnormalities. A prominent U wave is best appreciated in lead V3, a finding that may be seen in LVH. The negative U waves seen in leads V4–V6 suggest coronary ischemia.

FURTHER READING
Kishida H, Cole JS, Surawicz B: Negative U wave: A highly specific but poorly understood sign of heart disease. *Am J Cardiol* 49:2030–2036, 1982.
Lepeschkin E: The U wave of the electrocardiogram. *Mod Concepts Cardiovasc Dis* 38:39–45, 1969.

B-37

Clinical History
A 71-year-old man with congestive heart failure.

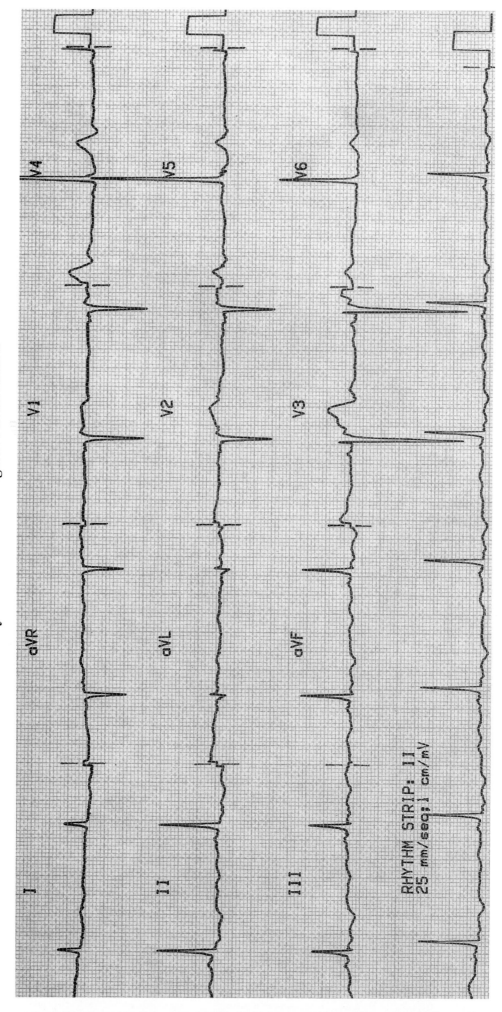

B-38

NARRATIVE INTERPRETATION

Rhythm:	**Sinus**
Rate:	**64**
Intervals:	**PR 0.16, QRS 0.08, QT 0.40**
Axis:	**0 degrees**

Abnormalities

Q waves leads II, III, aVF. R wave greater than S wave leads V1, V2, with upright T wave. "Coved" ST segments leads II, III, aVF. ST elevation leads aVL, V1–V3. T-wave inversion leads II, III, aVF.

Synthesis

Sinus rhythm. Recent (acute) inferior wall MI. Posterior wall MI of indeterminate age. Possible lateral wall acute MI. ST-T-wave abnormalities in leads II, III, aVL, aVF, suggesting acute myocardial injury.

TEST ANSWERS: 1, 91, (93), 94, 100.

Comment: This patient sustained an inferior and posterolateral wall MI with new Q waves in the inferior leads and an increase in R-wave amplitude in leads V1 and V2. This tracing illustrates that pathologic Q waves may not always be 0.04 ms in duration, especially in the inferior leads. They are, however, 25 percent of the amplitude of the associated R wave in leads II, III, and aVF. The ST-T-wave abnormalities in the inferior leads represent recent infarction. The prominent R waves in the right precordial leads with an upright T wave reflects involvement of the posterior wall. It must be classified as of indeterminate age because there are no corresponding acute ST changes in those leads or prior tracings for comparison. In reality, it was part of the acute inferior wall MI. The slight ST elevation in lead aVL should be commented on and reflects involvement of the lateral wall in the inferior and posterior infarction. There is no corresponding ST elevation in lead I to allow for a diagnosis of lateral wall MI. It is not always possible on the electrocardiogram to characterize every MI into s specific anatomical pattern.

FURTHER READING

Parker AB III, Waller BF, Gering LE: Usefulness of the 12-lead electrocardiogram in detection of myocardial infarction: Electrocardiographic-anatomic correlations. Part I. *Clin Cardiol* 19:55–61, 1996.

Parker AB III, Waller BF, Gering LE: Usefulness of the 12-lead electrocardiogram in detection of myocardial infarction: Electrocardiographic-anatomic correlations. Part II. *Clin Cardiol* 19:141–148, 1996.

B-38

Clinical History

A 48-year-old man 18 h after hospital admission for chest discomfort.

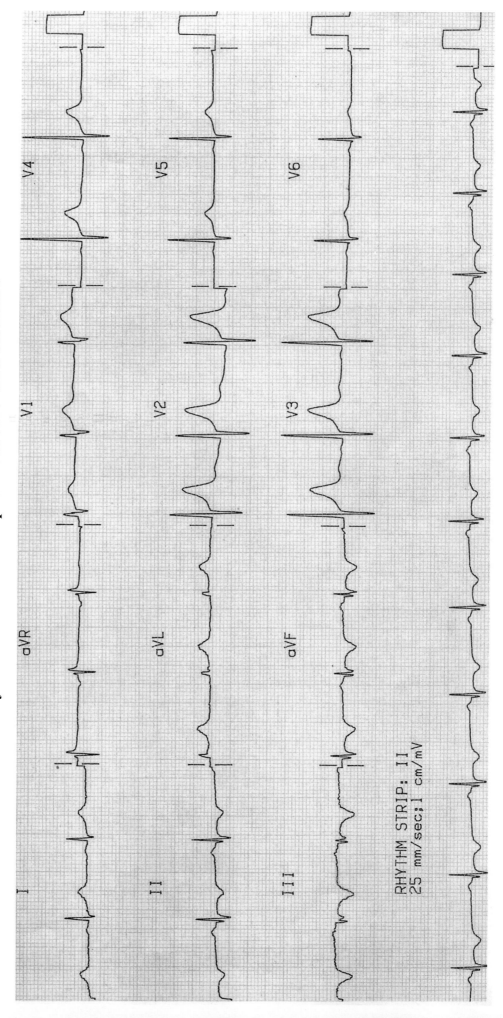

167

B-39

NARRATIVE INTERPRETATION

Rhythm:	**Sinus with first-degree AV block**
Rate:	**80**
Intervals:	**PR 0.24, QRS 0.08, QT 0.36**
Axis:	**−15 degrees**

Abnormalities
Prolonged PR interval. ST flat lead II, aVF. Slight ST depression leads V5–V6.

Synthesis
Sinus rhythm. First-degree AV block. Nonspecific ST abnormalities.

TEST ANSWERS: 1, 42, 106.

Comment: First-degree AV block is a common manifestation of relative digitalis toxicity. Prolongation of the PR interval is secondary to an increase in the AH interval, which reflects delay in AV conduction. In this patient, the serum digoxin level was in the "therapeutic" range. However, in this elderly female with underlying conduction system disease, the therapeutic blood level was "toxic."

B-39

Clinical History
A 90-year-old woman with congestive heart failure.

B-40

NARRATIVE INTERPRETATION

Rhythm:	**Sinus**
Rate:	**88**
Intervals:	**PR 0.20, QRS 0.14, QT 0.40**
Axis:	**+60 degrees**

Abnormalities

Broad, notched QRS in I, aVL, V5–V6. ST elevation leads II, III, aVF. Symmetric T-wave inversion leads II, III, aVF. Upright, symmetric T wave leads I, aVL.

Synthesis

Sinus rhythm. LBBB with associated ST-T-wave abnormalities. ST-T-wave abnormalities suggestive of acute inferior wall myocardial injury. Additional abnormal T waves in leads I, aVL.

TEST ANSWERS: 1, 74, 100, 101, 104.

Comment: This tracing demonstrates early, acute inferior wall myocardial injury in the presence of an underlying LBBB. The diagnosis of MI is usually very difficult in patients with LBBB. In this example however, the inferior ST-T-wave abnormalities are quite pronounced and are superimposed on the conduction abnormality.

Note also the upright T waves in leads I and aVL, findings that suggest lateral wall involvement of the MI, reciprocal change or additional ischemia. In uncomplicated LBBB, the T-wave vectors are directed in the opposite direction of the mean QRS vector and should be negative in leads I and aVL. In this example, the abnormal T waves in these leads are upright.

FURTHER READING

Hands ME, Cook EF, Stone PH, et al: Electrocardiographic diagnosis of myocardial infarction in the presence of complete left bundle branch block. *Am Heart J* 116:23–31, 1988.

Sgarbossa EB, Pinski SL, Barbagelta A, et al: Electrocardiographic diagnosis of evolving acute myocardial infarction in the presence of left bundle branch block. *N Engl J Med* 334:481–487, 1996.

B-40

Clinical History
A 78-year-old woman with hypotension.

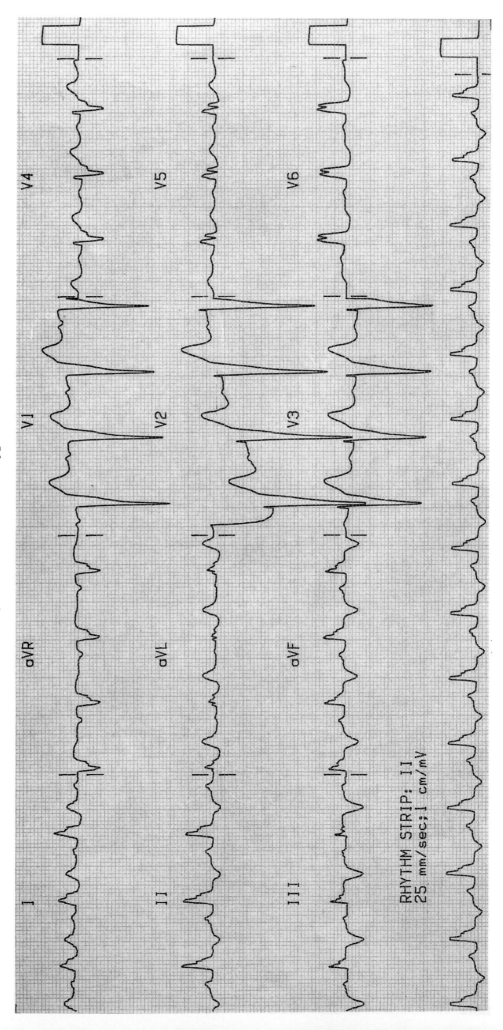

RHYTHM STRIP: II
25 mm/sec; 1 cm/mV

TEST C

C-1

NARRATIVE INTERPRETATION

Rhythm:	**Atrial flutter with 2:1 AV conduction**
Rate:	**Atrial rate 280, ventricular rate 140**
Intervals:	**PR −, QRS 0.06, QT 0.28**
Axis:	**0 degrees**

Abnormalities
Rapid heart rate with "sawtooth" configuration. Possible superimposed ST depression, leads II, II, aVF, V6.

Synthesis
Atrial flutter with 2:1 AV conduction. (Nonspecific ST abnormalities.)

TEST ANSWERS: 19, 50, (106).

Comment: Atrial flutter may be divided into type I (classic) or type II (very rapid). This tracing demonstrates classic atrial flutter with characteristic sawtoothed flutter waves in leads II, III, and aVF. In type I flutter, the atrial rate is between 240 and 340 bpm and may be interrupted with rapid atrial pacing. Type II atrial flutter is characterized by very rapid atrial rates of 340 to 433 bpm and cannot be controlled by atrial pacing.

It is appropriate to describe the 2:1 ratio of atrial to ventricular impulses as 2:1 AV *conduction* rather than *block*. The 2:1 conduction is a physiologic response of the AV node and should not imply a pathologic state, or *heart block*. Atrial flutter with 1:1 conduction may occur rarely from sympathetic stimulation or when antiarrhythmic agents slow the intrinsic atrial rate. Atrial flutter with 1:1 conduction can be a cardiac emergency because the resulting extremely rapid ventricular rate prevents physiologic cardiac filling and contraction.

It is difficult to exclude the presence of ST abnormalities superimposed on the flutter waves in this example.

C-1

Clinical History
A 55-year-old woman with palpitations.

aVR   V1   V4

aVL   V2   V5

aVF   V3   V6

I

II

III

RHYTHM STRIP: II
25 mm/sec; 1 cm/mV

C-2

NARRATIVE INTERPRETATION

Rhythm:	**Sinus**
Rate:	**96**
Intervals:	**PR 0.16, QRS 0.08, QT 0.38**
Axis:	**+15 degrees**

Abnormalities

APC. APC conducted aberrantly. ST depression leads I, II, III, aVL, aVF, V4–V6. T-wave inversion leads I, aVL, V4–V6. S wave lead V2 + R wave lead V5 greater than 35 mm. R wave aVL + S wave V3 greater than 20 mm in a woman. Abnormal P terminal force V1.

Synthesis

Sinus rhythm. APCs with normal and aberrant conduction. LVH by voltage criteria. Associated ST-T-wave abnormalities. Left atrial abnormality.

TEST ANSWERS: 1, 10, 11, 60, 78, 103.

Comment: This tracing demonstrates a number of findings, most of them related to LVH. A potential pitfall would be characterizing the wide complexes beats as ventricular in origin rather than as an aberrantly conducted atrial complexes. On close examination, a P wave is clearly seen to be deforming the preceding T wave, indicating that the complex is supraventricular. A normally conducted atrial premature complex is seen on the rhythm strip.

The configuration of the ST-T-wave abnormalities suggests they were most likely on the basis of LVH, rather than myocardial ischemia.

C-2

Clinical History

A 79-year-old hypertensive woman who presents to the emergency department with severe dyspnea.

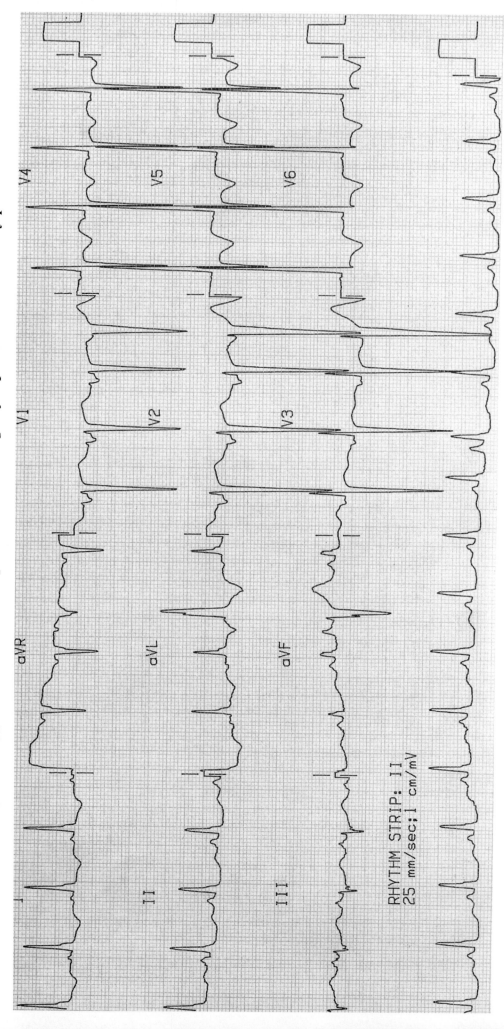

C-3

NARRATIVE INTERPRETATION

Rhythm:	**Sinus bradycardia**
Rate:	**55**
Intervals:	**PR 014, QRS 0.10, QT 0.44**
Axis:	**−45 degrees**

Abnormalities

Heart rate less than 60 bpm. VPCs. Axis leftward of −30 degrees. Abnormal P terminal force V1. Q waves leads II, III, aVF. rSr' lead V1. ST depression leads II, V5, V6. T-wave inversion leads II, III, aVF. T-wave flat lead V5. T-wave biphasic lead V6. T-wave upright lead V1.

Synthesis

Sinus bradycardia. VPCs. Left atrial abnormality. Inferior wall MI of indeterminate age. Nonspecific ST-T-wave abnormalities. Left-axis deviation. Left anterior fascicular block. rSr' pattern in lead V1, probably normal variant.

TEST ANSWERS: 3, 26, 60, 64, 72, 92, 98, 106.

Comment: This tracing demonstrates the combination of inferior wall MI and left anterior fascicular block, both of which may produce left-axis deviation. The terminal conduction delay in aVR, which occurs after that of aVL, suggests the counterclockwise vector loop of LAFB. Note that LAFB can diminish or mask the diagnostic Q waves of inferior infarction because the initial forces are directed inferiorly. The small Q wave in lead II in the presence of LAFB suggests that an inferior wall MI coexists.

The rSr' pattern in lead V1 represents a difficult differential diagnosis. This pattern could represent a normal variant, an incomplete RBBB, or result from the LAFB. In this example, this pattern is likely to represent a normal variant because the r and r' occur only in lead V1, are of low amplitude, and are less than the amplitude of the S wave.

FURTHER READING

Fisher ML, Mugmon MA, Carliner NH, et al: Left anterior fascicular block: Electrocardiographic criteria for its recognition in the presence of inferior myocardial infarction. *Am J Cardiol* 44:845–849, 1979.

Warner RA, Hill NE, Mookherjee S, Smulyan H: Electrocardiographic criteria for the diagnosis of combined inferior myocardial infarction and left anterior hemiblock. *Am Heart J* 51:718–722, 1983.

C-3

Clinical History

A 59-year-old asymptomatic man on his fifth hospital day.

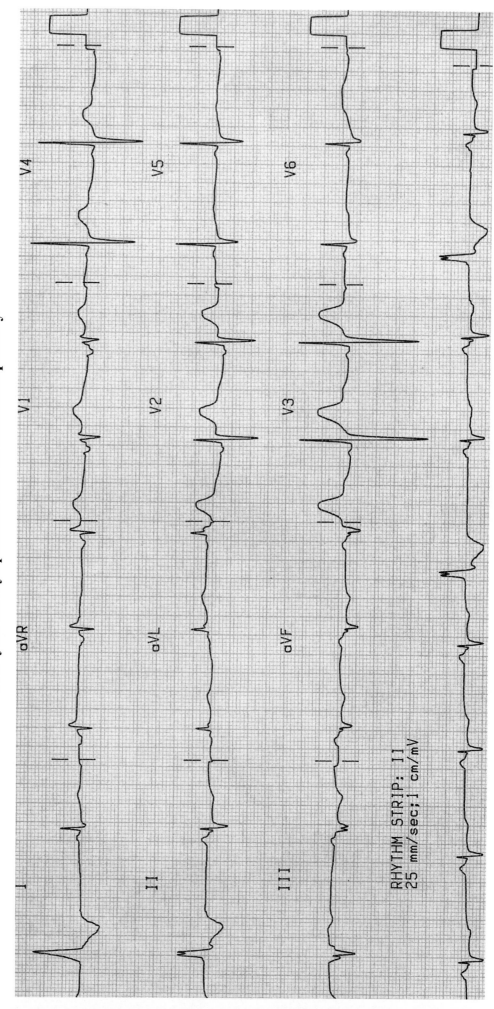

C-4

NARRATIVE INTERPRETATION

Rhythm:	**Accelerated AV junctional rhythm**
Rate:	**100**
Intervals:	**PR 0.10, QRS 0.08, QT 0.32**
Axis:	**−30 degrees**

Abnormalities
Inverted P waves II, III, aVF, with short PR interval. ST elevation leads I, II, III, aVL, aVF, V2–V6.

Synthesis
Accelerated AV junctional rhythm. ST-segment elevation suggestive of acute myocardial injury.

TEST ANSWERS: 23, 100.

Comment: Accelerated AV junctional rhythm is most often seen in patients with underlying cardiac disease. The rhythm may also be called *nonparoxysmal junctional tachycardia*, which distinguishes it from paroxysmal junctional tachycardia, a common form of reentrant supraventricular tachycardia. Accelerated AV junctional rhythm may be caused by acute MI, COPD, myocarditis, or occur after cardiac surgery.

Note the subtle ST elevation in the inferior leads, I, aVL, and across the precordium. This patient went on to develop an anteroapical and lateral wall MI. Q waves have not yet appeared; therefore, the best interpretation of this electrocardiogram is to comment on the ischemic ST abnormalities without localization of an acute Q wave MI. The ST elevation is "coved" and suggests myocardial injury. However, the generalized nature of the abnormalities might also raise the suspicion of pericarditis.

C-4

Clinical History

A 57-year-old man with chest discomfort.

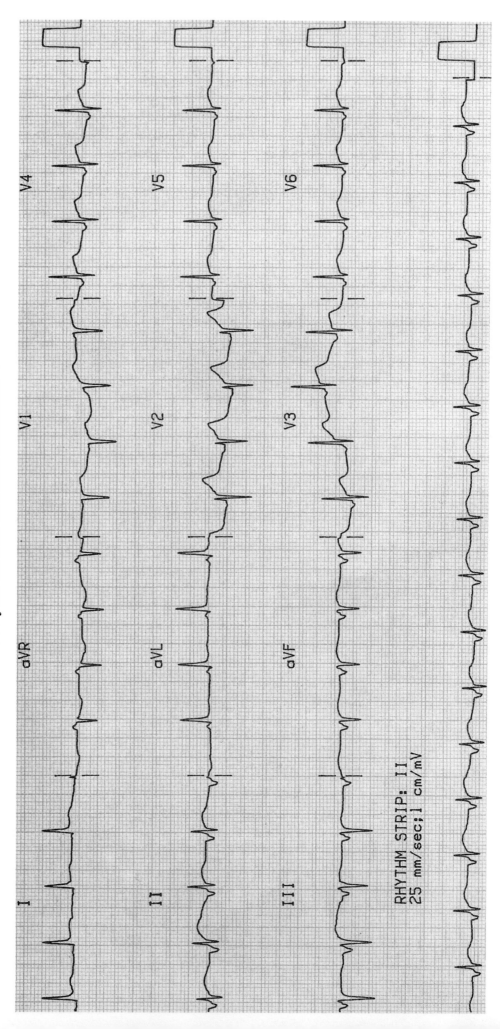

I

aVR

V1

V4

II

aVL

V2

V5

III

aVF

V3

V6

RHYTHM STRIP: II
25 mm/sec;1 cm/mV

C-5

NARRATIVE INTERPRETATION

Rhythm:	**Sinus**
Rate:	**75**
Intervals:	**PR 0.16, QRS 0.08, QT 0.36**
Axis:	**+30 degrees**

Abnormalities

APCs with aberrant conduction. ST elevation at J point leads II, III, aVF, V1–V4. T-wave inversion leads I, aVL. T wave flat leads V5–V6. S wave lead V1 + R wave lead V5 greater than 35 mm.

Synthesis

Sinus rhythm. APCs with aberrant conduction. Nonspecific T-wave abnormalities. Normal variant J-point elevation. LVH by voltage criteria.

TEST ANSWERS: 1, 11, 78, 96, (103), 106, (112).

Comment: The T wave represents ventricular repolarization and generally has the same direction as QRS depolarization. In normal individuals, the T-wave vector is directed leftward and inferiorly and is therefore upright in leads I, II, and V3–V6. T waves may be variable in leads III, aVL, aVF, V1, and V2. In this example there is also a slight ST elevation at the J point, which is probably within normal limits. Without clinical correlation, it would be difficult to completely exclude early myocardial injury.

APCs with variable degrees of aberrant conduction are noted on the rhythm strip. In the absence of underlying cardiac disease or tachyarrhythmias, these would generally not impact surgical care. It would be important however, for the surgical staff to be aware of the aberrant conduction of these complexes to avoid mistaking them for ventricular arrhythmias.

One minor point is the placement of lead V3, which appears to have been positioned too far laterally toward lead V4.

C-5

Clinical History

A 68-year-old asymptomatic man seen in preoperative evaluation.

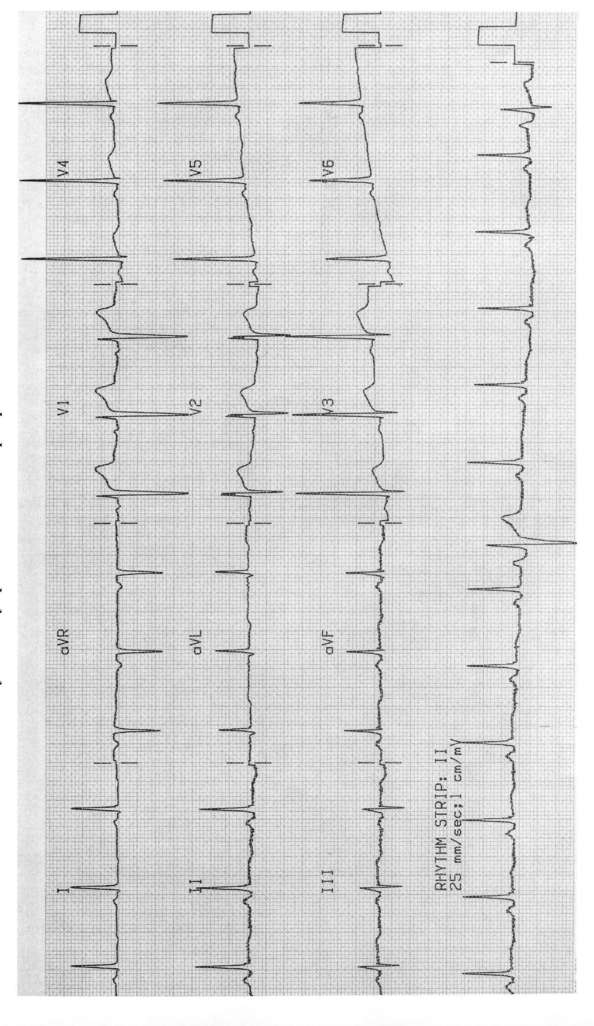

C-6

NARRATIVE INTERPRETATION

Rhythm:	**Atrial tachycardia with 2:1 AV conduction**
Rate:	**Atrial 170, ventricular 85**
Intervals:	**PR 0.20, QRS 0.10, QT 0.36**
Axis:	**0 degrees**

Abnormalities
Rapid atrial rate. T-wave inverted leads I, aVL, V5–V6. Ventricular pacemaker complex with capture.

Synthesis
Atrial tachycardia with 2:1 AV conduction. Nonspecific T-wave abnormalities. Ventricular pacemaker complex with appropriate capture.

TEST ANSWERS: 17, 35, (50), 51, 106.

Comment: This patient received a pacemaker and digoxin to treat sick sinus syndrome. The arrhythmia demonstrated here is characteristic of digitalis toxicity. PAT with 2:1 AV conduction (block) usually presents with an atrial rate of 200 to 250 bpm. In this example, the atrial rate is a bit slower. The 2:1 conduction ratio at this atrial rate is probably *nonphysiologic* secondary to the effect of digoxin, but this is difficult to confirm on the surface electrocardiogram. Note the prominent P waves in leads V1 and V2. The P wave following the QRS complex should not be mistaken for a T wave, which would normally occur further beyond the R wave.

A ventricular pacemaker capture is seen in the first complex. This is likely to be normal function, but it is impossible to determine the demand function without better visualizing the preceding beat.

C-6

Clinical History

A 72-year-old woman admitted to the coronary care unit (CCU).

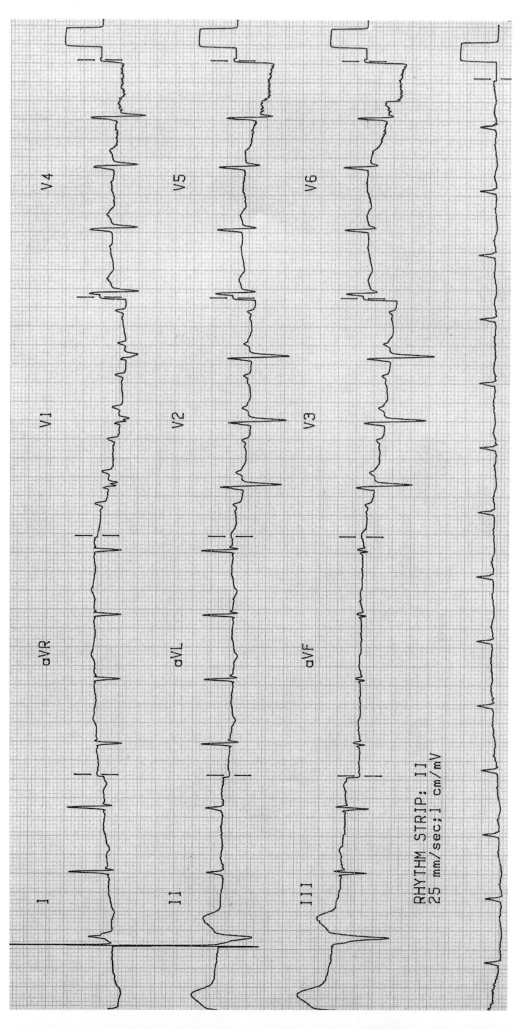

RHYTHM STRIP: II
25 mm/sec; 1 cm/mV

185

C-7

NARRATIVE INTERPRETATION

Rhythm:	**AV junctional rhythm**
Rate:	**55**
Intervals:	**PR –, QRS 0.10, QT –**
Axis:	**+60 degrees**

Abnormalities

Absent P waves. ST depression leads I, II, aVF, V3–V6. T-wave inversion leads I, II, aVL, V3–V6.

Synthesis

AV junctional rhythm. Diffuse nonspecific ST-T-wave abnormalities. Prominent U waves suggested.

TEST ANSWERS: 21, 106, (110).

Comment: This patient has suppression of sinus node function induced by a combination of excessive doses of verapamil and digoxin. This yielded an AV junctional rhythm. Inverted junctional P waves are absent because they are likely to be "buried" in the QRS complex. Remember that the inverted, retrograde P wave of AV junctional complexes can appear either before, within, or after the QRS complex because the position depends on the relative rates of antegrade and retrograde conduction.

The QT interval in this tracing is difficult to determine because there is considerable overlap of the T and U waves. The primary abnormality of repolarization may be the prominent U waves combined with digitalis-induced shortening of the QT interval.

C-7

Clinical History

A 78-year-old man treated with a calcium channel blocker and digoxin.

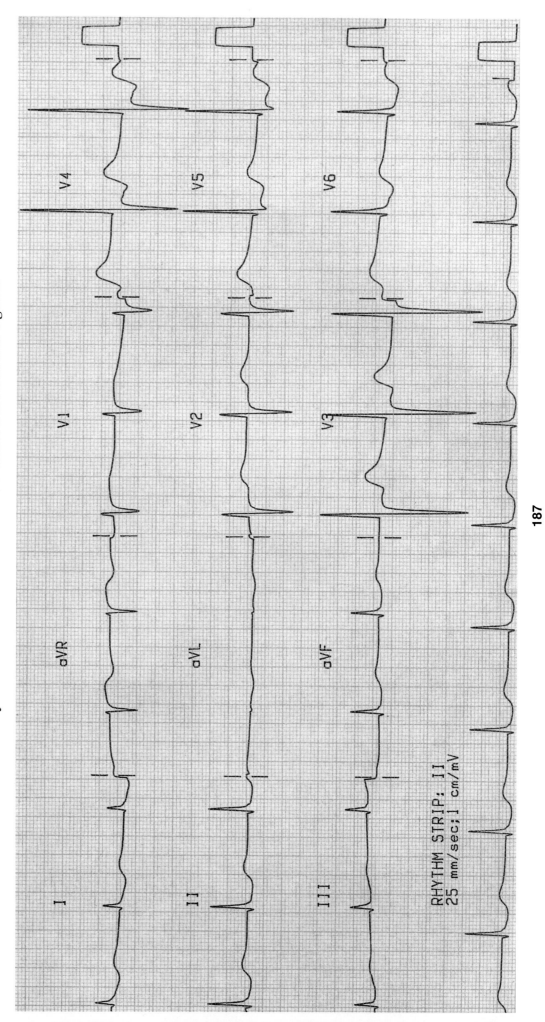

RHYTHM STRIP: II
25 mm/sec; 1 cm/mV

C-8

NARRATIVE INTERPRETATION

Rhythm:	**Sinus bradycardia**
Rate:	**56**
Intervals:	**PR 0.18, QRS 0.12, QT 0.44**
Axis:	**−15 degrees**

Abnormalities

Heart rate less than 60 bpm. Q wave leads II, III, aVF. ST elevation leads II, III, aVF. ST depression leads I, aVL. Slight ST elevation leads V5–V6. ST depression leads I, aVL. T-wave inversion leads III, aVF. T-wave biphasic lead II. Prolonged QRS with rSR' pattern and T-wave inversion leads V1–V3.

Synthesis

Sinus bradycardia. Inferior wall (inferolateral) MI with ST-T-wave abnormalities suggesting acute myocardial injury. RBBB with associated ST-T-wave abnormalities. ST-T-wave abnormalities in leads I and aVL, suggesting either reciprocal changes or lateral wall myocardial ischemia.

TEST ANSWERS: 3, 70, (85), 91, 100, 101, 104.

Comment: This patient was suffering from an acute inferior wall MI. Lateral (anterolateral) extension is also suggested by coved ST-segment elevation in the lateral precordial leads. In this patient, the RBBB was noted previously and T-wave inversion in leads V1–V3 would be expected; therefore, these findings are secondary rather than primary abnormalities. The acute ST-T-wave abnormalities in the inferior and lateral leads may be interpreted even in the presence of complete RBBB. The presence of a preexisting RBBB in a patient with acute MI does not suggest a higher likelihood of progression to complete heart block, and temporary pacemaker insertion is not indicated.

FURTHER READING

Hindman MC, Wagner GS, JaRo M, et al: The clinical significance of bundle branch block complicating acute myocardial infarction. I. Clinical characteristics, hospital mortality, and one-year follow-up. *Circulation* 58:679–688, 1978.

Hindman MC, Wagner GS, JaRo M, et al: The clinical significance of bundle branch block complicating acute myocardial infarction. II. Indications for temporary and permanent pacemaker insertion. *Circulation* 58:689–699, 1978.

C-8

Clinical History

A 77-year-old woman with 6 h of chest discomfort. She has been told of a *blockage* on her prior electrocardiogram.

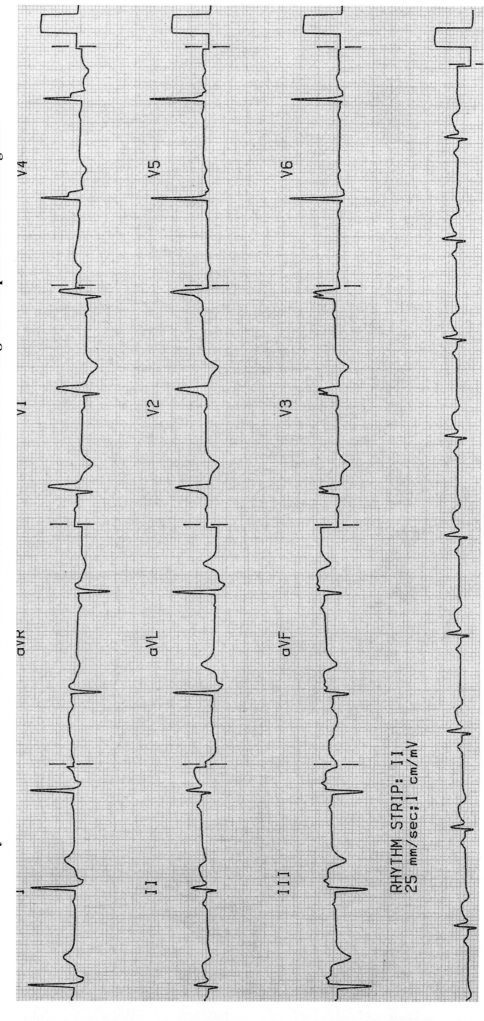

C-9

NARRATIVE INTERPRETATION

Rhythm:	**Sinus tachycardia**
Rate:	**106**
Intervals:	**PR 0.18, QRS 0.14, QT 0.36**
Axis:	**−45 degrees**

Abnormalities
Heart rate greater than 100 bpm. Broad, notched QRS complex with T-wave inversion leads I, aVL, V6. Axis leftward of −30 degrees. VPC. APC. (SV2 + RV5 greater than 45 mm).

Synthesis
Sinus tachycardia. LBBB. Left-axis deviation. VPC. APC. (Possible LVH).

TEST ANSWERS: 4, 10, 26, 74, (78), 104.

Comment: An interesting finding in this tracing is the narrow QRS morphology of the VPCs, present in the 10th and 13th complexes. This is not an infrequent finding in patients with LBBB. It is likely that the ectopic impulse originates from a location distal to the area of conduction delay and depolarizes the ventricles more rapidly, producing a narrower complex. A single atrial premature complex is present on the rhythm strip (16th complex).

Note that the precordial leads are recorded at one-half standard; therefore, precordial voltage is markedly increased. Some authors suggest that such increased voltage allows for a diagnosis of LVH, even in the presence of LBBB.

FURTHER READING
Howard RL, Dunn M: Left-axis deviation with left bundle branch block. *Am J Noninvas Cardiol* 1:98–101, 1987.

Kafka H, Burggraf GW, Milliken JA: Electrocardiographic diagnosis of left ventricular hypertrophy in the presence of left bundle branch block: An echocardiographic study. *Am J Cardiol* 55:103–106, 1985.

Klein RC, Vera Z, DeMaria JA, Mason DT: Electrocardiographic diagnosis of left ventricular hypertrophy in the presence of left bundle branch block. *Am Heart J* 108:502–506, 1984.

Vandenberg BF, Romhilt DW: Electrocardiographic diagnosis of left ventricular hypertrophy in the presence of bundle branch block. *Am Heart J* 122:818–822, 1991.

C-9

Clinical History

A 70-year-old woman with a history of congestive heart failure who has been admitted for abdominal surgery.

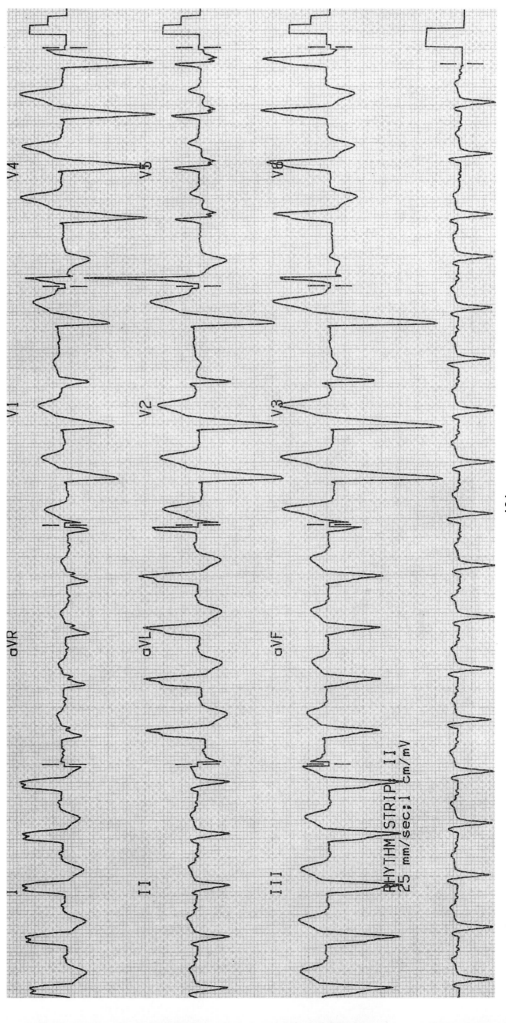

C-10

NARRATIVE INTERPRETATION

Rhythm:	**Sinus**
Rate:	**85**
Intervals:	**PR 0.16, QRS 0.08, QT 0.36**
Axis:	**−45 degrees**

Abnormalities

Axis leftward to −30 degrees. Q wave leads II, III, aVF. Tall R waves, with R wave greater than S wave leads V1–V2. ST elevation leads II, III, aVF. ST depression leads I, aVL, V1–V6. Deeply inverted T wave leads V1–V2.

Synthesis

Sinus rhythm. Left-axis deviation. Inferior wall MI with ST abnormalities of recent infarction. Posterior wall MI with ST abnormalities of recent infarction. ST depression in lateral leads suggesting possible lateral wall ischemia or reciprocal change.

TEST ANSWERS: 1, 64, 91, 93, 100, 101.

Comment: This tracing demonstrates an obvious acute inferior wall MI. The tall R waves with ST depression in the anterior precordial leads indicate that a posterior wall infarction is also present. The presence of significant Q waves inferiorly and tall R waves anteriorly indicates that a significant amount of myocardial necrosis has occurred. On angiography, this patient had occlusion of a dominant left circumflex artery with an extensive posterior-inferior infarction. The ST depression in the lateral leads may represent ischemia distant from the infarction or a reciprocal electrical phenomenon.

This ECG also demonstrates that inferior wall MI can produce left-axis deviation in the absence of left anterior fascicular block. LAFB is unlikely because the absence of a terminal R wave in lead aVR infers a normal clockwise loop. A counterclockwise vector loop should occur with LAFB.

FURTHER READING

Fisher ML, Mugmon MA, Carliner NH, et al: Left anterior fascicular block: Electrocardiographic criteria for its recognition in the presence of inferior myocardial infarction. *Am J Cardiol* 44:845–849, 1979.

Warner RA, Hill NE, Mookherjee S, Smulyan H: Electrocardiographic criteria for the diagnosis of combined inferior myocardial infarction and left anterior hemiblock. *Am Heart J* 51:718–722, 1983.

Warner RA, Hill NE, Mookherjee S, Smulyan H: Improved electrocardiographic criteria for the diagnosis of left anterior hemiblock. *Am J Cardiol* 51:723–726, 1983.

C-10

Clinical History

A 57-year-old man with 6 h of chest discomfort.

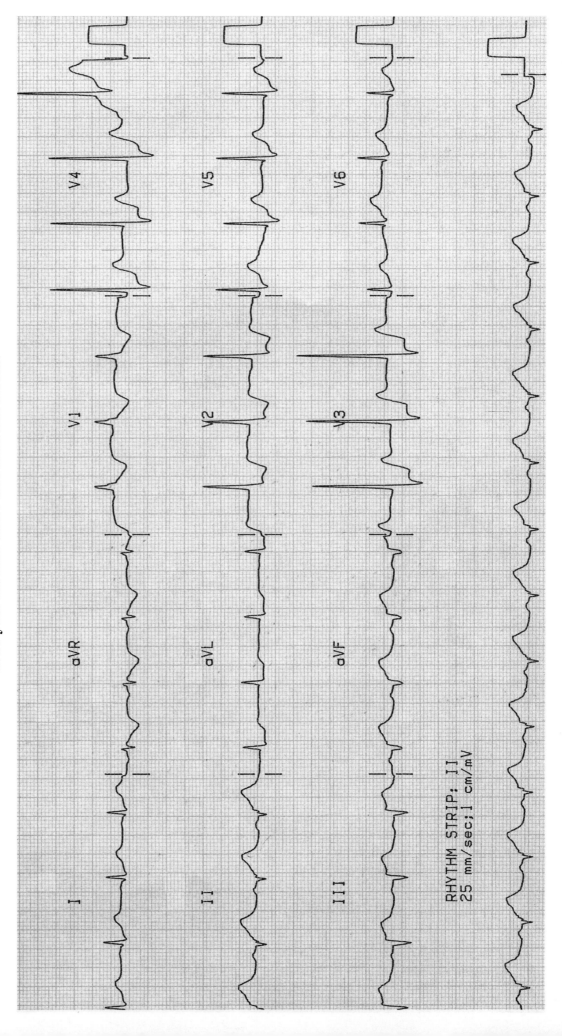

RHYTHM STRIP: II
25 mm/sec;1 cm/mV

C-11

NARRATIVE INTERPRETATION

Rhythm:	**Sinus**
Rate:	**66**
Intervals:	**PR 0.16, QRS 0.08, QT 0.36**
Axis:	**+15 degrees**

Abnormalities
Tall, broad R wave with upright T wave leads V1–V2.

Synthesis
Sinus rhythm. Posterior wall MI of indeterminate age.

TEST ANSWERS: 1, 94.

Comment: This patient was found on cardiac catheterization to have a posterior wall MI secondary to occlusion of the left circumflex coronary artery. A diagnosis of a coexistent inferior wall MI should not be made because of the absence of significant Q waves in the inferior leads. The rR' in lead V1 should not be mistaken for an incomplete RBBB because there are no other criteria to support this diagnosis.

FURTHER READING
Zema MJ, Kligfield P: Electrocardiographic tall R waves in the right precordial leads: Vectorcardiographic and electrocardiographic distinction of posterior myocardial infarction from prominent anterior forces in normal subjects. *J Electrocardiol* 17:129–138, 1984.

Zema MJ: Electrocardiographic tall R waves in the right precordial leads. *J Electrocardiol* 23:147–156, 1990.

C-11

Clinical History

A 43-year-old asymptomatic man with a history of *indigestion*.

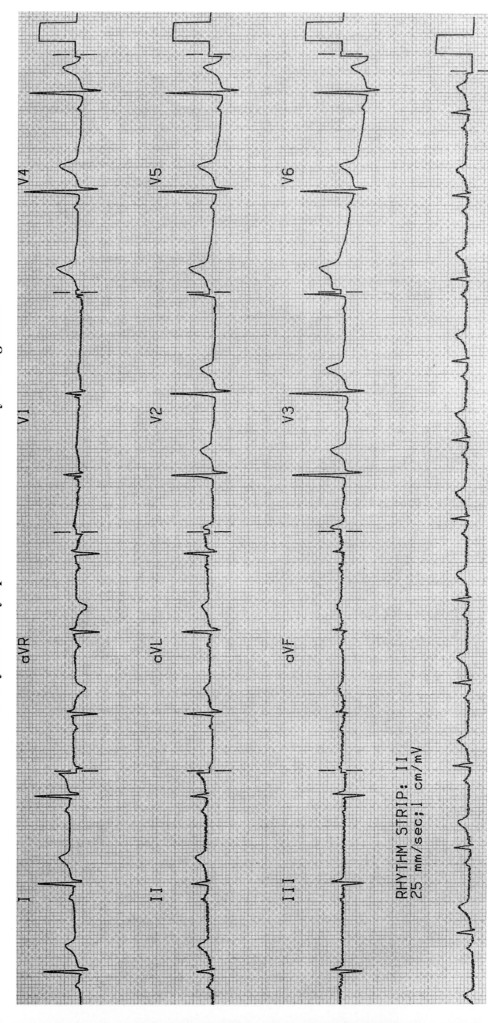

RHYTHM STRIP: II
25 mm/sec; 1 cm/mV

C-12

NARRATIVE INTERPRETATION

Rhythm:	**Sinus**
Rate:	**98**
Intervals:	**PR 0.18, QRS 0.11, QT 0.34**
Axis:	**−35 degrees**

Abnormalities

Axis leftward of −30 degrees. Abnormal P terminal force lead V1. S wave lead V2 + R wave lead V5 greater than 35 mm. Broad, slurred QRS leads I, aVL, V4–V6. Notching of R wave lead V4. Absent Q wave leads I, aVL, V6. Delayed intrinsicoid deflection of 0.06 s leads V5–V6. T-wave inversion leads I, aVL, V4–V6. VPC.

Synthesis

Sinus rhythm. VPC. Left-axis deviation. Left atrial abnormality. LVH. Incomplete LBBB. ST-T-wave abnormalities associated with LVH or conduction abnormality or both.

TEST ANSWERS: 1, 26, 60, 64, 75, 103, 104.

Comment: This tracing demonstrates most of the standard criteria for LVH, including increased QRS voltage, left-axis deviation, left atrial abnormality, and an increased QRS duration. An often confounding issue is whether there is coexistent incomplete LBBB. Suggestive criteria for incomplete LBBB in addition to LVH in this tracing are the absent septal Q waves, delayed intrinsicoid deflection in the left precordial leads, notching in lead V4, and slurring of the QRS in leads V5–V6. The absence of small Q waves in leads I and aVL and a late terminal R wave in lead aVR argue against a diagnosis of LAFB.

FURTHER READING

Barold SS, Linhart JW, Hildner FJ, et al: Incomplete left bundle branch block. *Circulation* 38:702–710, 1968.
Schamroth L, Bradlow BA: Incomplete left bundle branch block. *Br Heart J* 26:285–288, 1964.

C-12

Clinical History
A 56-year-old man with dyspnea.

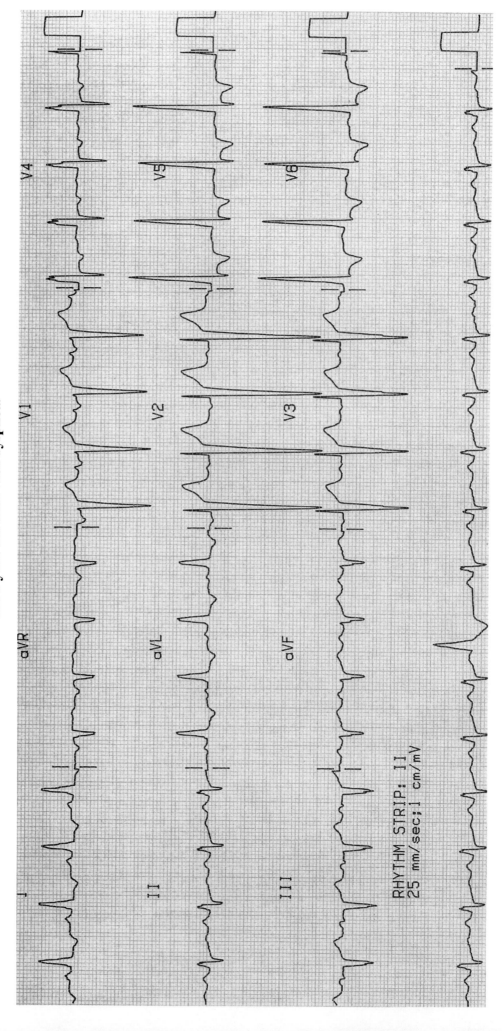

C-13

NARRATIVE INTERPRETATION

Rhythm:	**Sinus**
Rate:	**85**
Intervals:	**PR 0.16, QRS 0.08, QT 0.32**
Axis:	**+60 degrees**

Abnormalities
Q wave leads V1–V4. ST elevation leads I, aVL, V1–V5. ST depression leads II, III, aVF.

Synthesis
Sinus rhythm. Extensive anterior and lateral wall MI with ST-T-wave abnormalities of acute myocardial injury. ST-T-wave abnormalities in inferior leads suggesting either myocardial ischemia or reciprocal changes.

TEST ANSWERS: 1, 87, 89, 100, 101.

Comment: This patient sustained an extensive MI related to abuse of cocaine. On catheterization, he was found to have normal coronary arteries. This is not an unusual finding in young patients with MI after using cocaine. One hypothesis is that coronary spasm initiates formation of an intracoronary thrombus and acute MI, even in patients with no underlying coronary obstruction.

FURTHER READING
Zimmerman FH, Gustafson GM, Kemp HG Jr: Recurrent myocardial infarction associated with cocaine abuse in a young man with normal coronary arteries: Evidence of coronary artery spasm culminating in thrombosis. *J Am Coll Cardiol* 9:964–968, 1987.

C-13

Clinical History

A 37-year-old man with chest discomfort and dyspnea 2 h after inhaling cocaine.

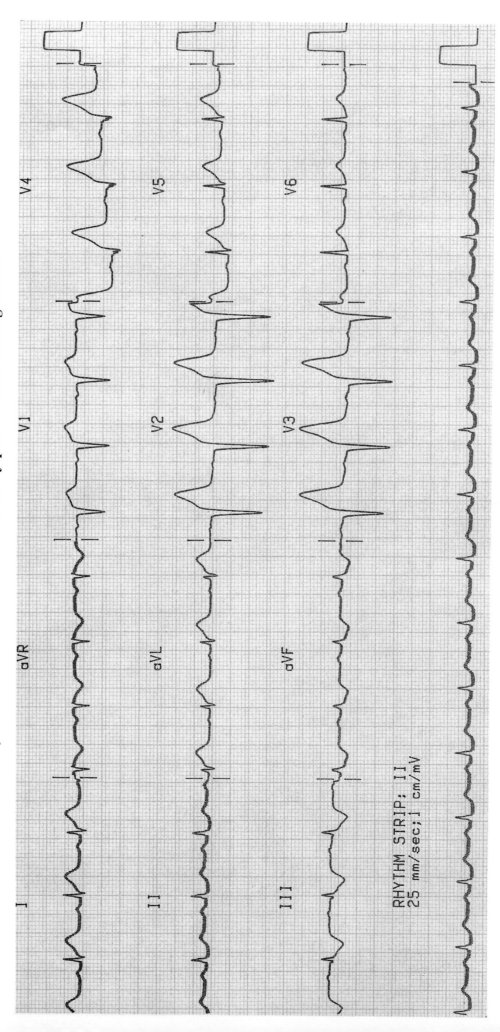

C-14

NARRATIVE INTERPRETATION

Rhythm:	**Sinus tachycardia**
Rate:	**135**
Intervals:	**PR 0.14, QRS 0.08, QT 0.26**
Axis:	**+90 degrees**

Abnormalities
Heart rate greater than 100 bpm.

Synthesis
Sinus tachycardia. Otherwise within normal limits.

TEST ANSWER: 4.

Comment: Patients with blunt chest trauma may suffer cardiac contusion. A variety of electrocardiographic abnormalities may result. The most common arrhythmia is sinus tachycardia, present in more than 70 percent of cases. Ventricular and atrial extrasystoles, intraventricular conduction abnormalities, and heart block are seen less frequently. Mechanical complications may also occur, including myocardial necrosis, valvular injury, coronary laceration, and hemopericardium. This patient suffered a mild cardiac contusion confirmed by elevation of cardiac enzymes.

FURTHER READING

Berk WA: ECG findings in nonpenetrating chest trauma: A review. *J Emerg Med* 5:209–215, 1987.

Macdonald RC, O'Neill CD, Ledingham IM: Myocardial contusion in blunt chest trauma. *Intensive Care Med* 7:265–268, 1981.

Tenzer ML: The spectrum of myocardial contusion: A review. *J Trauma* 25:620–627, 1985.

C-14

Clinical History

A 22-year-old man in the emergency department following a motor vehicle accident.

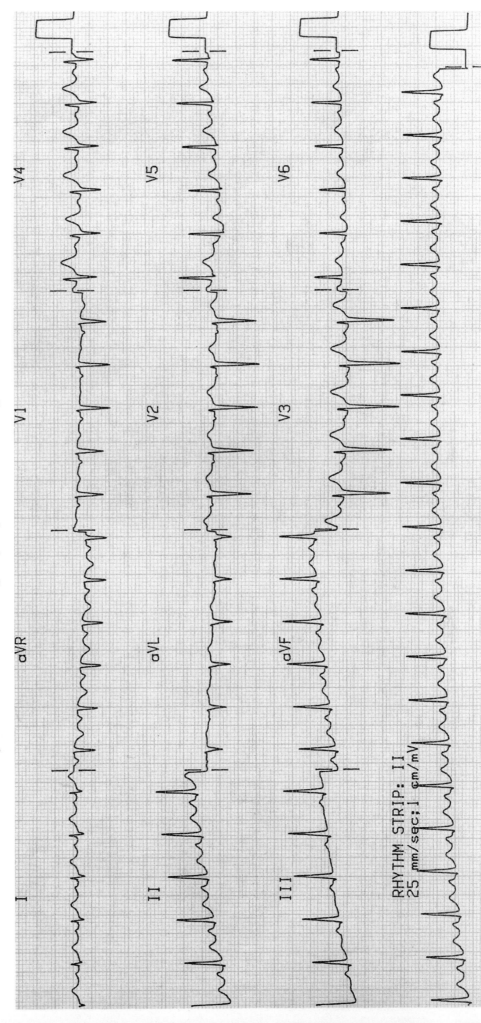

C-15

NARRATIVE INTERPRETATION

Rhythm:	**Sinus**
Rate:	**60**
Intervals:	**PR 0.16, QRS 0.08, QT 0.38**
Axis:	**+60 degrees**

Abnormalities

R waves V1–V3 less than 3 mm. Slight ST elevation with "coved" ST segment leads V2–V5. T-wave inversion leads V2–V5. T-wave biphasic leads I, II, III, aVF, V6.

Synthesis

Sinus rhythm. Poor R-wave progression. Probable recent anteroseptal wall MI. ST-T-wave abnormalities in leads V2–V6 suggesting recent myocardial injury. Nonspecific T-wave abnormalities leads I, II, III, aVF.

TEST ANSWERS: 1, 66, (81), 100, 106.

Comment: This patient suffered an MI a number of hours before being taken to the emergency department. By this time, more pronounced ST elevation has started to return toward baseline and T-wave inversion has occurred. Although profound ST elevation is no longer apparent, subtle elevation remains with downward concavity, or "coving." Myocardial necrosis has resulted in loss of anterior R forces; hence, poor R-wave progression is observed in leads V1–V3. The ST-T-wave abnormalities reflect extensive involvement, although criteria for an extensive, anterior, Q wave MI are not met.

FURTHER READING

Bar FW, Brugada P, Dassen WRM, et al: Prognostic value of Q waves, R/S ratio, loss of R-wave voltage, ST-T-segment abnormalities, electrical axis, low voltage and notching: Correlation of electrocardiogram and left ventriculogram. *J Am Coll Cardiol* 4:17–27, 1984.

DePace NL, Colby J, Hakki A, et al: Poor R-wave progression in the precordial leads: Clinical implications for the diagnosis of myocardial infarction. *J Am Coll Cardiol* 2:1073–1079, 1983.

C-15

Clinical History

A 69-year-old man seen in the emergency department 12 h after an episode of chest discomfort.

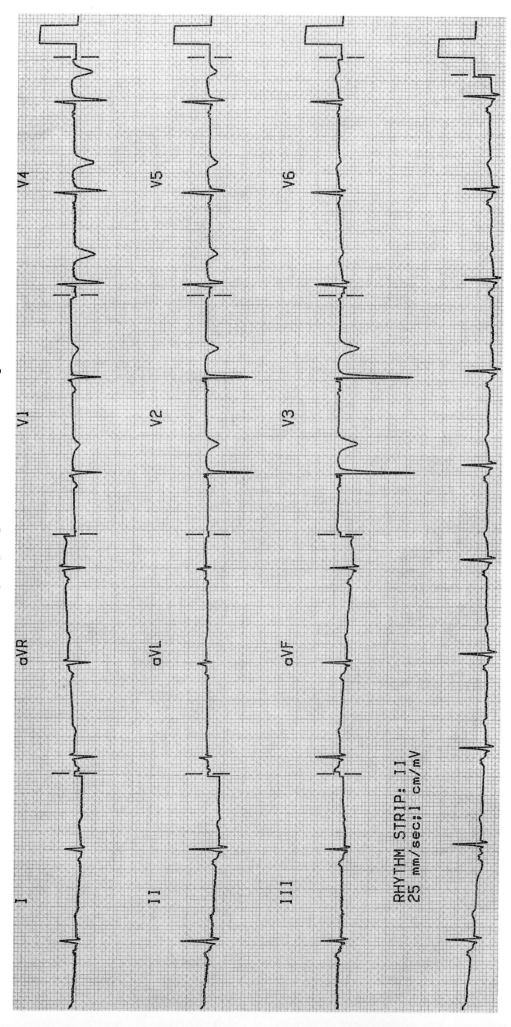

C-16

NARRATIVE INTERPRETATION

Rhythm:	**Sinus**
Rate:	**84**
Intervals:	**PR 0.14, QRS 0.09, QT 0.36**
Axis:	**+15 degrees**

Abnormalities

Q wave leads II, III, aVF. Slight ST elevation and "coving" leads II, III, aVF. ST depression lead V6. T-wave inversion leads II, III, aVF, V6. R wave lead aVL greater than 11 mm. R wave lead aVL + S wave lead V3 greater than 20 mm in a woman. VPCs. Abnormal P terminal force lead V1.

Synthesis

Sinus rhythm. VPCs. Inferior wall MI with ST-T-wave abnormalities suggesting recent myocardial injury. LVH by voltage criteria. ST-T-wave abnormalities associated with LVH. Left atrial abnormality.

TEST ANSWERS: 1, 26, 60, 78, 91, 100, 103.

Comment: The reader should not mistakenly identify the slurred upstroke seen in lead I or aVL as a delta wave and consider this tracing a "pseudoinfarction" pattern of WPW. The PR interval, albeit somewhat short, is still within normal limits and there are no other supporting criteria of WPW. This patient sustained an inferior wall MI with evolving ST-T-wave abnormalities evident in the inferior limb leads.

Another finding in this electrocardiogram is LVH, likely secondary to long-standing hypertension. The slight ST elevation in the anterior precordial leads and ST depression and T-wave inversion in lead V6 are probably secondary to LVH, rather than the infarction.

C-16

Clinical History

A 55-year-old asymptomatic woman on her second hospital day.

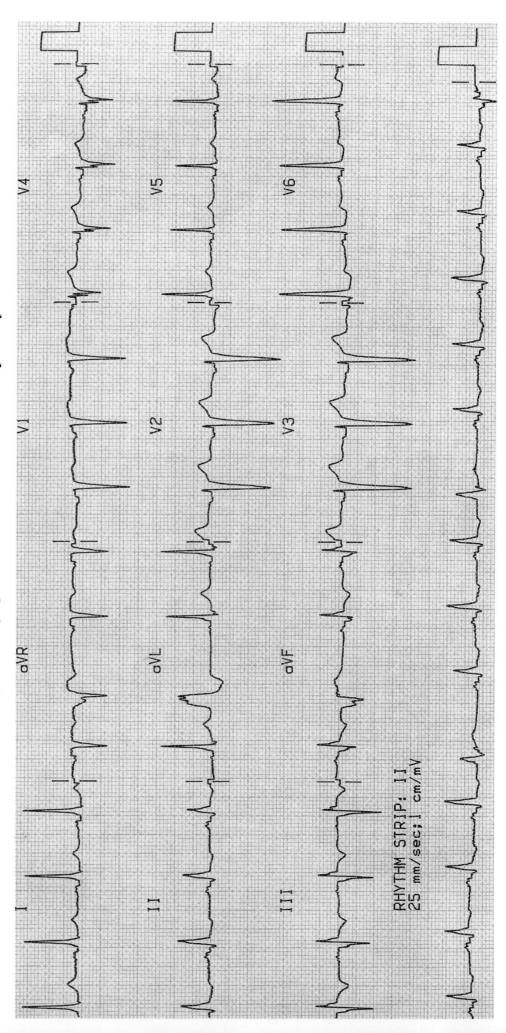

C-17

NARRATIVE INTERPRETATION

Rhythm:	**Sinus**
Rate:	**85**
Intervals:	**PR 0.16, QRS 0.10, QT 0.36**
Axis:	**−45 degrees**

Abnormalities

Axis leftward of −30 degrees. Abnormal P terminal force, lead V1. R wave lead aVL greater than 11 mm. R wave lead I + S wave lead III, greater than 25 mm. RSR' pattern lead V1.

Synthesis

Sinus rhythm. Left-axis deviation. Left anterior fascicular block. Probable LVH. Incomplete RBBB. Left atrial abnormality.

TEST ANSWERS: 1, 60, 64, 71, 72, 78.

Comment: This is a controversial tracing with regard to the limb lead criteria for left ventricular hypertrophy because of the presence of LAFB. Isolated left anterior fascicular block can increase the R wave voltage in leads I and aVL and use of standard criteria may lead to a spurious diagnosis of LVH. A suggested criterion for the diagnosis of LVH in the presence of LAFB is if the sum of the S wave in lead III added to the maximal precordial R + S voltage in any precordial lead is greater than 30 mm. Another suggested criterion for LVH and LAFB is an R wave in aVL greater than 13 mm. Neither criterion is met in this example, so it is reasonable to consider LVH as *probable.*

FURTHER READING

Gertsch M, Theler A, Foglia E: Electrocardiographic detection of left ventricular hypertrophy in the presence of left anterior fascicular block. *Am J Cardiol* 61:1098–1101, 1988.

Milliken JA: Isolated and complicated left anterior fascicular block: A review of suggested electrocardiographic criteria. *J Electrocardiol* 16:199–212, 1983.

C-17

Clinical History
A 56-year-old man with hypertension.

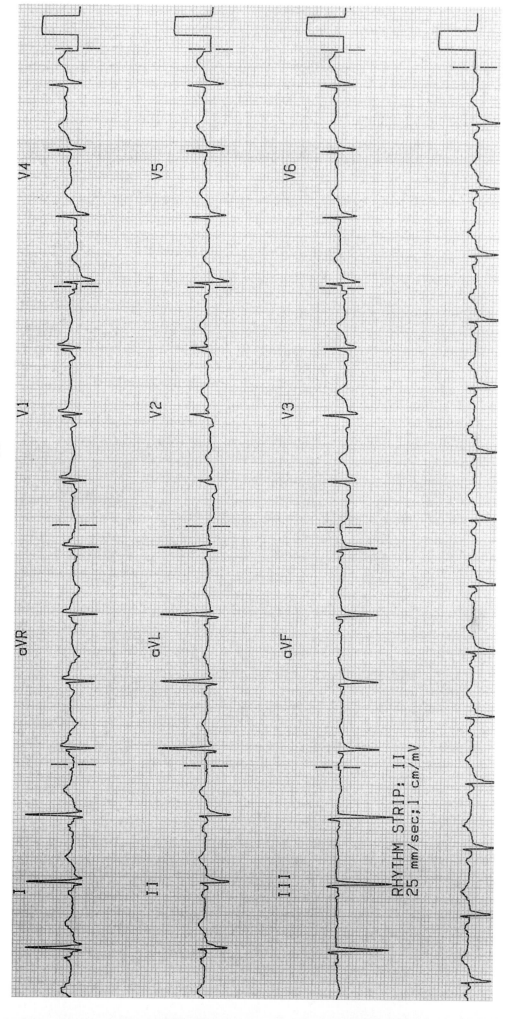

C-18

NARRATIVE INTERPRETATION

Rhythm:	**Atrial fibrillation**
Rate:	**62 (average)**
Intervals:	**PR –, QRS 0.08, QT 0.36**
Axis:	**–15 degrees**

Abnormalities
Tall R waves with R/S greater than 1 in leads V1–V3. T-wave inverted leads V4–V6.

Synthesis
Atrial fibrillation with a controlled ventricular response. Posterior wall MI of indeterminate age. Nonspecific T-wave abnormalities.

TEST ANSWERS: 20, 51, 94, 106.

Comment: This patient had suffered a posterior wall MI a number of years previously. This diagnosis may be made on the basis of tall R waves in leads V1 and V2. The differential diagnosis of tall R waves in the right precordial leads includes RVH, posterior wall MI, normal variant, and misplacement of the chest leads. Other conditions producing tall R waves are AV nodal bypass tract patterns and RBBB.

FURTHER READING
Benchimol A, Desser KB: The electrovectorcardiographic diagnosis of posterior wall myocardial infarction. In: Fisch C (ed), *Complex Electrocardiography I.* Philadelphia, Davis, 1973, pp. 184–197.
Zema MJ, Kligfield P: Electrocardiographic tall R waves in the right precordial leads: Vectorcardiographic and electrocardiographic distinction of posterior myocardial infarction from prominent anterior forces in normal subjects. *J Electrocardiol* 17:129–138, 1984.
Zema MJ: Electrocardiographic tall R waves in the right precordial leads. *J Electrocardiol* 23:147–156, 1990.

C-18

Clinical History
A 78-year-old man with dyspnea.

C-19

NARRATIVE INTERPRETATION

Rhythm:	**Accelerated AV junctional rhythm**
Rate:	**90**
Intervals:	**PR 0.12, QRS 0.12, QT 0.36**
Axis:	**−30 degrees**

Abnormalities

Inverted P waves leads II, III, aVF with PR interval at lower limit of normal. VPC. Broad, notched QRS with rSR' and T-wave inversion lead V1.

Synthesis

Accelerated AV junctional rhythm. VPC. RBBB with associated ST-T-wave changes. Normalization of conduction in post-VPC complex.

TEST ANSWERS: (9), 23, 26, 70, 104.

Comment: This rhythm is likely to be an accelerated AV junctional rhythm on the basis of the inverted P waves in the inferior leads and a relatively short PR interval. An ectopic atrial rhythm cannot be excluded as the PR interval is borderline.

An interesting feature of this electrocardiogram is seen in the sixth complex. Note, after the post-extrasystolic pause that the conduction is normalized with loss of the terminal conduction delay from the RBBB. The conduction abnormality returns with the subsequent complex. The development of a new RBBB after coronary bypass surgery does not appear to indicate an adverse prognosis.

FURTHER READING

Thomas JL, Dickstein RA, Parker FB Jr, et al: Prognostic significance of the development of left bundle conduction defects following aortic valve replacement. *J Thorac Cardiovasc Surg* 84:382–386, 1982.

Tuzcu EM, Emre A, Goormastic M, et al: Incidence and prognostic significance of intraventricular conduction abnormalities after coronary bypass surgery. *J Am Coll Cardiol* 16:607–610, 1990.

Wexelman W, Lichstein E, Cunningham JN, et al: Etiology and clinical significance of new fascicular conduction defects following coronary bypass surgery. *Am Heart J* 111:923–927, 1986.

C-19

Clinical History

A 77-year-old man in the recovery unit after open heart surgery. Previous electrocardiograms are normal.

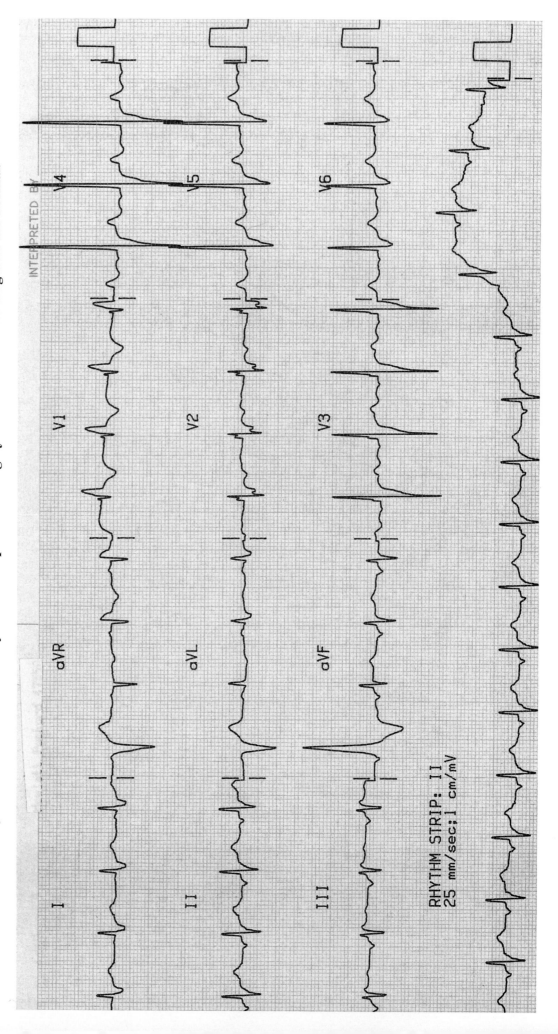

C-20

NARRATIVE INTERPRETATION

Rhythm:	**Sinus bradycardia with sinus pause**
Rate:	**57**
Intervals:	**PR 0.20, QRS 0.08, QT 0.36**
Axis:	**+45 degrees**

Abnormalities

Heart rate less than 60 bpm. Sinus pause. "Low" atrial escape complexes. ST depression leads I, II, aVF, V3–V6. T-wave inversion lead III. T-wave biphasic lead aVF.

Synthesis

Sinus bradycardia with sinus pause. "Low" atrial escape complexes. Nonspecific ST-T-wave abnormalities.

TEST ANSWERS: 3, 7, 106.

Comment: This patient demonstrates sinus bradycardia with an apparent sinus pause after the fifth complex on the rhythm strip. A subsidiary pacemaker in a "low" atrial site takes over at a slightly slower intrinsic heart rate. The sinus node then again regains control after two complexes. The escape complexes should not be characterized as AV junctional because the P wave remains upright with a normal PR interval in the lead II rhythm strip.

This tracing represents a true sinus pause rather than sinus arrhythmia with a wandering atrial pacemaker. Sinus arrhythmia is absent because the rhythm is regular with an abrupt pause, thereby producing escape complexes. In contrast, wandering atrial pacemaker would be characterized by regular R-to-R intervals with a different P-wave configuration and normal PR interval.

C-20

Clinical History
A 77-year-old asymptomatic woman.

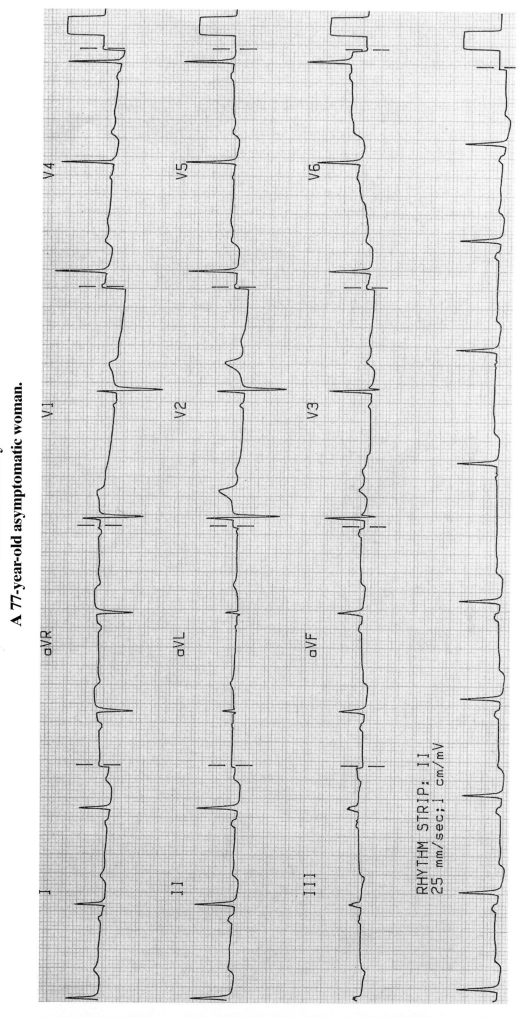

RHYTHM STRIP: II
25 mm/sec; 1 cm/mV

213

C-21

NARRATIVE INTERPRETATION

Rhythm:	**Multifocal atrial tachycardia**
Rate:	**138**
Intervals:	**PR –, QRS 0.10, QT 0.34**
Axis:	**–45 degrees**

Abnormalities

Rapid heart rate with variable P-wave morphologies and PR intervals. Axis leftward of –30 degrees. QS wave leads V3–V4. RS wave leads V1–V2. R wave aVL greater than 11 mm. R wave aVL + S wave lead V3 greater than 20 mm in a woman. R wave lead I + S wave lead III greater than 25 mm. ST elevation leads II, III, aVF, V2–V5. ST depression leads I, aVL. VPCs.

Synthesis

Multifocal atrial tachycardia. VPCs. LVH by multiple limb lead voltage criteria. Associated nonspecific ST abnormalities leads I, aVL. Left-axis deviation. Left anterior fascicular block. Anterior wall MI of indeterminate age. ST abnormalities of acute myocardial injury (cannot be excluded).

TEST ANSWERS: 14, 26, 64, 72, 78, (83), 84, 100, 103.

Comment: There are quite a number of abnormalities in this tracing. The rhythm is multifocal atrial tachycardia characterized by a minimum of three different P-wave configurations with varying PP and PR intervals.

Left ventricular hypertrophy and left anterior fascicular block are both present. Either finding may produce a "pseudoinfarction" pattern by diminishing R-wave voltage in the anterior precordial leads. It would be unusual however, for either LVH or LAFB to produce QS waves in lead V4 and it is correct to make a diagnosis of MI. Interestingly, the ST changes present in this example were chronic and probably secondary to LVH. The ST elevation is suspicious for acute myocardial injury, however, and deserves mention.

FURTHER READING

Goldberger AL: ECG simulators of myocardial infarction. Part I. Pathophysiology and differential diagnosis of pseudoinfarct Q wave patterns. *PACE* 5:106–119, 1982.
Goldberger AL: ECG simulators of myocardial infarction. Part II. Pathophysiology and differential diagnosis of pseudoinfarct ST-T-wave patterns. *PACE* 5:414–430, 1982.

C-21

Clinical History

A 77-year-old woman in the ICU with respiratory arrest.

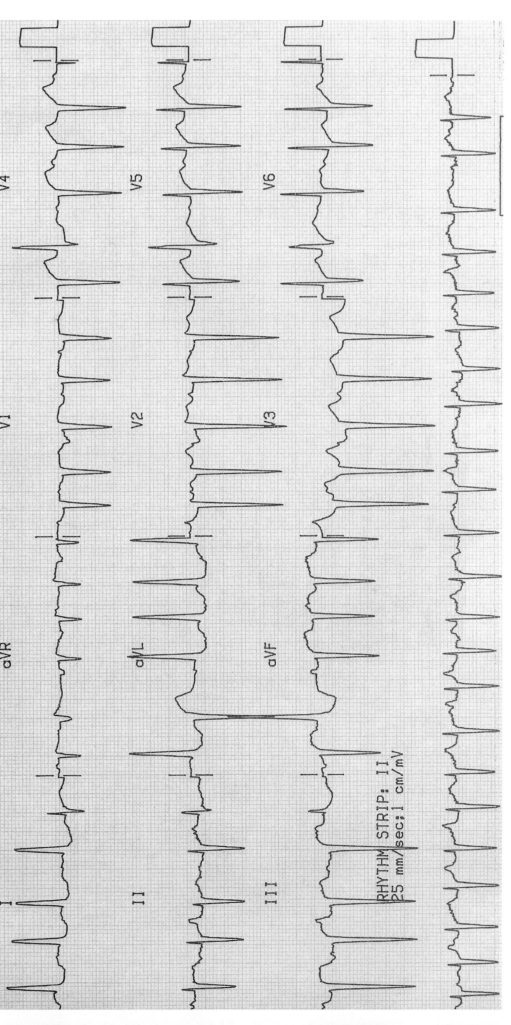

C-22

NARRATIVE INTERPRETATION

Rhythm:	**Sinus arrhythmia**
Rate:	**90 (average)**
Intervals:	**PR 0.16, QRS 0.08, QT 0.36**
Axis:	**0 degrees**

Abnormalities

Variation in sinus rate. Q wave lead III with small Q wave leads II, aVF. ST elevation leads II, III, aVF, V1–V2. ST depression leads I, aVL, V4–V6. T-wave inversion lead aVL.

Synthesis

Sinus arrhythmia. Inferior wall MI with ST abnormalities suggesting acute myocardial injury. ST-T-wave abnormalities suggesting either reciprocal change or myocardial ischemia.

TEST ANSWERS: 2, 91, 100, 101.

Comment: Sinus arrhythmia may be divided into two types, respiratory and nonrespiratory. Respiratory sinus arrhythmia occurs most often in the setting of sinus bradycardia and results from vagal influences that vary with the respiratory cycle. Nonrespiratory sinus arrhythmia is most often seen in patients with organic heart disease. The profound vagal influences characteristic of acute inferior wall MI may produce a marked nonrespiratory sinus arrhythmia, a finding seen in the current example. Other causes of nonrespiratory sinus arrhythmia include medications such as digoxin or morphine.

Note the ST elevation in leads V1–V2 in conjunction with the acute inferior wall MI. A number of investigators suggest that this represents concomitant right ventricular MI. Right ventricular leads may be useful to confirm this diagnosis.

FURTHER READING

Lopez-Sendon J, Coma-Canella I, Alcasena S, et al: Electrocardiographic findings in acute right ventricular infarction: Sensitivity and specificity of electrocardiographic alterations in right precordial leads, V4R, V3R, V1, V2, and V3. *J Am Coll Cardiol* 6:1273–1279, 1985.

Robalino BD, Whitlow PL, Underwood DA, Salcedo EE: Electrocardiographic manifestations of right ventricular infarction. *Am Heart J* 118:138–144, 1989.

Shah PK: New insights into the electrocardiogram of acute myocardial infarction. In: Gersh BJ, Rahimtoola SH (eds), *Acute Myocardial Infarction.* New York, Elsevier, 1991, pp. 128–143.

C-22

Clinical History

A 51-year-old man with chest discomfort.

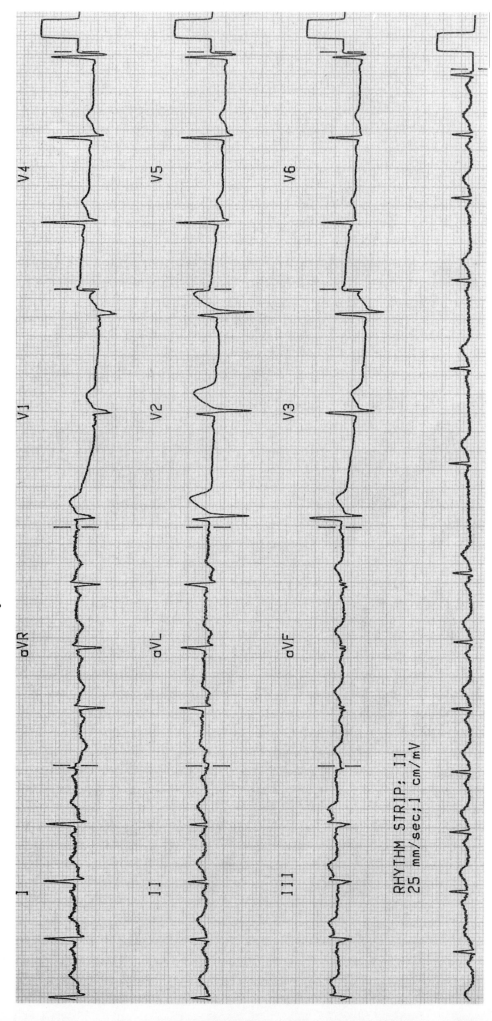

C-23

NARRATIVE INTERPRETATION

> **Rhythm:** **Sinus**
> **Rate:** **84**
> **Intervals:** **PR variable, QRS 0.13, QT 0.40**
> **Axis:** **−75 degrees**

Abnormalities

Gradual prolongation of PR interval with failure to conduct P wave. Axis leftward of −30 degrees. Prolonged QRS duration. rSR' V1–V3 with associated T-wave inversion leads V1–V3. R wave lead aVL greater than 11 mm. R wave lead I + S wave lead III greater than 25 mm. ST depression leads I, aVL. T-wave inversion leads I, aVL.

Synthesis

Sinus rhythm with second-degree AV block, Mobitz type I (Wenckebach). Left-axis deviation. Left anterior fascicular block. RBBB with associated ST-T-wave changes. LVH with associated ST-T-wave abnormalities.

TEST ANSWERS: 1, 43, 64, 70, 72, 78, 103, 104.

Comment: Note the Wenckebach sequence with eventual failure to conduct a P wave. Prolongation of the PR interval causes the P waves to be "lost" in the T wave of the preceding QRS complex. The superimposition of the P wave seems to produce ST elevation in some complexes, but this patient had no evidence of MI.

This tracing also demonstrates the phenomenon of "masquerading" bundle branch block. Note the right bundle branch pattern in the right precordial leads and a left bundle branch block type pattern in the limb leads. A right bundle branch block is the primary conduction abnormality. The limb lead findings result from the combination of marked left-axis deviation, left anterior fascicular block, and LVH. In RBBB, the first 0.6 s may be interpreted normally. The marked increase in limb lead voltage reflects the combined influence of LVH and LAFB. Marked LVH was confirmed by echocardiography.

FURTHER READING

Rosenbaum MB, Yesuron J, Lazzaari JO, Elizari MV: Left anterior hemiblock obscuring the diagnosis of right bundle branch block. *Circulation* 48:298–303, 1973.

C-23

Clinical History

A 78-year-old man in the CCU with severe congestive heart failure.

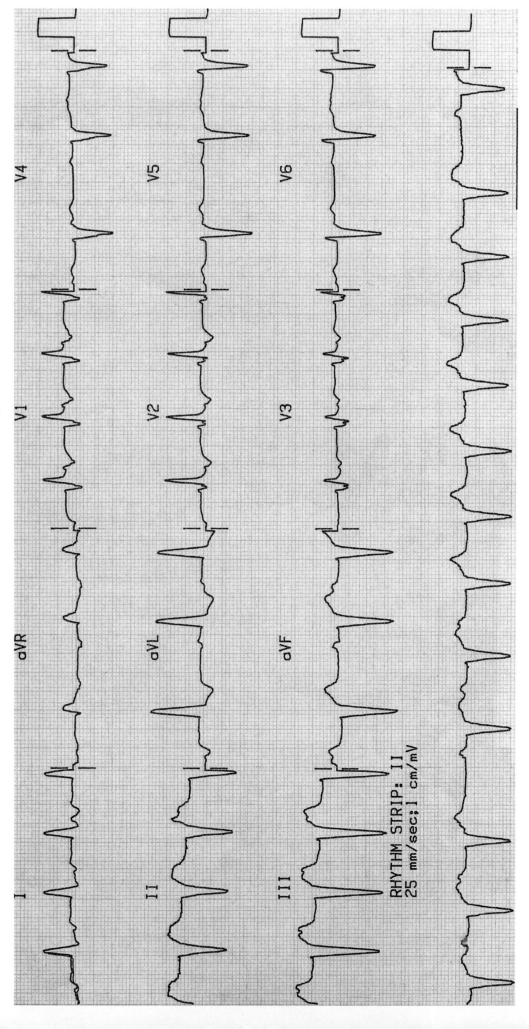

I aVR V1 V4

II aVL V2 V5

III aVF V3 V6

RHYTHM STRIP: II
25 mm/sec; 1 cm/mV

C-24

NARRATIVE INTERPRETATION

Rhythm:	**Atrial fibrillation**
Rate:	**92 (average)**
Intervals:	**PR −, QRS 0.08, QT 0.30**
Axis:	**−15 degrees**

Abnormalities
VPCs. Aberrantly conducted beats.

Synthesis
Atrial fibrillation with a controlled ventricular response. Aberrantly conducted beats. VPCs. Otherwise within normal limits.

TEST ANSWERS: 20, 26, 51, 77.

Comment: This tracing demonstrates that VPCs and aberrantly conducted complexes may resemble each other and coexist. The differentiation of beats of ventricular origin and those conducted aberrantly of supraventricular origin is particularly difficult in patients with atrial fibrillation. Because the cycle lengths are constantly changing, there is a tendency for aberrant conduction by virtue of *Ashman's phenomenon*. This states that aberrant ventricular conduction is favored by a long-short sequence because the ventricular refractory period is proportional to the preceding cycle length. When the preceding cycle length, and hence, refractory period is longer, the next impulse is more likely to be conducted aberrantly.

The ninth complex on the rhythm strip that follows a long-short cycle most likely represents aberrant conduction. Conversely, the wide complex in the next-to-last beat on the rhythm strip is most likely a VPC. It is identical to a complex in the limb leads that occurs without a long-short sequence.

FURTHER READING

Gulamhusein S, Yee R, Ko PT, Klein GJ: Electrocardiographic criteria for differentiating aberrancy and ventricular extrasystole in chronic atrial fibrillation: Validation by intracardiac recordings. *J Electrocardiol* 18:41–50, 1985.
Marriott HJL, Sandler IA: Criteria, old and new, for differentiating between ectopic ventricular beats and aberrant ventricular conduction in the presence of atrial fibrillation. *Prog Cardiovasc Dis* 9:18–28, 1966.

C-24

Clinical History
A 61-year-old man with palpitations.

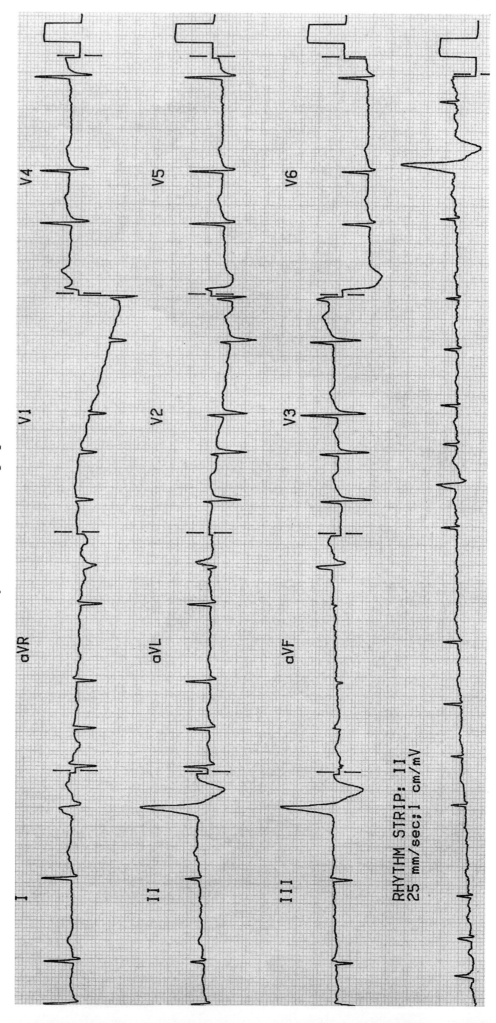

I
aVR
V1
V4

II
aVL
V2
V5

III
aVF
V3
V6

RHYTHM STRIP: II
25 mm/sec; 1 cm/mV

C-25

NARRATIVE INTERPRETATION

Rhythm:	**Sinus bradycardia**
Rate:	46
Intervals:	**PR 0.20, QRS 0.08, QT 0.44**
Axis:	**+45 degrees**

Abnormalities
Heart rate less than 60 bpm. Notched P wave. VPCs. Echo complexes.

Synthesis
Sinus bradycardia. VPCs. Retrograde atrial activation with echo complexes. Nonspecific atrial abnormality.

TEST ANSWERS: 3, 26, 54, 55, 62.

Comment: The basic rhythm of this electrocardiogram is sinus bradycardia. Note the VPCs that are "sandwiched" between two sinus beats. Be careful not to characterize these as interpolated VPCs. The narrow complex beat following the VPC has an inverted P wave and occurs earlier than the next expected sinus beat. This indicates that this complex is an *echo* or reciprocal beat. The VPC has depolarized the atria in a retrograde fashion and the impulse returns to depolarize the ventricles.

Another minor finding is the slightly wide and notched P wave, seen best on the rhythm strip. This is considered a nonspecific atrial abnormality.

FURTHER READING

Saunders JL, Calatayud JB, Schulz KJ, et al: Evaluation of ECG criteria for P-wave abnormalities. *Am Heart J* 74:757–765, 1967.

Thomas P, DeJong D: The P wave in the electrocardiogram in the diagnosis of heart disease. *Br Heart J* 16:241–254, 1954.

C-25

Clinical History

A 61-year-old asymptomatic man.

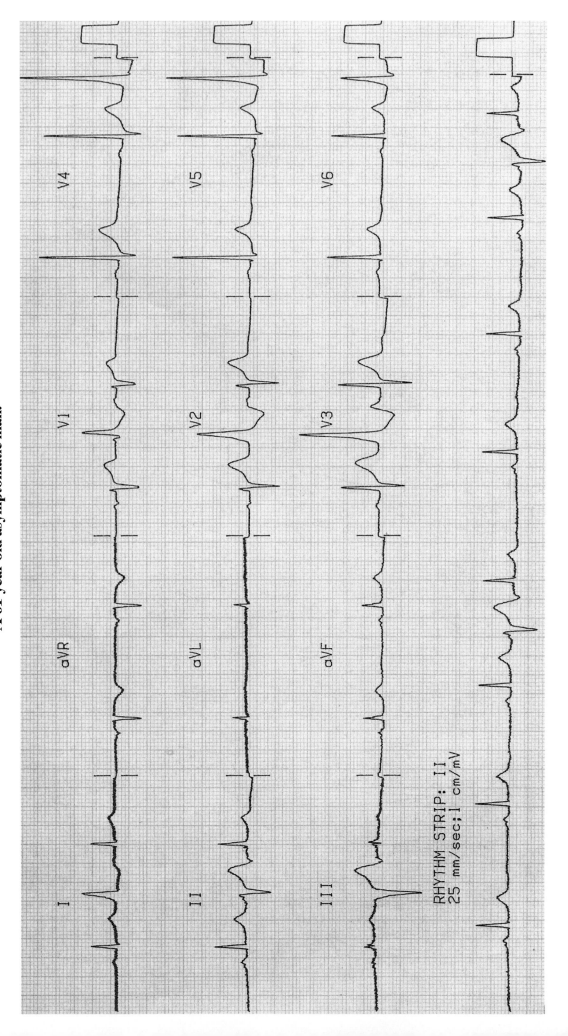

I

aVR

V1

V4

II

aVL

V2

V5

III

aVF

V3

V6

RHYTHM STRIP: II
25 mm/sec; 1 cm/mV

C-26

NARRATIVE INTERPRETATION

Rhythm:	**Sinus**
Rate:	**70**
Intervals:	**PR 0.14, QRS 0.06, QT 0.36**
Axis:	**0 degrees**

Abnormalities

Complexes with shortened PR interval with delta waves and change in QRS axis and configuration. T-wave inversion leads V1–V3 with slight ST elevation in nonpreexcited complexes.

Synthesis

Sinus rhythm. Intermittent ventricular preexcitation (WPW). Nonspecific ST-T-wave abnormalities in nonpreexcited complexes (cannot exclude myocardial injury).

TEST ANSWERS: 1, 49, (100), 106.

Comment: This tracing demonstrates intermittent ventricular preexcitation (WPW pattern). The 2nd, 5th, 8th, and 11th complexes of the 12-lead ECG demonstrate normal conduction, whereas the 3rd, 9th, 10th, 12th, and 13th complexes clearly show delta waves, a shortened PR interval, and a change in QRS morphology. Note the *pseudoinfarction* pattern in leads V1–V3 with apparent QS waves that mimic anteroseptal MI. The WPW pattern results from preexcitation of the ventricles via an accessory bypass tract. In classic WPW, there is conduction over an accessory bundle of Kent. Alternative forms include conduction over a paranodal pathway of James or Mahaim fibers. The term *Wolff-Parkinson-White syndrome* should be reserved for patients with this pattern who also have tachyarrhythmias.

Interestingly, the pattern in the right chest leads in the nonpreexcited complexes suggests coronary heart disease with T-wave inversion and slight ST elevation. Further workup revealed this patient had no evidence of coronary heart disease.

FURTHER READING

Klein GJ, Yee R, Sharma AD: Longitudinal electrophysiologic assessment of asymptomatic patients with the Wolff-Parkinson-White electrocardiographic pattern. *N Engl J Med* 320:1229–1233, 1989.

Reddy GV, Schamroth L: The localization of bypass tracts in the Wolff-Parkinson-White syndrome from the surface electrocardiogram. *Am Heart J* 113:984–993, 1987.

C-26

Clinical History

A 45-year-old woman with atypical chest pain. She has been told she has a history of a *silent* myocardial infarction (MI).

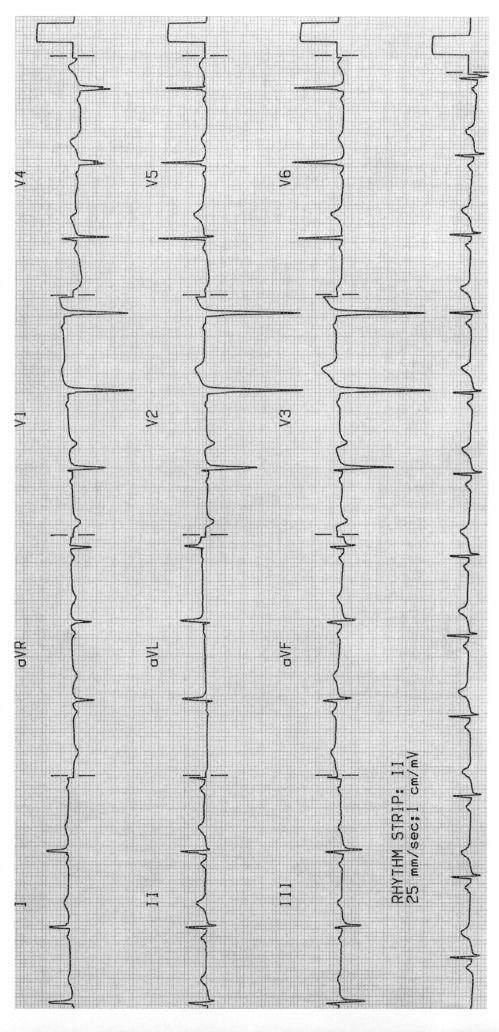

C-27

NARRATIVE INTERPRETATION

Rhythm:	**Sinus with first-degree AV block**
Rate:	**71**
Intervals:	**PR 0.22, QRS 0.16, QT 0.44**
Axis:	**0 degrees**

Abnormalities

Prolonged PR interval. Abnormal P terminal force lead V1. Broad, notched QRS leads I, aVL, V5–V6. T-wave upright leads I, aVL, V5–V6. VPC. Ventricular pacemaker functioning on demand with appropriate capture, rate 72. Pacemaker pseudofusion complexes.

Synthesis

Sinus rhythm. First-degree AV block. VPC. Ventricular pacemaker on demand with capture. Pacemaker pseudofusion complexes. LBBB. Left atrial abnormality. ST nonspecific T-wave abnormalities.

TEST ANSWERS: 1, 26, 35, 42, 60, 74, (104), 106.

Comment: The underlying rhythm is sinus with first-degree AV block and LBBB. Normally, the T waves are inverted with the opposite polarity from the bundle branch block. Thus, T-wave inversion would be expected in leads I and aVL and in the left precordial leads. In this example, the T waves are upright in these leads. Although this is a nonspecific finding, it is important to recognize because an unexpected change in T-wave polarity may be a sign of myocardial ischemia. In this patient, the T waves were chronic and were associated only with the conduction abnormality.

Note the *pseudofusion* pacemaker complexes (beats 3–7) on the rhythm strip. These are classified as pseudofusion rather than true fusion complexes because the pacemaker does not actually depolarize the ventricles. Despite the pacemaker spike, the QRS morphology is unchanged from baseline. This does not represent pacemaker failure to sense and is simply a manifestation of an intrinsic sinus rate that is nearly identical to the programmed rate of the pacemaker. Only after the pause induced by the VPC does the pacemaker truly capture the ventricles.

C-27

Clinical History
An 88-year-old asymptomatic man.

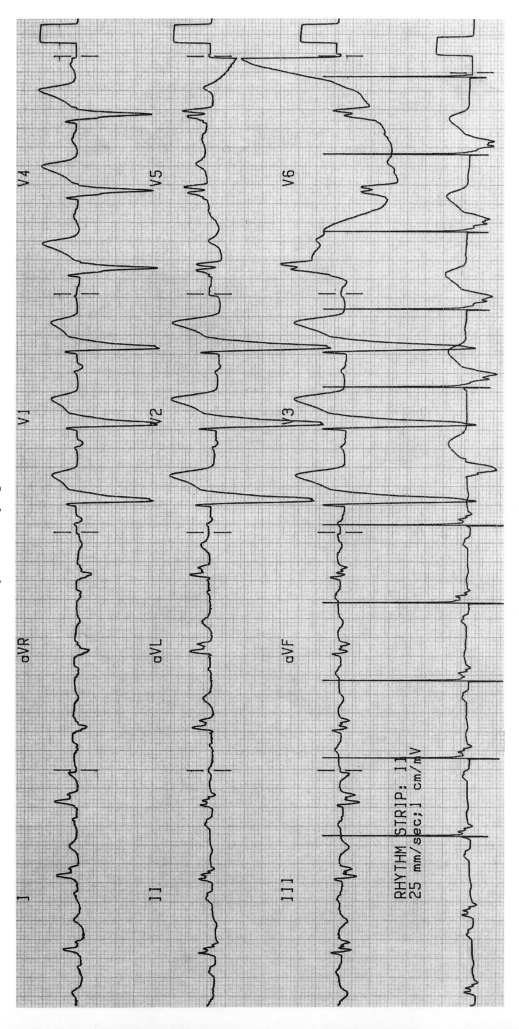

C-28

NARRATIVE INTERPRETATION

Rhythm: Sinus
Rate: 68
Intervals: PR 0.16, QRS 0.08, QT 0.46
Axis: −15 degrees

Abnormalities

Q wave leads II, III, aVF, V4–V6. QS lead V3. Slight ST elevation leads II, III, aVF, V3–V6. ST depression lead aVL. T-wave inverted lead aVL. T-wave flat lead I. R wave aVL + S wave lead III greater than 20 mm in a woman. Prolonged QTc. VPC.

Synthesis

Sinus rhythm. VPC. Inferior wall MI of indeterminate age. Anterolateral wall MI of indeterminate age. Anterior wall MI of indeterminate age. ST abnormalities suggestive of ventricular aneurysm. LVH. Nonspecific T-wave abnormalities. QTc prolongation.

TEST ANSWERS: 1, 26, 78, 84, 86, 92, 95, 106, 109.

Comment: This tracing illustrates the complex Q-wave patterns of patients with multiple infarctions. This patient sustained a prior inferolateral wall infarction with persistent ST elevation in the infarct leads indicating probable aneurysm formation. There was also a second anterior infarction. The clinical history allows the reader to exclude recent myocardial injury. The T-wave abnormalities in leads I and aVL are most likely related to coronary heart disease, but are best categorized as nonspecific. An additional finding is prolongation of the QT interval, probably secondary to coronary disease.

FURTHER READING

Heinbuch S, Koenig W, Gehring J: Assessment of global and regional myocardial function using the Minnesota Q/QS codes. *J Electrocardiol* 26:137–145, 1993.

Pahlm US, Chaitman, BR, Rautaharju PM, et al: Comparison of the various electrocardiographic scoring codes for estimating anatomically documented sizes of single and multiple infarcts of the left ventricle. *Am J Cardiol* 81:809–815, 1998.

C-28

Clinical History

An 82-year-old asymptomatic woman with a long history of coronary heart disease who is seen in the office.

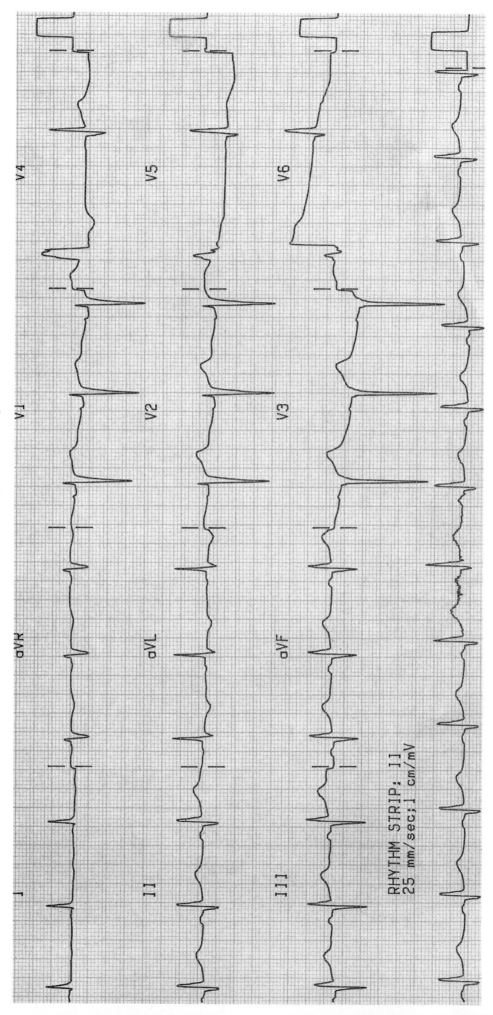

C-29

NARRATIVE INTERPRETATION

Rhythm:	**Sinus**
Rate:	**64**
Intervals:	**PR 0.14, QRS 0.06, QT 0.36**
Axis:	**0 degrees**

Abnormalities
R wave greater than S wave with upright T wave leads V1–V2.

Synthesis
Sinus rhythm. Posterior MI of indeterminate age.

TEST ANSWERS: 1, 94.

Comment: The tall R waves in the anterior precordial leads should alert the reader to the potential diagnosis of a posterior wall MI. In lead V1, note the upright T wave and an R/S ratio greater than 1. An R/S ratio greater than 1 in lead V2 is present in up to 10 percent of normal persons, but this would be highly unusual in lead V1 in the absence of pathology.

At the time of clinical evaluation, this electrocardiogram was interpreted as suggestive but not diagnostic of posterior wall MI of indeterminate age. Nevertheless, the patient was admitted to the hospital for clinical evaluation. The wisdom of this decision and the definitive diagnosis became apparent a number of hours later (see next tracing).

C-29

Clinical History
A 38-year-old man with intermittent chest discomfort.

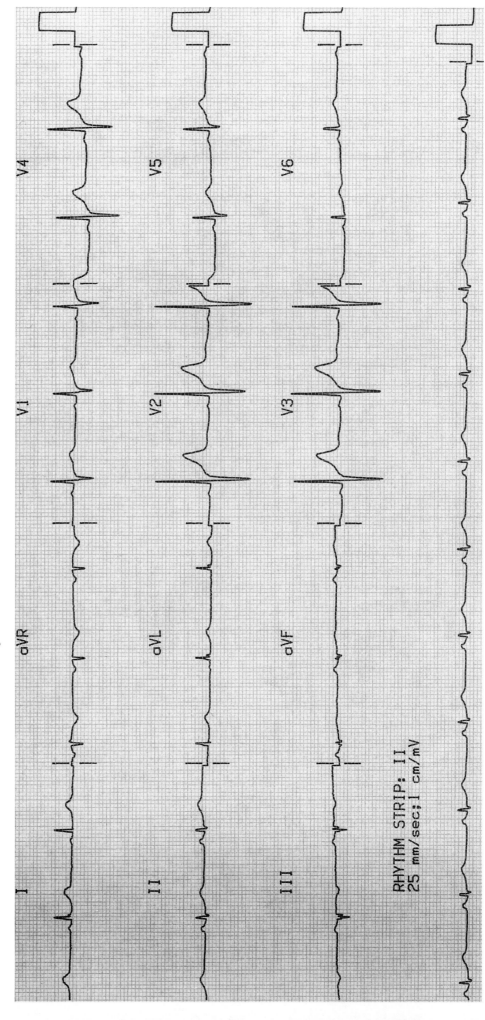

I
aVR
V1
V4

II
aVL
V2
V5

III
aVF
V3
V6

RHYTHM STRIP: II
25 mm/sec; 1 cm/mV

C-30

NARRATIVE INTERPRETATION

Rhythm:	**Sinus**
Rate:	**80**
Intervals:	**PR 0.14, QRS 0.08, QT 0.36**
Axis:	**−45 degrees**

Abnormalities

APCs. Axis leftward of −30 degrees. Q wave leads II, III, aVF. R wave greater than S wave with upright T wave leads V1–V2. ST depression leads I, aVL, V4–V5. ST elevation leads II, III, aVF. T-wave inversion leads II, III, aVF, V6.

Synthesis

Sinus rhythm. APCs. Inferior wall MI with ST-T-wave abnormalities suggesting acute myocardial injury. Acute posterior wall MI. Left-axis deviation. Left anterior fascicular block. ST-T-wave abnormalities suggesting myocardial ischemia or reciprocal change.

TEST ANSWERS: 1, 10, 64, 72, 91, 93, 100, 101.

Comment: This patient demonstrates an obvious acute inferior wall MI. A more subtle finding is involvement of the posterior wall in the infarction. When compared with the previous tracing, the R-wave voltage in leads V1 and V2 is greater and it is appropriate to diagnose an acute posterior MI.

Criteria are also now present for combined inferior wall MI and LAFB. Note the terminal R wave in lead aVR occurring after the terminal R wave in aVL. The "notching" of the QRS in the inferior leads also supports the diagnosis of combined inferior wall MI and LAFB.

The QRS complexes in the limb leads, on this and the previous tracing are small, but do not reach criteria for abnormally low voltage.

FURTHER READING

Fisher ML, Mugmon MA, Carliner NH, et al: Left anterior fascicular block: Electrocardiographic criteria for its recognition in the presence of inferior myocardial infarction. *Am J Cardiol* 44:845–849, 1979.

Louridas G, Patakas D, Angomachalelis N: Concomitant presence of left anterior hemiblock and inferior myocardial infarction: Electrocardiographic recognition of each entity. *J Electrocardiol* 14:365–370, 1981.

Warner RA, Hill NE, Mookherjee S, Smulyan H: Electrocardiographic criteria for the diagnosis of combined inferior myocardial infarction and left anterior hemiblock. *Am Heart J* 51:718–722, 1983.

C-30

Clinical History

A 38-year-old man with recurrent chest discomfort. Tracing taken 6 h after previous electrocardiogram.

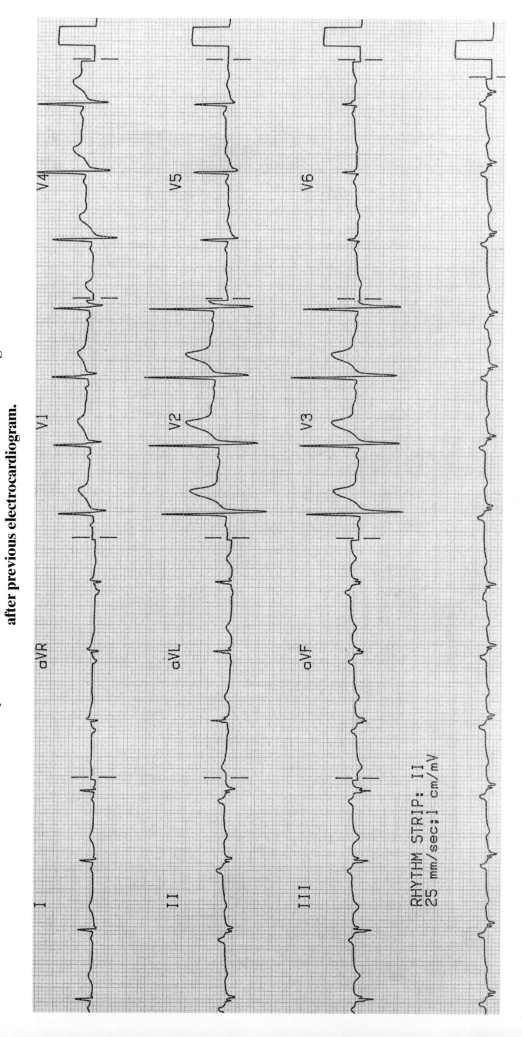

C-31

NARRATIVE INTERPRETATION

Rhythm:	**Sinus**
Rate:	96
Intervals:	**PR 0.16, QRS 0.08, QT 0.40**
Axis:	+15 degrees

Abnormalities

VPCs. Paired and multiform VPCs. Ventricular tachycardia on rhythm strip. Abnormal P terminal force V1. Diffuse T-wave flattening, limb leads. S wave lead V2 + R wave lead V5 greater than 35 mm.

Synthesis

Sinus rhythm. Frequent VPCs with paired, multiform VPCs. Ventricular tachycardia (multiform triplet) on rhythm strip. Left atrial abnormality. LVH. Nonspecific T-wave abnormalities.

TEST ANSWERS: 1, 27, 28, 30, 60, 78, 106.

Comment: This patient had congestive heart failure and massive cardiomegaly on the basis of an idiopathic dilated cardiomyopathy. Interestingly, voltage criteria for LVH are borderline. Chronic ventricular ectopy, which is often multiform, is commonly seen in patients with left ventricular dysfunction. Ventricular ectopy is the most common and likely the earliest manifestation of digitalis toxicity.

FURTHER READING

Fisch C, Knoebel SB: Digitalis cardiotoxicity. *J Am Coll Cardiol* 5:91A–98A, 1985.

Smith TW, Antman EM, Friedman PL, et al: Digitalis glycosides: Mechanisms and manifestations of toxicity. *Prog Cardiovasc Dis* 27:21–56, 1984.

C-31

Clinical History

A 68-year-old man with cardiomegaly and dyspnea. Medications include digoxin.

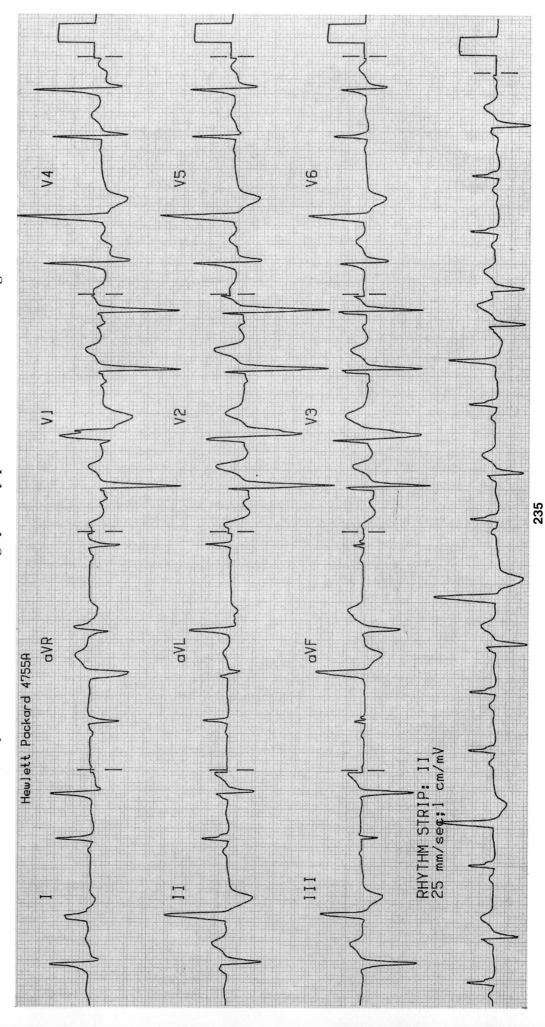

C-32

NARRATIVE INTERPRETATION

Rhythm:	**Sinus**
Rate:	**78**
Intervals:	**PR 14, QRS 0.12, QT 0.40**
Axis:	**−45 degrees**

Abnormalities

Axis leftward of −30 degrees. Abnormal P terminal force lead V1. R wave aVL greater than 11 mm. R wave aVL + S wave V3 greater than 28 mm in a man. R wave lead I + S wave lead III greater than 25 mm. Prolonged QRS interval. ST depression leads I, aVL, V5–V6. T-wave inversion leads I, aVL. Flat T wave leads V5–V6. VPC. JPC.

Synthesis

Sinus rhythm. VPC. JPC. Left-axis deviation. LAFB. LVH by voltage criteria with associated ST-T-wave abnormalities. Intraventricular conduction delay. Left atrial abnormality.

TEST ANSWERS: 1, 25, 26, 60, 64, 72, 76, 78, 103.

Comment: This patient had significant cardiomegaly and echocardiographic LVH secondary to aortic stenosis. LVH is indicated by multiple voltage criteria, an intraventricular conduction delay, ST-T-wave abnormalities, and left atrial enlargement. Note however, that LVH alone is unlikely to produce this degree of left axis shift and LAFB, must be considered. In uncomplicated LAFB, the QRS duration is less than 0.12 s. Here, the QRS duration is prolonged further due to concomitant LVH. Additional supporting criteria for LAFB superimposed on LVH are the small Q waves in leads I and aVL, and the late, slurred R wave in aVR.

FURTHER READING

Gertsch M, Theler A, Foglia E: Electrocardiographic detection of left ventricular hypertrophy in the presence of left anterior fascicular block. *Am J Cardiol* 61:1098–1101, 1988.

Milliken JA: Isolated and complicated left anterior fascicular block: A review of suggested electrocardiographic criteria. *J Electrocardiol* 16:199–212, 1983.

Perloff JK, Roberts NK, Cabeen WR Jr: Left-axis deviation: A reassessment. *Circulation* 60:12–21, 1979.

C-32

Clinical History
A 72-year-old man with aortic stenosis.

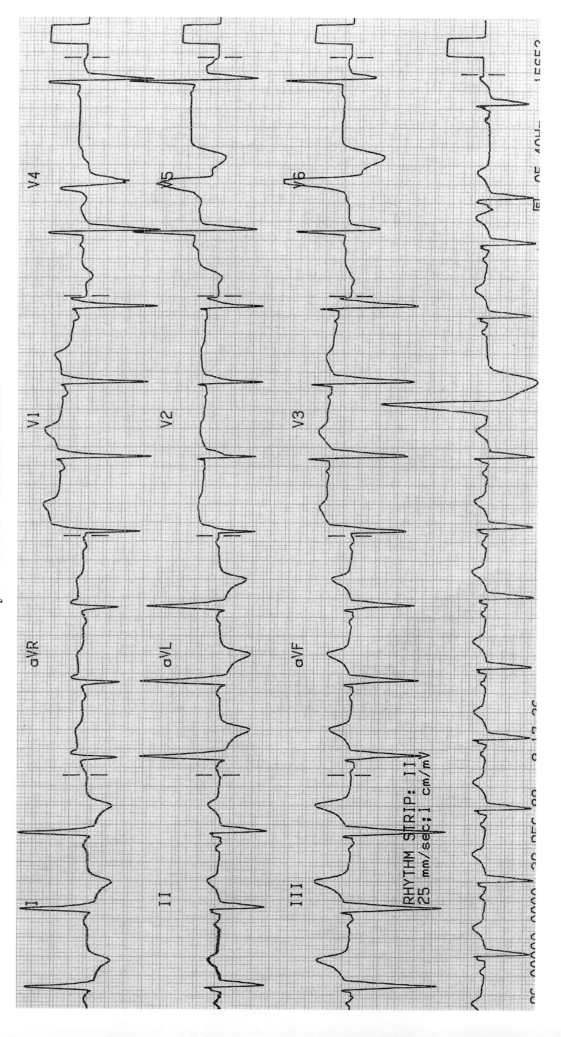

C-33

NARRATIVE INTERPRETATION

Rhythm:	**Atrial flutter with 2:1 AV conduction**
Rate:	**Atrial 270, ventricular 135**
Intervals:	**PR −, QRS 0.08, QT 0.32**
Axis:	**Indeterminate**

Abnormalities
Generalized ST depression.

Synthesis
Atrial flutter with 2:1 AV conduction. Generalized ST-segment depression, possibly artifactual from superimposition of inverted flutter (P) waves.

TEST ANSWERS: 19, 50, (106).

Comment: The rhythm disturbance is fairly obvious with characteristic "sawtooth" inverted flutter waves evident in leads II, III, and aVF. A more difficult determination is whether or not there are additional ST or T-wave abnormalities. There is an inverted flutter wave superimposed on the ST segment immediately following the QRS, and the author has concluded that these findings are likely artifactual. The determination of abnormal ST-T-wave findings in patients with atrial flutter often requires comparison with additional tracings or after conversion to sinus rhythm (see next tracing).

C-33

Clinical History

A 43-year-old man with palpitations.

aVR   V1   V4

II   aVL   V2   V5

III   aVF   V3   V6

RHYTHM STRIP: II
25 mm/sec; 1 cm/mV

239

C-34

NARRATIVE INTERPRETATION

Rhythm:	**Sinus**
Rate:	**68**
Intervals:	**PR 0.18, QRS 0.08, QT 0.42**
Axis:	**+60 degrees**

Abnormalities
Generalized T-wave flattening. Prolonged QTc interval.

Synthesis
Sinus rhythm. Nonspecific T-wave abnormalities. Prolonged QTc.

TEST ANSWERS: 1, 106, 109.

Comment: This tracing represents the postcardioversion electrocardiogram from the previous tracing. The marked ST findings seen in the previous tracing are no longer present, confirming that they were artifactual from superimposition of flutter waves. Overall T-wave voltage is low, a nonspecific finding. Also note the slight QT prolongation, likely secondary to treatment with quinidine.

C-34

Clinical History

A 43-year-old asymptomatic man. Medications include quinidine and digoxin.

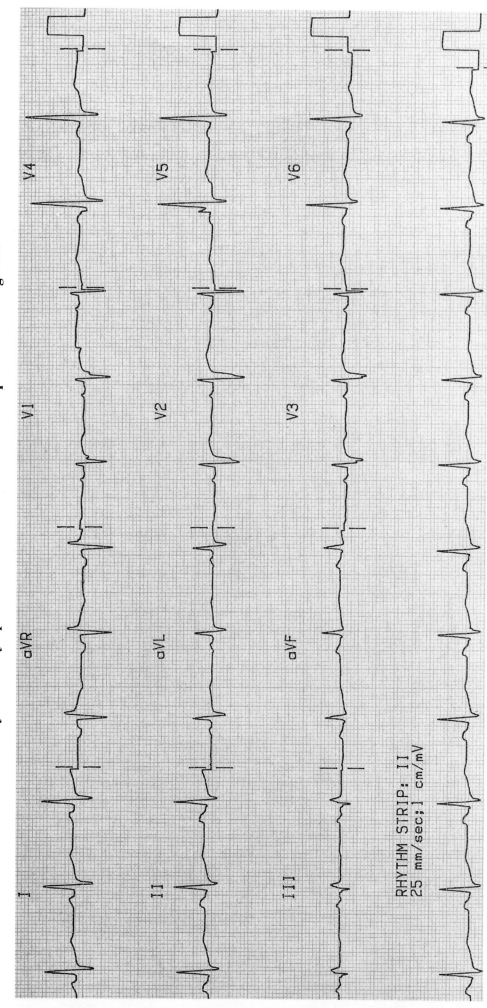

C-35

NARRATIVE INTERPRETATION

Rhythm:	**Sinus**
Rate:	77
Intervals:	**PR 0.18, QRS 0.08, QT 0.38**
Axis:	**+60 degrees**

Abnormalities
PR depression leads II, aVF. ST elevation with upward concavity leads I, II, aVF, V2–V6.

Synthesis
Sinus rhythm. PR depression and generalized ST elevation suggestive of early acute pericarditis.

TEST ANSWERS: 1, 63, 105.

Comment: PR depression, often most prominent in the inferior leads, is an early finding in acute pericarditis. Diffuse ST elevation with upward concavity is also characteristic of pericarditis, but this finding is often difficult to differentiate from a normal variant. ST elevation in pericarditis is typically diffuse, but may be localized to a few leads. In such circumstances, it may be difficult to differentiate these abnormalities from those of acute myocardial injury. The ST elevation associated with MI however, characteristically demonstrates downward concavity (coving).

FURTHER READING
Gintzon LE, Laks MM: The differential diagnosis of acute pericarditis from the normal variant: New electrocardiographic criteria. *Circulation* 65:1004–1009, 1982.
Spodick DH: Differential characteristics of the electrocardiogram in early repolarization and acute pericarditis. *N Engl J Med* 295:523–526, 1976.

C-35

Clinical History

A 34-year-old female nurse with chest pain on inspiration.

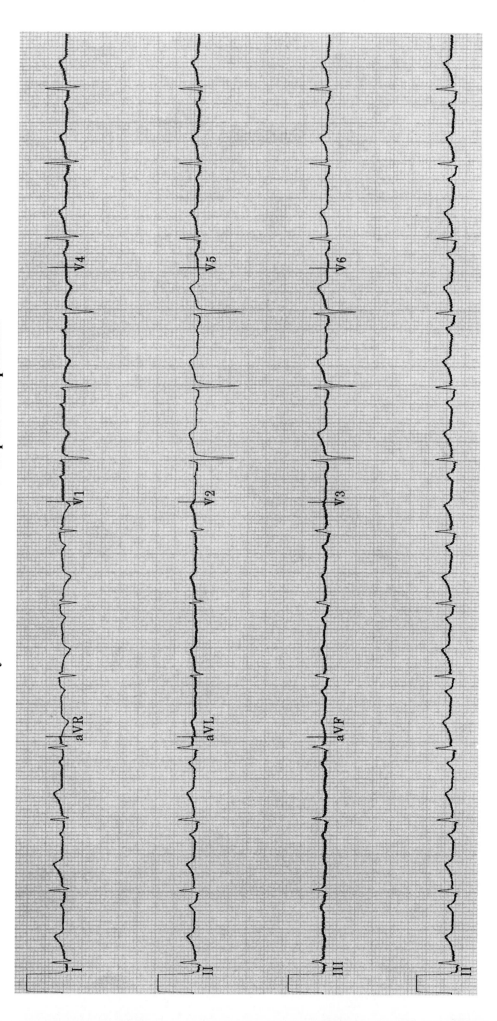

C-36

NARRATIVE INTERPRETATION

Rhythm:	**Sinus**
Rate:	99
Intervals:	**PR 014, QRS 0.08, QT 0.36**
Axis:	**−35 degrees**

Abnormalities

Axis leftward of −30 degrees. Q waves leads II, III, aVF. ST elevation leads II, III, aVF, V2–V6. Slight ST elevation leads I, aVL. T-wave inversion leads III, aVF. R wave lead aVL greater than 11 mm. R wave lead I + S wave lead III greater than 25 mm.

Synthesis

Sinus rhythm. Inferior wall MI with ST-T-wave abnormalities in leads II, III, aVF suggestive of recent myocardial injury. Additional ST abnormalities leads I, aVL, V2–V6 suggestive of anterolateral myocardial injury. Left-axis deviation. Probable left anterior fascicular block. LVH by voltage criteria.

TEST ANSWERS: 1, 64, 72, 78, 91, 100.

Comment: It is often difficult to determine whether left anterior fascicular block coexists with an inferior MI. Either diagnosis may produce left-axis deviation. In LAFB, the initial forces are directed inferiorly followed by superiorly oriented terminal forces. This produces initial R waves and terminal S waves in leads II, III and aVF. In this example, the extensive loss of viable myocardium from the inferior wall MI produced deep Q waves, obscuring the initial inferior vector of the LAFB. Following a tiny R wave, small terminal S waves appear, making LAFB a likely diagnosis.

FURTHER READING

Fisher ML, Mugmon MA, Carliner NH, et al: Left anterior fascicular block: Electrocardiographic criteria for its recognition in the presence of inferior myocardial infarction. *Am J Cardiol* 44:845–849, 1979.

Louridas G, Patakas D, Angomachalelis N: Concomitant presence of left anterior hemiblock and inferior myocardial infarction: Electrocardiographic recognition of each entity. *J Electrocardiol* 14:365–370, 1981.

Milliken JA: Isolated and complicated left anterior fascicular block: A review of suggested electrocardiographic criteria. *J Electrocardiol* 16:199–212, 1983.

Warner RA, Hill NE, Mookherjee S, Smulyan H: Electrocardiographic criteria for the diagnosis of combined inferior myocardial infarction and left anterior hemiblock. *Am Heart J* 51:718–722, 1983.

C-36

Clinical History

A 74-year-old man with recurrent chest discomfort on his third day in the CCU.

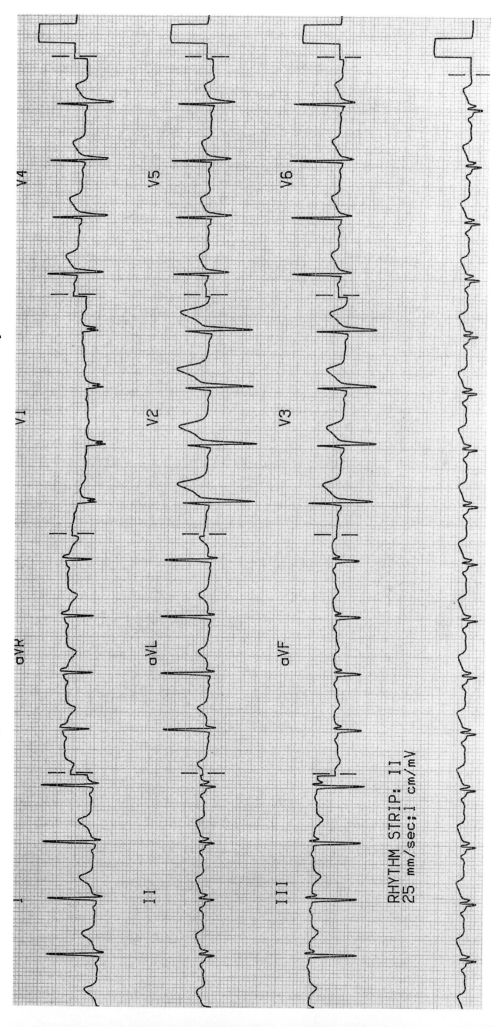

C-37

NARRATIVE INTERPRETATION

Rhythm:	**Sinus with first-degree AV block**
Rate:	96
Intervals:	**PR 0.21, QRS 0.12, QT 0.36**
Axis:	**+120 degrees**

Abnormalities

Axis rightward of +90 degrees. Prolonged PR interval. Abnormal P terminal force lead V1. Q wave leads II, III, aVF. ST elevation leads II, III, aVF. Broad, notched R wave with rR' pattern and T-wave inversion lead V1.

Synthesis

Sinus rhythm. First-degree AV block. Right-axis deviation. Left atrial abnormality. RBBB with associated ST-T-wave abnormalities. Left posterior fascicular block. Inferior wall MI with ST-T-wave abnormalities suggestive of acute myocardial injury.

TEST ANSWERS: 1, 42, 60, 65, 70, 73, 91, 100, 104.

Comment: This patient has a number of conduction abnormalities in the presence of an acute MI. Diagnostic Q waves are not yet present, but there are early Q waves and ST-segment abnormalities indicative of acute inferior wall MI. The combination of a MI with multiple conduction abnormalities is particularly ominous. The posterior fascicle derives its blood supply from both the left anterior descending and posterior descending coronary arteries. One series found a 20 percent incidence of progression to complete heart block in patients with acute MI and concomitant bifascicular bundle branch block and first-degree AV block.

FURTHER READING

Alpert JS: Conduction disturbances: Temporary and permanent pacing in patients with acute myocardial infarction. In: Gersh BJ, Rahimtoola SH (eds), *Acute Myocardial Infarction.* New York, Elsevier, 1991, pp. 249–258.

Hindman MC, Wagner GS, JaRo M, et al: The clinical significance of bundle branch block complicating acute myocardial infarction. I. Clinical characteristics, hospital mortality, and one-year follow-up. *Circulation* 58:679–688, 1978.

Hindman MC, Wagner GS, JaRo M, et al: The clinical significance of bundle branch block complicating acute myocardial infarction. II. Indications for temporary and permanent pacemaker insertion. *Circulation* 58:689–699, 1978.

C-37

Clinical History

A 63-year-old woman with severe dyspnea and chest discomfort.

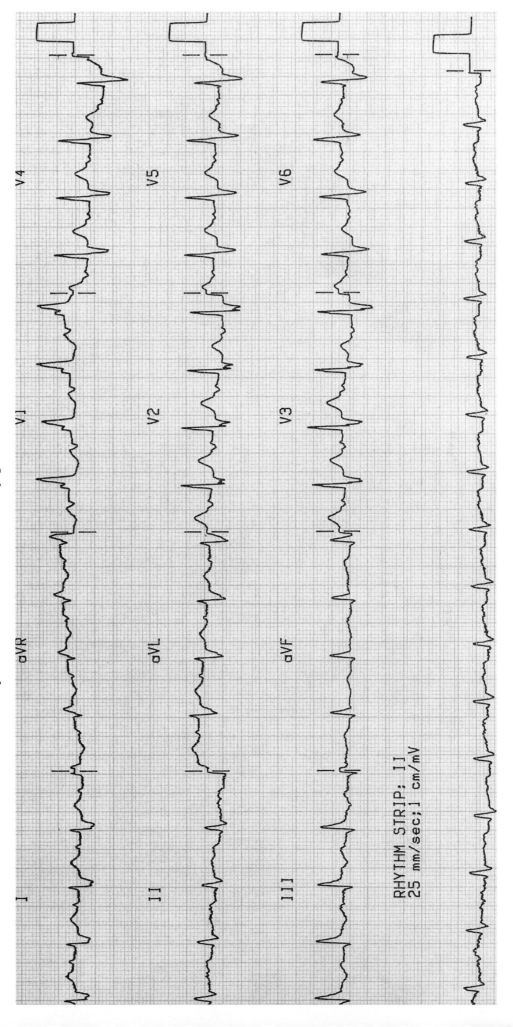

C-38

NARRATIVE INTERPRETATION

Rhythm:	**Sinus**
Rate:	**84**
Intervals:	**PR 0.18, QRS 0.08, QT 0.36**
Axis:	**−15 degrees**

Abnormalities

R wave lead aVL greater than 11 mm. R wave lead I + S wave lead III greater than 25 mm. S wave lead V1 + R wave lead V5 greater than 35mm. ST depression lead V6. T-wave inversion leads I, II, aVL, V4–V6.

Synthesis

Sinus rhythm. LVH. Associated ST-T-wave abnormalities.

TEST ANSWERS: 1, 78, 103.

Comment: This patient had marked cardiomegaly secondary to chronic mitral insufficiency. Note that LVH is present by traditional precordial voltage criteria as well as by two different limb lead criteria. Interestingly, the newer gender-specific Cornell criteria fail to indicate LVH. Compared to precordial lead standards, limb lead criteria are less sensitive, but highly specific for diagnosing LVH.

FURTHER READING

Casale PN, Devereux RB, Kligfield P, et al: Electrocardiographic detection of left ventricular hypertrophy: Development and prospective validation of improved criteria. *J Am Coll Cardiol* 6:572–580, 1985.

Romhilt DW, Estes EH: A point score system for the ECG diagnosis of left ventricular hypertrophy. *Am Heart J* 75:752–758, 1968.

Romhilt DW, Bove KE, Norris RJ, et al: A critical appraisal of the electrocardiographic criteria for the diagnosis of left ventricular hypertrophy. *Circulation* 40:185–195, 1969.

C-38

Clinical History
A 61-year-old man with a systolic murmur.

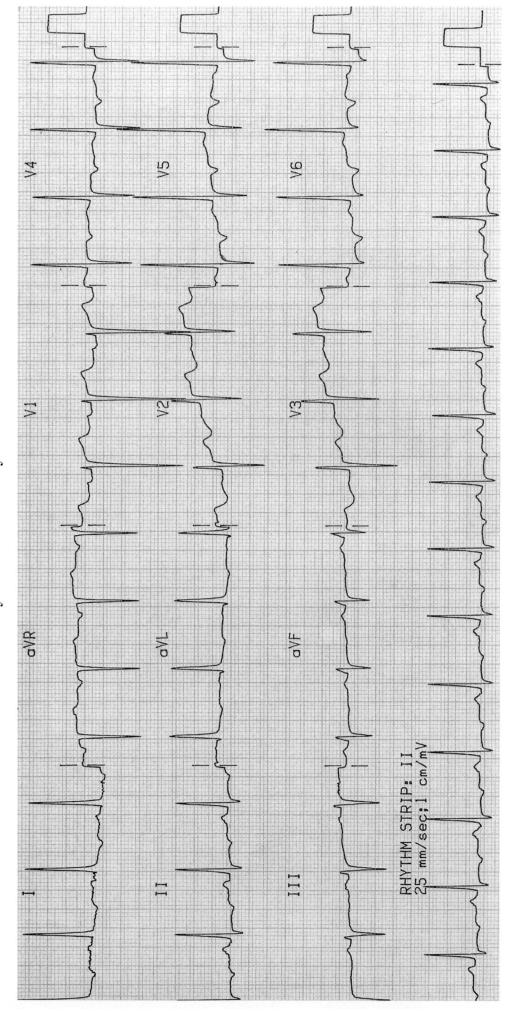

C-39

NARRATIVE INTERPRETATION

Rhythm:	**Sinus**
Rate:	**99**
Intervals:	**PR 0.16, QRS 0.11, QT 0.30**
Axis:	**−45 degrees**

Abnormalities

Prolonged QRS with rsR' leads V1–V3 and T-wave inversions leads V1–V3. Axis leftward of −30 degrees. APCs.

Synthesis

Sinus rhythm. APCs. Left-axis deviation. Left anterior fascicular block. Incomplete RBBB with associated ST-T-wave changes.

TEST ANSWERS: 1, 10, 64, 71, 72, 104.

Comment: Despite the conduction abnormalities, this patient had no evidence of clinical cardiac disease. The RBBB is characterized as *incomplete* because the QRS duration does not quite reach 0.12 s. A left anterior fascicular block is also present. RBBB and LAFB occur rarely in young, normal individuals. In one study of 23,700 healthy airmen, this electrocardiographic diagnosis was found in 0.1 percent. In patients with underlying cardiac disease, bifascicular block may indicate an adverse prognosis. It is important to note however, that the excess mortality is not a result of progression to complete AV block.

FURTHER READING

Barrett PA, Peter CT, Swan HJC, et al: The frequency and prognostic significance of electrocardiographic abnormalities in clinically normal individuals. *Prog Cardiovasc Dis* 23:299–319, 1981.

Liao Y, Emidy LA, Dyer A, et al: Characteristics and prognosis of incomplete right bundle branch block: An epidemiologic study. *J Am Coll Cardiol* 7:492–499, 1986.

McAnulty JH, Rahimtoola SH, Murphy E, et al: Natural history of "high risk" bundle branch block. *N Engl J Med* 307:137–143, 1982.

C-39

Clinical History

A 41-year-old asymptomatic man seen preoperatively for minor surgery.

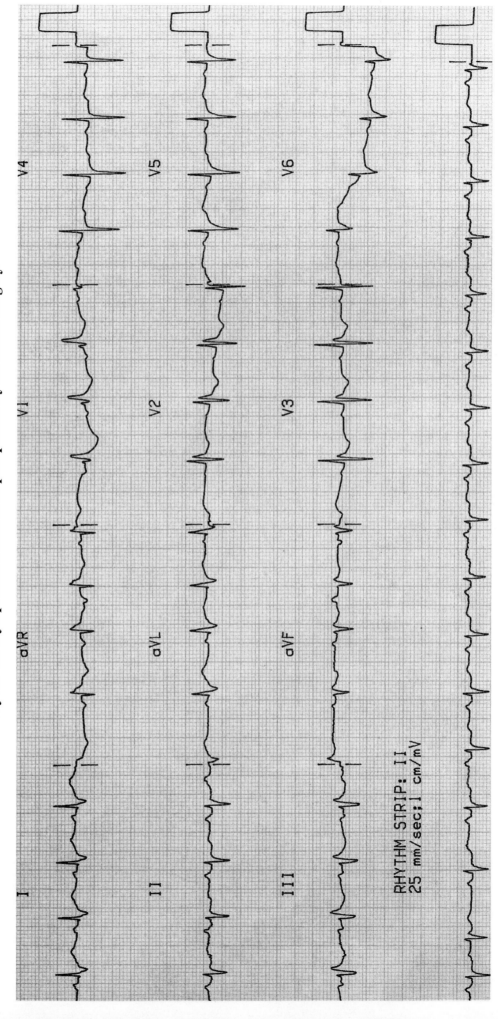

C-40

NARRATIVE INTERPRETATION

Rhythm:	**Ectopic atrial rhythm**
Rate:	**58**
Intervals:	**PR 0.14, QRS 0.08, QT 0.42**
Axis:	**+60 degrees**

Abnormalities
Retrograde P waves with slow heart rate.

Synthesis
Ectopic atrial rhythm. Otherwise within normal limits.

TEST ANSWER: 9.

Comment: Inverted P waves are easily seen in leads II, III, and aVF, a finding that excludes a sinus mechanism. The inverted P wave and normal PR interval suggests an ectopic atrial focus. One cannot exclude however, an AV junctional rhythm with antegrade AV conduction delay. Older textbooks of electrocardiography have referred to the rhythm displayed in the present example as *coronary sinus rhythm*, a term no longer in use.

C-40

Clinical History

A 45-year-old asymptomatic woman in the recovery room after minor surgery.

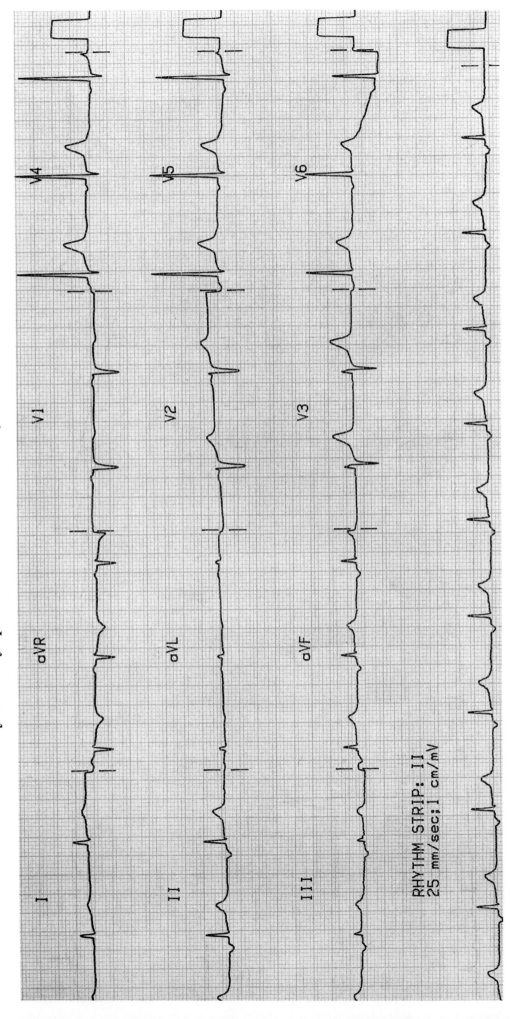

TEST D

D-1

NARRATIVE INTERPRETATION

Rhythm:	**Sinus**
Rate:	**80**
Intervals:	**PR 0.16, QRS 0.12, QT 0.40**
Axis:	**0 degrees**

Abnormalities
Broad, notched QRS complex with ST depression and T-wave inversion leads I, aVL, V4–V6.

Synthesis
Sinus rhythm. Left bundle branch block with associated ST-T wave abnormalities.

TEST ANSWERS: 1, 74, 104.

Comment: Most individuals with LBBB have underlying cardiovascular disease. One study of 25,522 patients who underwent cardiac catheterization found 550 with LBBB. The most common diagnoses in patients with LBBB were coronary heart disease (49 percent), valvular and congenital heart disease (9 percent), cardiomyopathy (8.5 percent), and hypertension (8 percent). In this angiographic study, 12 percent of patients had no demonstrable cardiovascular abnormalities.

FURTHER READING
Jain AC, Mehta MC: Etiologies of left bundle branch block and correlations with hemodynamic and angiographic findings. *Am J Cardiol* 91:1375–1378, 2003.

D-1

Clinical History
An 89-year-old asymptomatic woman.

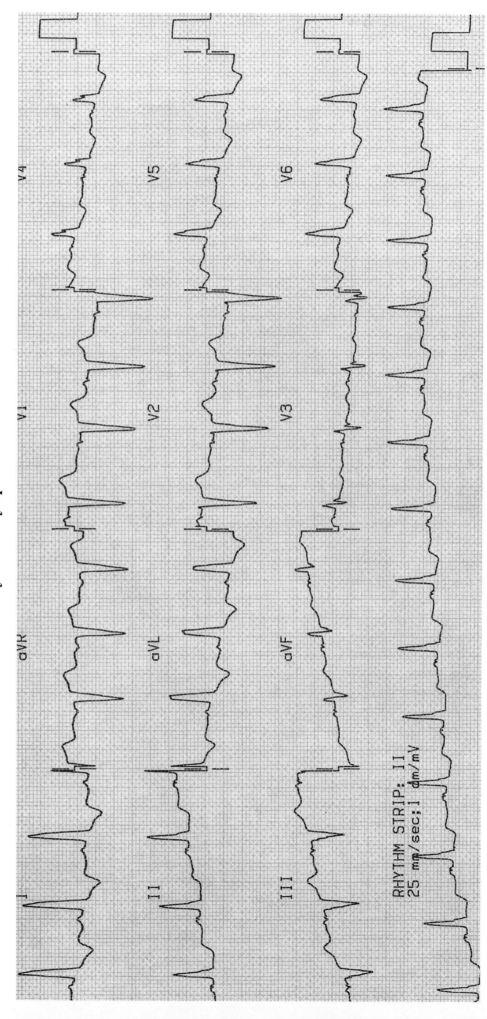

RHYTHM STRIP: II
25 mm/sec; 1 dm/mV

D-2

NARRATIVE INTERPRETATION

Rhythm:	**Sinus bradycardia, AV junctional escape complexes (rhythm)**
Rate:	**Sinus rate 50, AV junctional rate 45**
Intervals:	**PR 0.16, QRS 0.08, QT 0.36**
Axis:	**+60 degrees**

Abnormalities

Heart rate less than 60 bpm. APC followed by second premature complex and sinus pause. AV junctional escape complexes (rhythm). ST depression leads V4–V5. T-wave inversion leads II, III, aVF, V4–V6.

Synthesis

Sinus bradycardia. APC with probable reciprocal (echo) complex. Sinus pause with AV junctional escape complexes (rhythm). Period of isorhythmic AV dissociation on rhythm strip. Nonspecific ST-T-wave abnormalities.

TEST ANSWERS: 3, 7, 10, (22), 24, 53, 54, 106.

Comment: When first looking at the rhythm strip, one could easily mistake this rhythm as a wandering atrial pacemaker to the AV junction. This is probably not the case. The more likely mechanism is explained by an intrinsic rhythm of sinus bradycardia at a rate of 50 and junctional escape complexes. Note the atrial premature in the fifth complex of the tracing, followed by a reciprocal, "echo" beat. The sinus node is depolarized in a retrograde fashion and is temporarily suppressed. A subsidiary pacemaker in the AV junction then takes over until the sinus pacemaker recovers and regains control. A period of isorhythmic AV dissociation is evident on the rhythm strip where the P waves and QRS complexes occur in close proximity, but are unrelated.

258

D-2

Clinical History
A 68-year-old asymptomatic man.

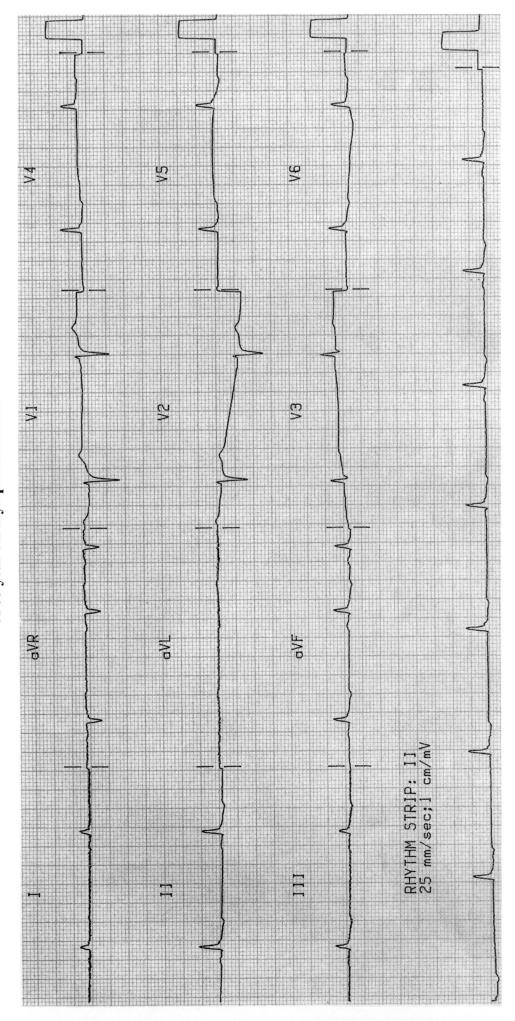

259

D-3

NARRATIVE INTERPRETATION

> **Rhythm:** **Atrial fibrillation**
> **Rate:** **100 (average)**
> **Intervals:** **PR –, QRS 0.10, QT 0.30**
> **Axis:** **+105 degrees**

Abnormalities

Axis rightward of +90 degrees. qR pattern V1. R-wave voltage less than 3 mm leads V1–V3. T-wave inversion leads II, III, aVF.

Synthesis

Atrial fibrillation with a moderate ventricular response. Right-axis deviation. RVH. Nonspecific ST-wave abnormalities. Poor R-wave progression.

TEST ANSWERS: 20, 50, 65, 66, 79, 106.

Comment: This patient had a history of an atrial septal defect, pulmonary hypertension, and right ventricular enlargement. The right-axis deviation is characteristic of an ostium secundum type of atrial septal defect and is usually accompanied by an rSR' pattern in lead V1. The qR pattern in lead V1 seen in this example is a very specific sign of RVH. The poor R-wave progression and deep S waves in leads V4–V6 are also likely secondary to RVH.

D-3

Clinical History

A 69-year-old woman with dyspnea and a history of cardiac surgery for congenital heart disease.

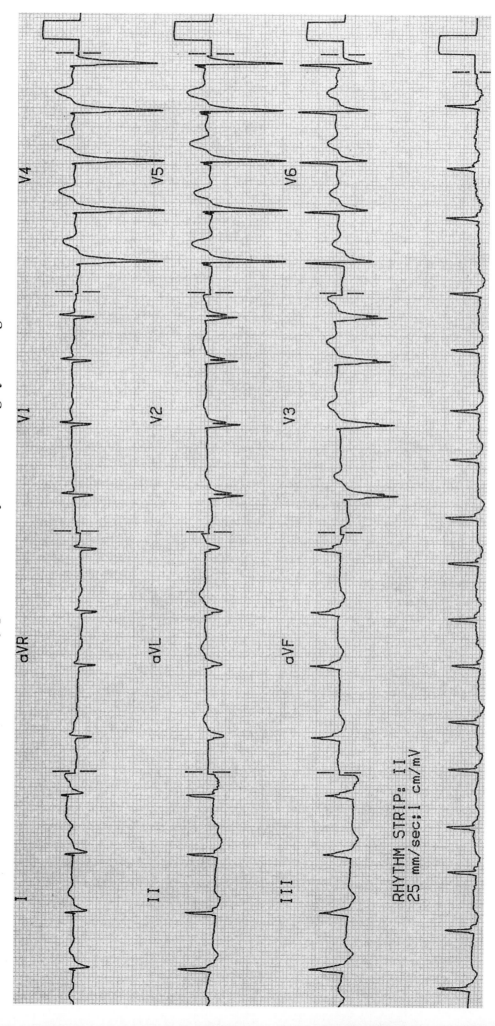

D-4

NARRATIVE INTERPRETATION

> **Rhythm:** **Atrial fibrillation**
> **Rate:** 90 (average)
> **Intervals:** PR −, **QRS 0.08, QT 0.26**
> **Axis:** **+75 degrees**

Abnormalities

ST depression leads I, II, III, aVF, V4–V6. T-wave inversion leads II, III, aVF, V4–V6. S wave lead V2 + R wave lead V5 greater than 35 mm. R wave leads V1–V3 less than 3 mm. VPC. Prominent U waves, in leads V4–V6.

Synthesis

Atrial fibrillation with a controlled ventricular response. VPC. LVH with associated ST-T-wave abnormalities. Poor R-wave progression. Prominent U waves.

TEST ANSWERS: 20, 26, 51, 66, 78, 103, 110.

Comment: This patient had LVH secondary to chronic mitral regurgitation. A number of findings associated with LVH are seen, including increased voltage in the precordial leads, generalized ST-T-wave abnormalities and poor R-wave progression. The prominent U waves are also most likely secondary to LVH.

Some of the ST depression seen in this example is likely due to treatment with digoxin. Note also the relatively short QT interval, another digoxin effect.

The configuration of the wide complex beat in this example suggests that it is of ventricular origin. A monophasic QRS complex in lead V1 is unlikely to be supraventricular with aberrancy.

FURTHER READING

Wellens HJJ, Barr FWHM, Lie KI: The value of the electrocardiogram in the differential diagnosis of a tachycardia with a widened QRS complex. *Am J Med* 84:27–33, 1978.

D-4

Clinical History

A 67-year-old woman following mitral valve replacement. The patient is prescribed digoxin.

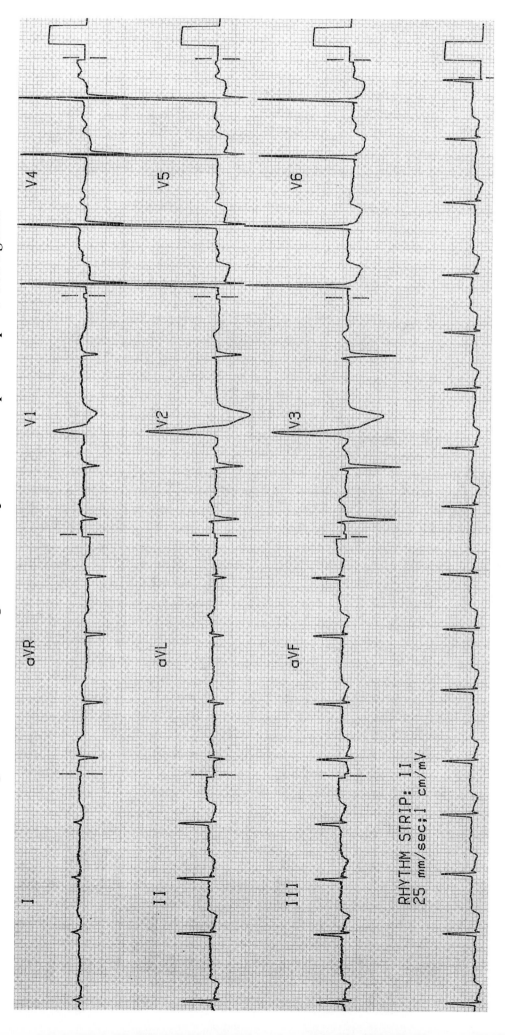

D-5

NARRATIVE INTERPRETATION

Rhythm:	**Sinus bradycardia**
Rate:	**45**
Intervals:	**PR 0.18, QRS 0.08, QT 0.44**
Axis:	**+15 degrees**

Abnormalities

Heart rate less than 60 bpm. Q wave leads I, aVL, V4–V5. "Micro" R waves leads V1–V3. ST "coved" with slight elevation leads I, aVL, V1–V5. T-wave inversion leads I, II, aVL, V3–V6. R wave lead aVL + S wave lead V3 greater than 28 mm in a man.

Synthesis

Sinus bradycardia. Extensive anterior and lateral wall MI with ST-T-wave changes suggestive of recent myocardial injury. Increased voltage for LVH.

TEST ANSWERS: 3, (66), 78, (85), 87, 89, 100, (101).

Comment: This patient sustained an extensive anterior and lateral wall MI 36 hours prior to this tracing. Q waves appear in the lateral limb leads, as well as in leads V4 and V5. A micro R wave remains in the anterior precordial leads. The small Q wave in lead V6 cannot be truly categorized as pathologic despite the clinical picture and is therefore not mentioned as an abnormality.

264

D-5

Clinical History

A 46-year-old man in the coronary care unit (CCU).

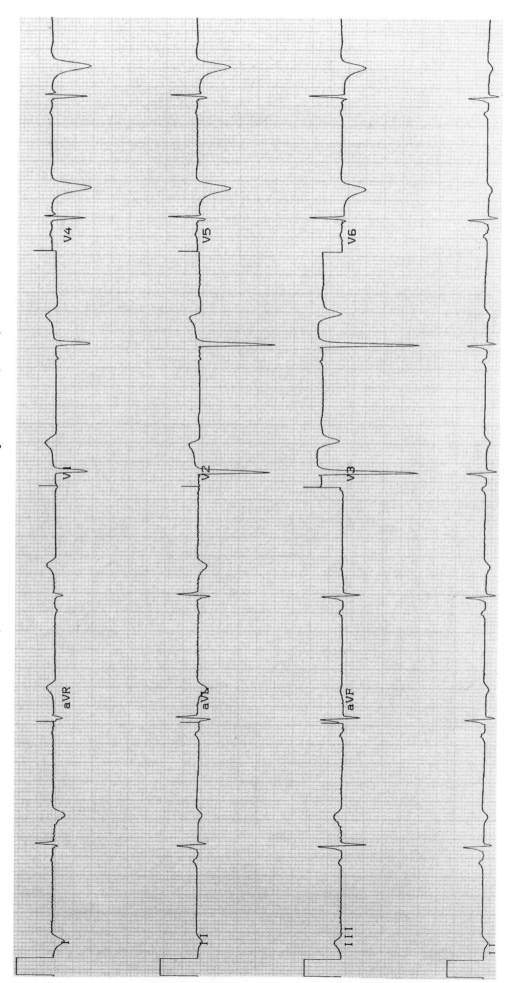

D-6

NARRATIVE INTERPRETATION

Rhythm:	**Sinus with first-degree AV block**
Rate:	**84**
Intervals:	**PR 0.24, QRS 0.13, QT 0.34**
Axis:	**−45 degrees**

Abnormalities
Prolonged PR interval. APCs. Blocked APC. Axis leftward of −30 degrees. Broad, slurred R wave leads I, aVL, V6 with ST depression and T-wave inversion.

Synthesis
Sinus rhythm. First-degree AV block. APCs. Blocked APC on rhythm strip. LBBB with associated ST-T-wave abnormalities. Left-axis deviation.

TEST ANSWERS: 1, 10, 12, 42, 64, 74, 104.

Comment: At first glance, the rhythm strip might appear to demonstrate a Wenckebach sequence with a pause followed by a short PR interval. On closer inspection however, the pause is not preceded by progressive prolongation of the PR intervals or shortening of the RR intervals. The cause of the pause is revealed by carefully reviewing the pattern of atrial ectopy. Note that the T wave prior to the pause is slightly more prominent than other complexes and results from a nonconducted APC. The sinus mechanism resets shortly thereafter. The relatively short PR interval of the next beat is likely due to transient improvement of AV conduction following the pause.

Left-axis deviation and LBBB are noted. LBBB may occur with a normal, left, or right frontal plane axis.

FURTHER READING
Howard RL, Dunn M: Left-axis deviation with left bundle branch block. *Am J Noninvas Cardiol* 1:98–101, 1987.

D-6

Clinical History

An 80-year-old man with a history of aortic valve replacement. He is treated with digoxin.

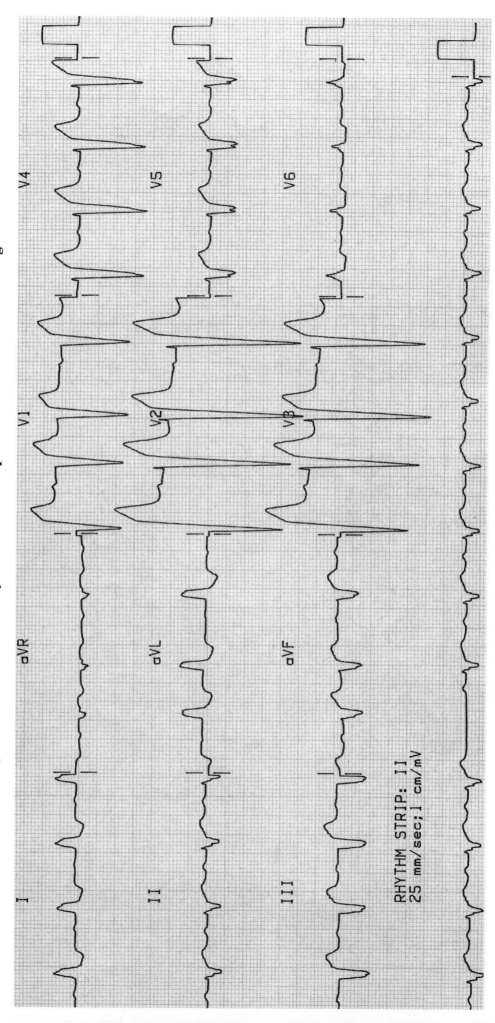

267

D-7

NARRATIVE INTERPRETATION

Rhythm:	**Atrial flutter with 2:1 AV conduction**
Rate:	**Atrial rate 144, ventricular rate 72**
Intervals:	**PR −, QRS 0.12, QT 0.28**
Axis:	**−45 degrees**

Abnormalities

Axis leftward of –30 degrees. QRS prolongation. R wave aVL + S wave V3 greater than 28 mm in a man. R wave aVL greater than 11 mm. ST depression leads I, aVL, V6. Probable T-wave inversion leads I, aVL, V6. VPC.

Synthesis

Atrial flutter with 2:1 AV conduction. VPC. Left-axis deviation. LAFB. LVH. Intraventricular conduction delay. ST-T-wave abnormalities associated with either ventricular conduction abnormality, hypertrophy, or both.

TEST ANSWERS: 19, 26, 50, 64, 72, 76, 78, 103, 104, (106).

Comment: At first examination, it might be difficult for the reader to differentiate atrial flutter from supraventricular tachycardia. The inverted P waves in leads II, III, and aVF could easily be mistaken for T waves related to the preceding QRS complex. However, a ventricular rate approximating 150 bpm should always make one suspect atrial flutter with 2:1 AV conduction. In clinical practice, it is often impossible to differentiate these two entities without "uncovering" the underlying flutter waves. Methods to accomplish this include performing carotid sinus pressure or using medications that inhibit conduction at the AV node (see next tracing).

Left-axis deviation is present in this example due to a combination of LAFB and LVH. The QRS duration is greater than usually expected for uncomplicated LAFB because of the contribution of ventricular hypertrophy. Remember that LVH alone is unlikely to produce left-axis deviation to the degree seen here. The small Q waves in leads I and aVL support LAFB and are inconsistent with LBBB.

D-7

Clinical History
A 55-year-old man with palpitations.

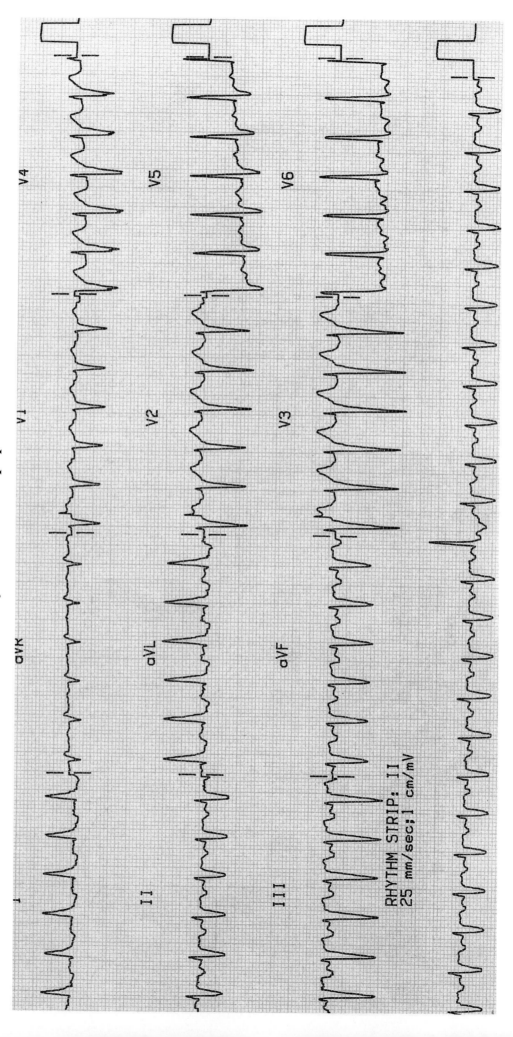

D-8

NARRATIVE INTERPRETATION

Rhythm:	**Atrial flutter with variable AV conduction**
Rate:	**Atrial 144, ventricular 85 (variable)**
Intervals:	**PR –, QRS 0.12, QT 0.30**
Axis:	**–45 degrees**

Abnormalities

Axis leftward of –30 degrees. Prolonged QRS duration. R wave aVL + S wave lead V3 greater than 28 mm in a man. Flat T wave leads I, aVL, V6.

Synthesis

Atrial flutter with variable AV conduction. Left-axis deviation. LAFB. LVH by voltage. Intraventricular conduction delay. ST-T-wave abnormalities associated with either ventricular conduction abnormality, hypertrophy, or both.

TEST ANSWERS: 19, 51, 64, 72, 76, 78, 103, 104, (106).

Comment: The patient in the previous example has been given a medication that inhibits AV conduction. The flutter waves are now obvious and the correct diagnosis is made easy. Useful bedside tools to differentiate atrial flutter from supraventricular tachycardia include carotid sinus pressure or the Valsalva maneuver. These may convert SVT to sinus rhythm, but they will only slow the ventricular rate of atrial flutter. Intravenous administration of AV blocking agents such as adenosine, verapamil, diltiazem, or short-acting beta-blockers such as esmolol is also helpful in making a rapid diagnosis. Note in the previous example, the 2:1 conduction ratio was a physiologic response of the AV node. In this tracing, the conduction response is now nonphysiologic after treatment with verapamil.

D-8

Clinical History

A 55-year-old man with palpitations administered 5 mg of verapamil HCl intravenously in the emergency department.

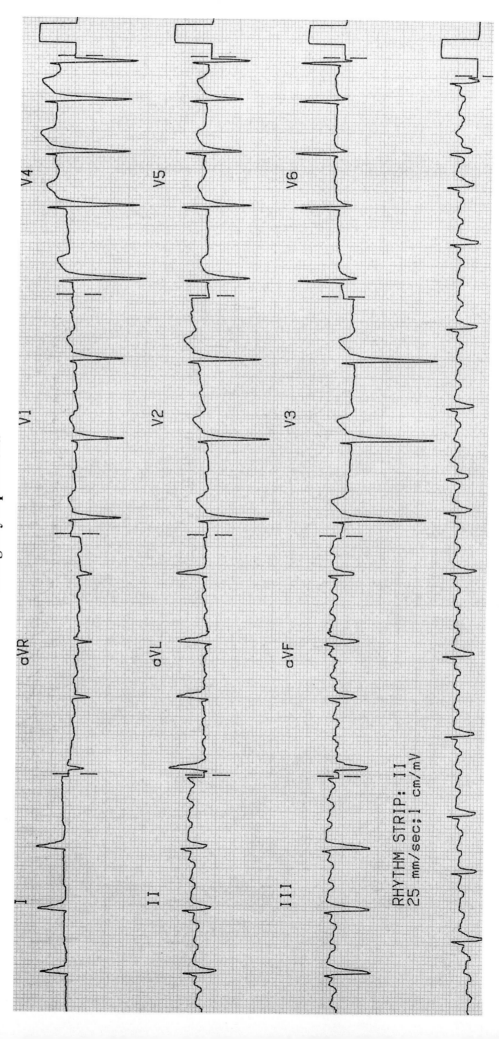

D-9

NARRATIVE INTERPRETATION

Rhythm:	**Accelerated AV junctional rhythm**
Rate:	65
Intervals:	**PR −, QRS 0.08, QT 0.36**
Axis:	**+15 degrees**

Abnormalities
P waves not evident. ST depression leads I, II, aVL, aVF, V2–V6. VPC.

Synthesis
Accelerated AV junctional rhythm. VPC. Diffuse nonspecific ST abnormalities.

TEST ANSWERS: 23, 26, 106.

Comment: This tracing demonstrates a characteristic rhythm of digitalis toxicity. Digitalis excess may manifest as depression of spontaneous pacemakers, inhibition of conduction, or with ectopic rhythms. Nonparoxysmal junctional tachycardia, otherwise known as *accelerated AV junctional rhythm*, is diagnosed here on the basis of absent P waves and a relatively fast rate for an AV junctional rhythm.

Another digitalis effect is diffuse ST depression, seen throughout this tracing. Ventricular ectopy is also present and it is important to remember that this is the most common cardiac arrhythmia associated with digitalis toxicity.

FURTHER READING
Fisch C, Knoebel SB: Digitalis cardiotoxicity. *J Am Coll Cardiol* 5:91A–98A, 1985.
Smith TW, Antman EM, Friedman PL, et al: Digitalis glycosides: Mechanisms and manifestations of toxicity. *Prog Cardiovasc Dis* 27:21–56, 1984.

Clinical History

A 75-year-old woman with a history of heart failure. She is prescribed digoxin.

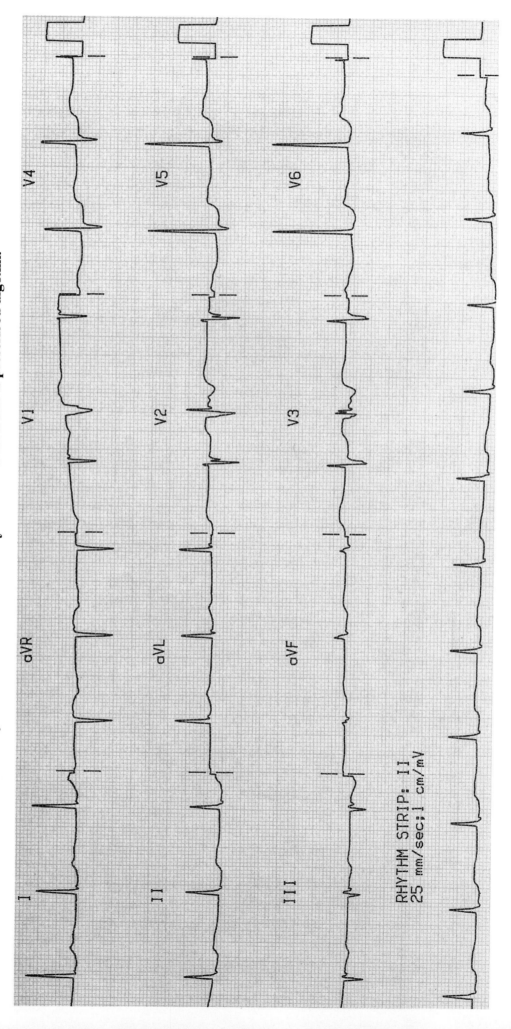

D-10

NARRATIVE INTERPRETATION

Rhythm:	**Sinus tachycardia**
Rate:	**102**
Intervals:	**PR 0.14, QRS 0.08, QT 0.40**
Axis:	**−15 degrees**

Abnormalities
Heart rate greater than 100 bpm. ST depression leads I, II, aVF, V5–V6. T-wave inversion leads I, II, III, aVF, V2–V6. QT prolonged for heart rate. APCs.

Synthesis
Sinus tachycardia. APCs. Diffuse, nonspecific ST-T-wave abnormalities. QTc prolongation.

TEST ANSWERS: 4, 10, (11), (102), 106, 109.

Comment: Electrocardiographic abnormalities frequently occur in patients with cerebrovascular accidents. These include disorders of conduction and repolarization as well as a variety of cardiac arrhythmias. Two studies of a total of 250 patients with acute stroke found QT prolongation in 33 percent, ST-T-wave abnormalities in 45 percent, and abnormal U waves in 18 percent. Supraventricular ectopy, seen in the present tracing, is reported in 5 to 13 percent of patients with acute stroke. The ST-T-wave abnormalities in patients with central nervous system events often cannot be distinguished from those seen in myocardial ischemia. Moreover, coronary and cerebral ischemic events may occur simultaneously.

FURTHER READING
Fass AE, Zimmerman FH: Electrocardiographic abnormalities associated with cerebrovascular accidents. In: Weintraub MI, Fass AE (eds), *Heart and Brain: Interactions of Cardiac and Neurologic Disease.* Santa Ana, CA, PMA Publishing, 1991, pp. 163–170.

D-10

Clinical History

A 59-year-old woman admitted to the ICU after a cerebral vascular accident.

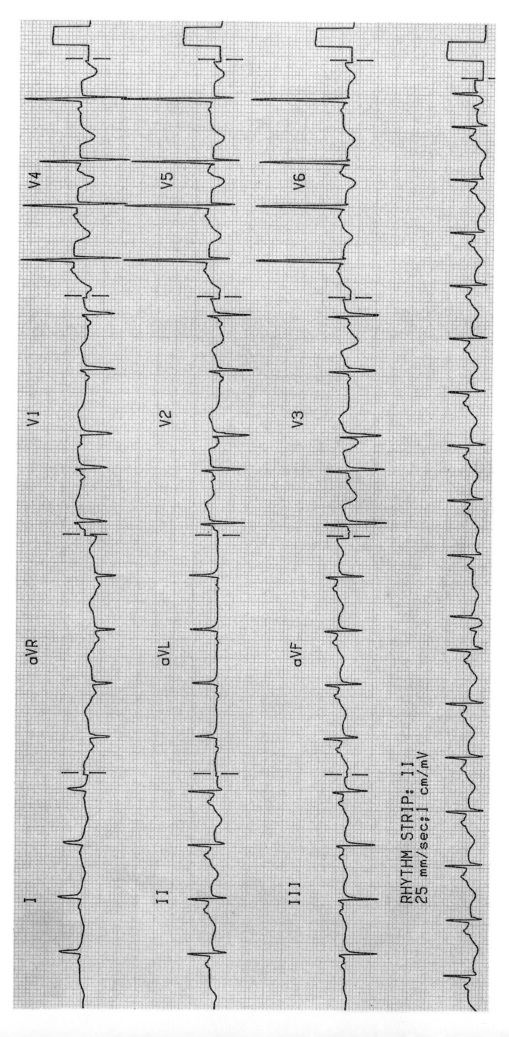

D-11

NARRATIVE INTERPRETATION

> **Rhythm:** Sinus
> **Rate:** 79
> **Intervals:** PR 0.14, QRS 0.14, QT 0.40
> **Axis:** −60 degrees

Abnormalities

Axis leftward of −30 degrees. Broad, notched QRS with RsR′ and T-wave inversion leads V1–V2. Q wave leads II, III, aVF. R wave lead V5 greater than 35 mm.

Synthesis

Sinus rhythm. RBBB with associated ST-T-wave changes. Left-axis deviation. Left anterior fascicular block. Inferior wall MI of indeterminate duration. Probable LVH.

TEST ANSWERS: 1, 64, 70, 72, 78, 92, 104.

Comment: Remember that in RBBB, the initial forces (0.06 s) are unaffected by the conduction abnormality, and standard diagnostic criteria for Q wave MI still apply. The Q waves in the inferior leads are diagnostic of this patient's prior inferior wall MI. The tall, broad, initial R wave in lead V1 might also suggest a coexisting posterior wall MI. However, this diagnosis is very difficult in the presence of RBBB, particularly with coexisting left anterior fascicular block.

LAFB may be diagnosed by analyzing the first 0.06 s of the QRS complex. LVH is also indicated by unusually tall R waves in the left precordial leads.

276

D-11

Clinical History

A 72-year-old man seen in routine follow-up. He has a history of hypertension and coronary heart disease.

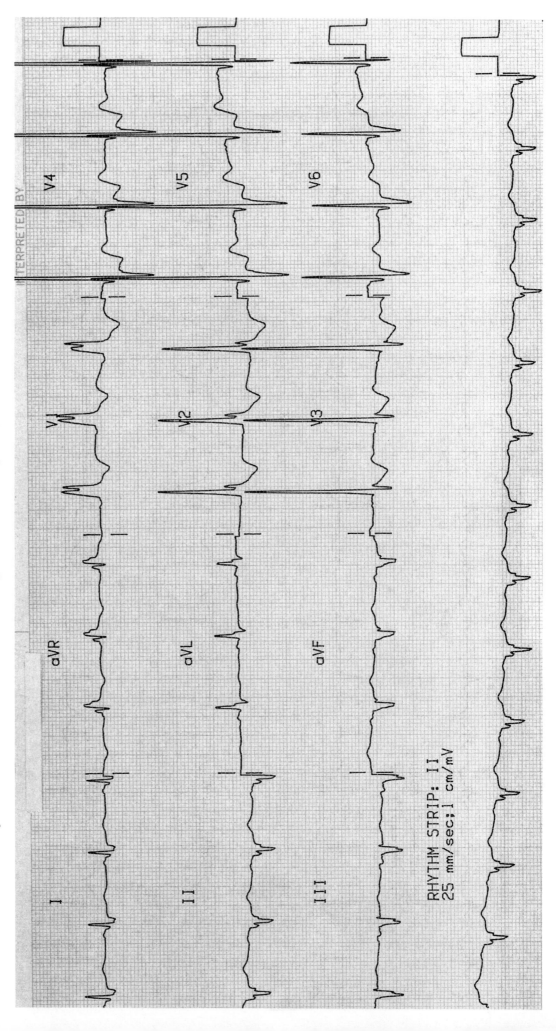

D-12

NARRATIVE INTERPRETATION

Rhythm: Sinus
Rate: 110
Intervals: PR 0.16, QRS 0.12, QT 0.36
Axis: −15 degrees

Abnormalities
Heart rate greater than 100 bpm. Broad QRS with slurred R waves, ST depression and T-wave inversion leads I, aVL, V6. (Prominent ST-segment elevation leads V1–V4.)

Synthesis
Sinus tachycardia. LBBB with associated ST-T-wave changes. (Possible superimposed abnormalities suspicious for myocardial injury. Clinical correlation required.)

TEST ANSWERS: 4, 74, (100), 104.

Comment: The electrocardiographic diagnosis of acute MI is often impossible in patients with LBBB. The ST elevation seen primarily in the right precordial leads in this example is not diagnostic of myocardial injury and may be found in uncomplicated LBBB. Some authors report that ST elevation greater than 7 mm in a direction opposite the main QRS complex is suggestive of acute infarction. In this example, the ST elevation seen in leads V1–V5 is somewhat suspicious for myocardial injury and warrants some comment. In reality, it was due to the conduction abnormality alone. In the absence of serial tracings, clinical correlation, or other supporting evidence, this diagnosis cannot be definitive.

FURTHER READING
Hands ME, Cook EF, Stone PH, et al: Electrocardiographic diagnosis of myocardial infarction in the presence of complete left bundle branch block. *Am Heart J* 116:23–31, 1988.
Sgarbossa EB, Pinski SL, Barbagelta A, et al: Electrocardiographic diagnosis of evolving acute myocardial infarction in the presence of left bundle branch block. *N Engl J Med* 334:481–487, 1996.
Wackers FJT: The diagnosis of myocardial infarction in the presence of left bundle branch block. *Cardiol Clin* 5:393–401, 1987.

D-12

Clinical History

An 82-year-old woman presenting in pulmonary edema.

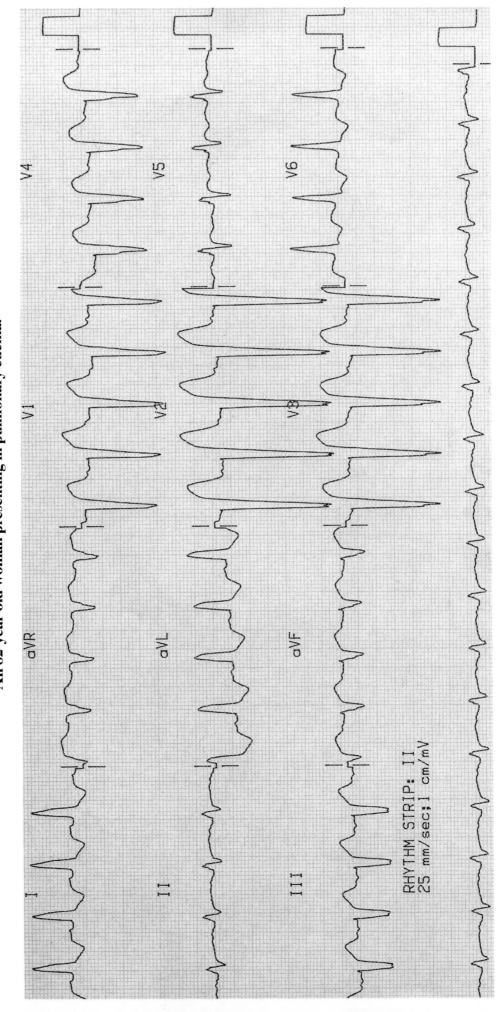

RHYTHM STRIP: II
25 mm/sec; 1 cm/mV

D-13

NARRATIVE INTERPRETATION

Rhythm:	**Sinus**
Rate:	**70**
Intervals:	**PR 0.16, QRS 0.08, QT 0.34**
Axis:	**−15 degrees**

Abnormalities

S wave lead V2 + R wave lead V5 greater than 35 mm. R wave lead aVL greater than 11 mm. R wave lead I + S wave lead III greater than 25 mm. R wave lead aVL + S wave lead V3 greater than 20 mm in a woman. ST depression leads I, aVL, V4–V6. T-wave inversion leads I, II, aVL, V4–V6.

Synthesis

Sinus rhythm. LVH with associated ST-T-wave abnormalities.

TEST ANSWERS: 1, 78, 103.

Comment: Multiple limb lead criteria for LVH are present in this example. If one were not careful however, the concomitant precordial lead criteria for LVH could easily be overlooked. Note the standardization at the far right of the tracing indicating that the precordial leads are recorded at one-half standard.

D-13

Clinical History

An 80-year-old woman admitted for elective hip surgery.

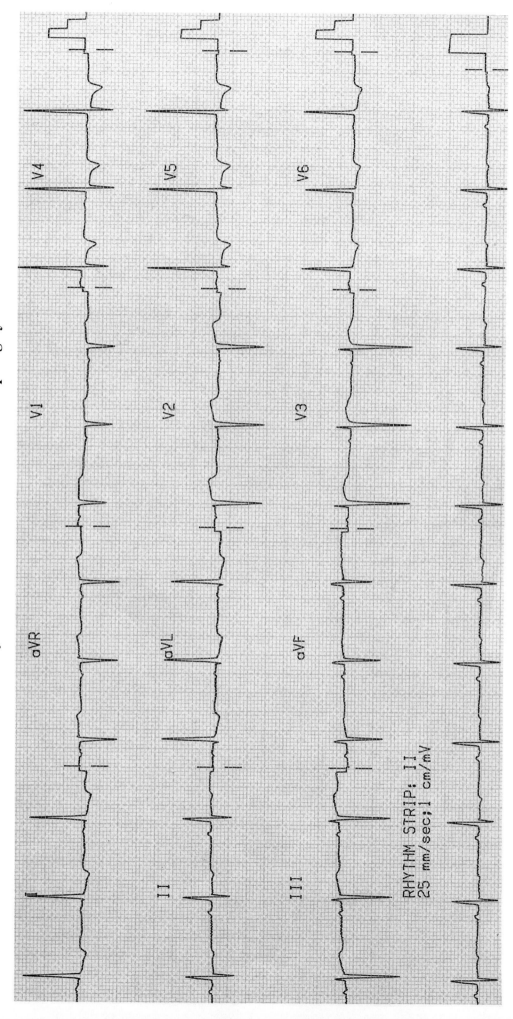

D-14

NARRATIVE INTERPRETATION

Rhythm:	**Sinus**
Rate:	**86**
Intervals:	**PR 0.20, QRS 0.08, QT 0.34**
Axis:	**+120 degrees**

Abnormalities
Axis rightward of +90 degrees. QR lead V1. R wave less than S wave lead V6. Abnormal P terminal force lead V1. T-wave inversion lead III. Biphasic T wave lead II, aVF.

Synthesis
Sinus rhythm. Right-axis deviation. RVH. Left atrial abnormality. Nonspecific ST-T-wave abnormalities.

TEST ANSWERS: 1, 60, 65, 79, 106.

Comment: This tracing demonstrates many diagnostic features of RVH. There is marked right-axis deviation. A qR pattern, seen in lead V1, is a very specific criterion for RVH. The S wave is slightly greater than the R wave in lead V6. Right atrial hypertrophy is suggested in lead II but does not quite meet definitive criteria. Causes of RVH commonly seen in clinical practice include primary pulmonary hypertension, cor pulmonale, mitral stenosis, and right ventricular volume overload from left-to-right intracardiac shunts.

FURTHER READING
Surawicz B: Electrocardiographic diagnosis of chamber enlargement. *J Am Coll Cardiol* 8:711–724, 1986.

D-14

Clinical History
A 42-year-old woman with dyspnea.

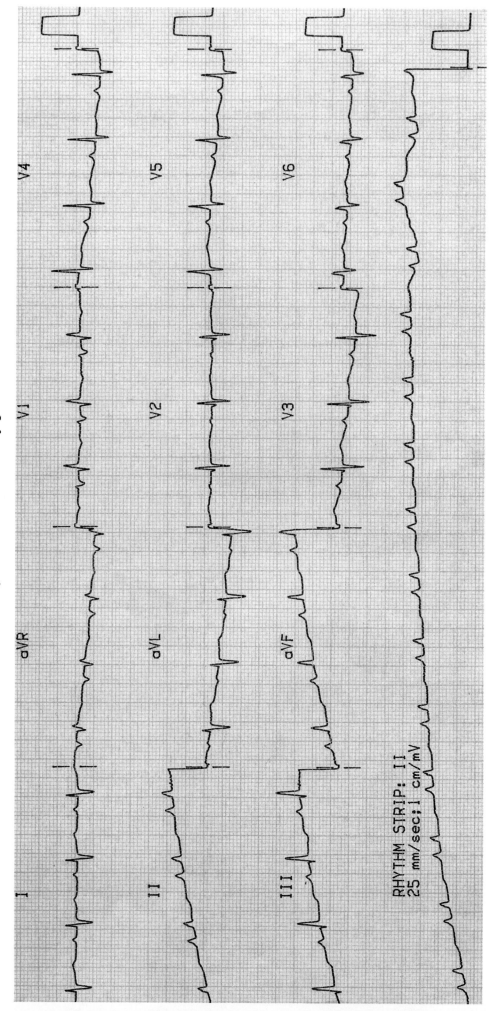

D-15

NARRATIVE INTERPRETATION

Rhythm:	**Supraventricular tachycardia**
Rate:	**155**
Intervals:	**PR –, QRS 0.06, QT 0.28**
Axis:	**+30 degrees**

Abnormalities
Rapid heart rate. ST depression leads II, III, aVF, V3–V6.

Synthesis
Supraventricular tachycardia. Nonspecific ST-segment abnormalities.

TEST ANSWERS: 18, 106.

Comment: This example demonstrates supraventricular tachycardia. The most common mechanism for SVT in adults is AV nodal reentrant tachycardia. The P wave in this form of SVT is either hidden in the QRS complex or is evident slightly thereafter. The reentry circuit is located in the AV node and has two separate pathways with different conduction properties. The reentrant mechanism postulates that a premature stimulus blocks in the pathway with the longer refractory period and conducts in the pathway with the shorter refractory period. The impulse then conducts retrograde via the recovered limb and a new cycle is begun.

The nonspecific ST-segment abnormalities seen during SVT may be seen in individuals with otherwise normal hearts and do not necessarily reflect myocardial ischemia.

FURTHER READING
Bar FW, Brugada P, Dassen WRM, Wellens HJJ: Differential diagnosis of tachycardia with narrow QRS complex (shorter than 0.12 s). *Am J Cardiol* 54:555–560, 1984.

Ganz LI, Friedman PL: Supraventricular tachycardia. *N Engl J Med* 332:162–173, 1995.

Kalbfleisch SJ, El-Atassi R, Calkins H, et al: Differentiation of paroxysmal narrow QRS complex tachycardias using the 12-lead electrocardiogram. *J Am Coll Cardiol* 21:85–89, 1993.

D-15

Clinical History

A 55-year-old woman with sudden onset of lightheadedness.

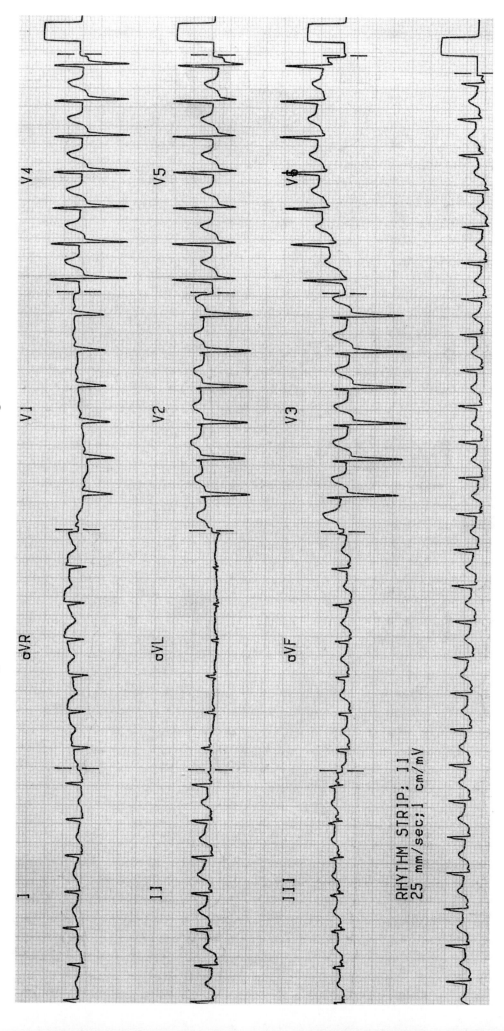

D-16

NARRATIVE INTERPRETATION

Rhythm:	**Atrial fibrillation**
Rate:	**116 (average)**
Intervals:	**PR –, QRS 0.08, QT 0.36**
Axis:	**+60 degrees**

Abnormalities
Rapid, irregular heart rate.

Synthesis
Atrial fibrillation with rapid ventricular response. Otherwise within normal limits.

TEST ANSWERS: 20, 50.

Comment: The relationship between heavy alcohol consumption and the development of atrial fibrillation of new onset has been termed the "holiday heart syndrome." Whereas this relationship has not been corroborated in all studies, there is little doubt that alcohol may play a role in the genesis of atrial arrhythmias in patients without other demonstrable cardiac disease. Note that the fibrillatory waves appear somewhat organized or "coarse," particularly in lead V1. Some authors have noted a correlation between coarse fibrillatory waves and an abnormal P terminal force indicative of left atrial enlargement after resumption of sinus rhythm (see next tracing).

FURTHER READING
Koskinen P, Kupari M, Leinonen H, Luomanmaki K: Alcohol and new onset atrial fibrillation: A case-control study. *Br Heart J* 57:468–473, 1987.

D-16

Clinical History

A 44-year-old man with palpitations after drinking heavily.

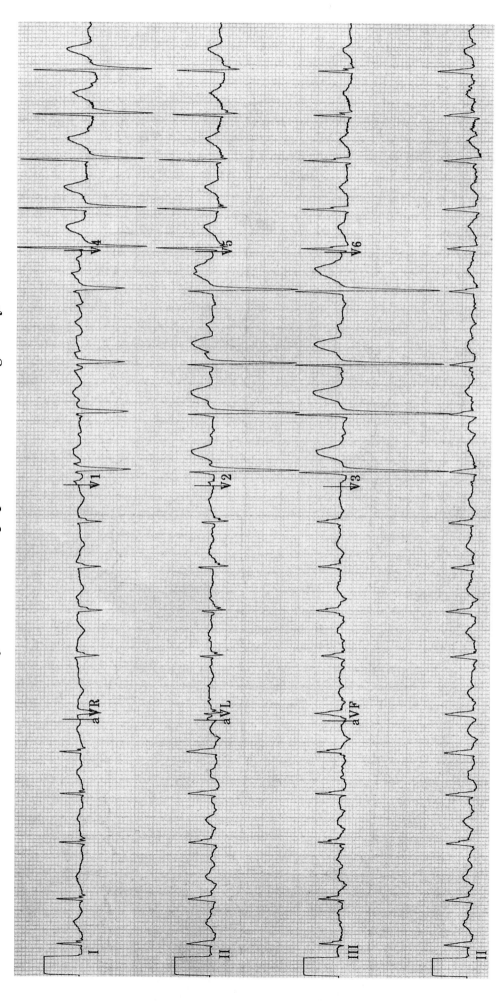

287

D-17

NARRATIVE INTERPRETATION

Rhythm:	**Sinus**
Rate:	**60**
Intervals:	**PR 0.20, QRS 0.08, QT 0.54**
Axis:	**+45 degrees**

Abnormalities
Abnormal P terminal force lead V1. Prolonged QT interval for heart rate.

Synthesis
Sinus rhythm. Left atrial abnormality. Prolonged QTc interval.

TEST ANSWERS: 1, 60, 109.

Comment: The patient described in the previous tracing was converted to sinus rhythm with intravenous digoxin and procainamide. Although the rhythm has normalized, there is now marked prolongation of the QT interval. This may predispose to malignant ventricular arrhythmias, including *torsades de pointes*. This arrhythmia is defined by ventricular tachycardia with cycles of differing polarity, such that it appears to be *turning around the point* of the baseline of the electrocardiogram.

FURTHER READING
Stratmann HG, Kennedy HL: Torsades de pointes associated with drugs and toxins: Recognition and management. *Am Heart J* 113:1470–1482, 1987.

D-17

Clinical History

A 44-year-old man treated with an antiarrhythmic agent for new-onset atrial fibrillation.

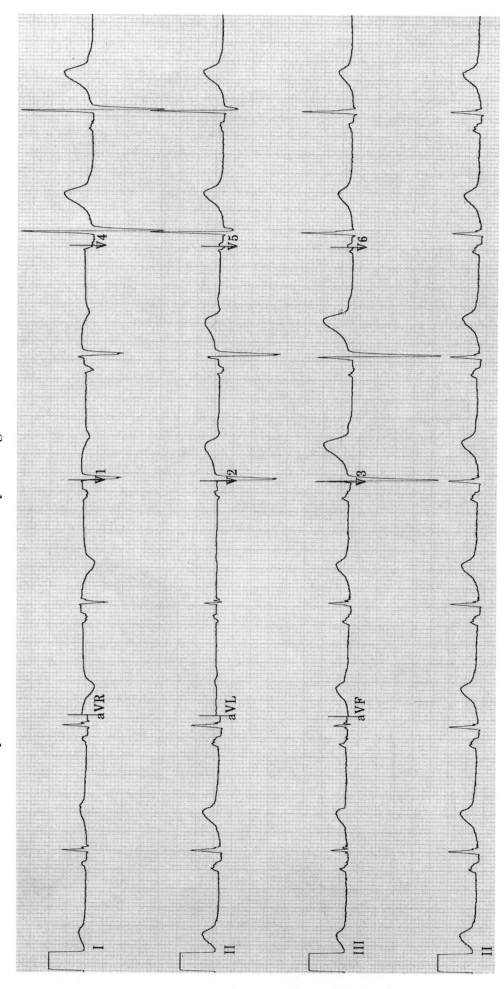

D-18

NARRATIVE INTERPRETATION

Rhythm:	**Sinus with first-degree AV block**
Rate:	**70**
Intervals:	**PR 0.24, QRS 0.08, QT 0.36**
Axis:	**+45 degrees**

Abnormalities
Prolonged PR interval.

Synthesis
Sinus rhythm. First-degree AV block. Otherwise within normal limits.

TEST ANSWERS: 1, 42.

Comment: This patient had clinical evidence of Lyme disease with a characteristic rash of erythema migrans. He also had evidence of Lyme carditis on the basis of new onset, first-degree AV block. Lyme carditis is reported in 4 to 10 percent of cases of acute Lyme disease, with AV block being the most common manifestation of cardiac involvement. Of patients who do develop conduction system disease, up to 98 percent will demonstrate first-degree AV block at some point in their illness. High-grade AV block may also develop and require insertion of a temporary pacemaker. The conduction abnormalities generally resolve over 1 to 2 weeks.

FURTHER READING

Cox J, Krajden M: Cardiovascular manifestations of Lyme disease. *Am Heart J* 122:1449–1455, 1991.
Rubin DA, Sorbera C, Nikitin P, et al: Prospective evaluation of heart block complicating early Lyme disease. *PACE* 15:252–255, 1992.

D-18

Clinical History

A 41-year-old man seen for evaluation of a forearm rash. He has a history of a tick bite 3 weeks earlier.

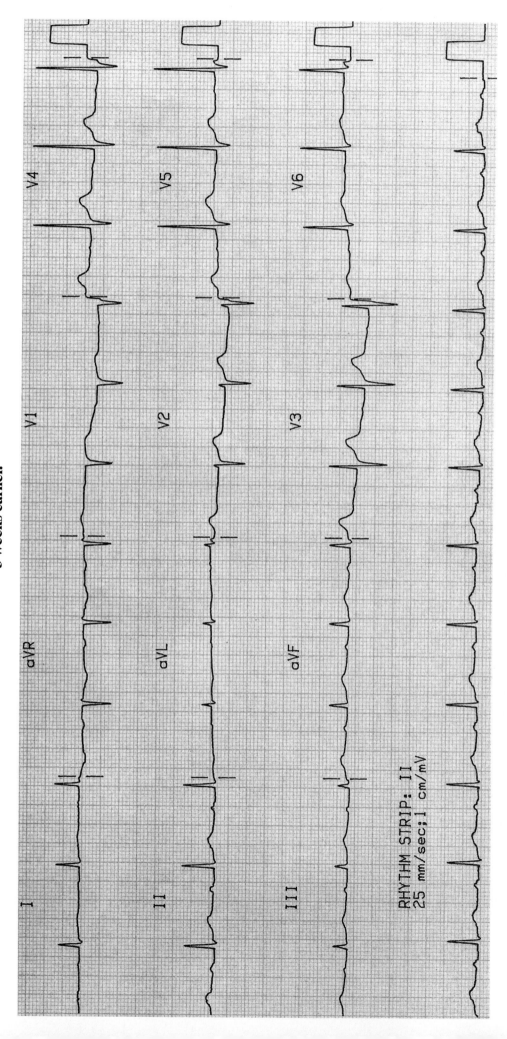

D-19

NARRATIVE INTERPRETATION

Rhythm:	**Sinus**
Rate:	**90**
Intervals:	**PR 0.16, QRS 0.08, QT 0.38**
Axis:	**+15 degrees**

Abnormalities
APCs. Abnormal P terminal force lead V1. ST segment straight with slight downward concavity leads V1–V3. T-wave inversion leads V1–V3.

Synthesis
Sinus rhythm. APCs. ST-T-wave abnormalities suggestive of recent myocardial injury (or ischemia). Left atrial abnormality.

TEST ANSWERS: 1, 10, 60, 100, (102).

Comment: This patient developed a non-Q-wave anterior wall MI. The configuration of the ST segment in leads V1–V3 suggests that these abnormalities reflect myocardial injury. It is difficult to differentiate recent injury from ischemia on the basis of a single electrocardiogram. However, the slight ST elevation and coving suggests that some degree of myocardial injury is likely.

A number of characteristic findings for left atrial enlargement are also seen in this electrocardiogram. Note the abnormal P terminal force in lead V1 as well as the notched P waves and leftward P axis in the limb leads.

FURTHER READING
Hazen MS, Marwick TH, Underwood DA: Diagnostic accuracy of the resting electrocardiogram in detection and estimation of left atrial enlargement: An echocardiographic correlation in 551 patients. *Am Heart J* 122:823–828, 1991.

D-19

Clinical History

A 76-year-old woman admitted to the CCU.

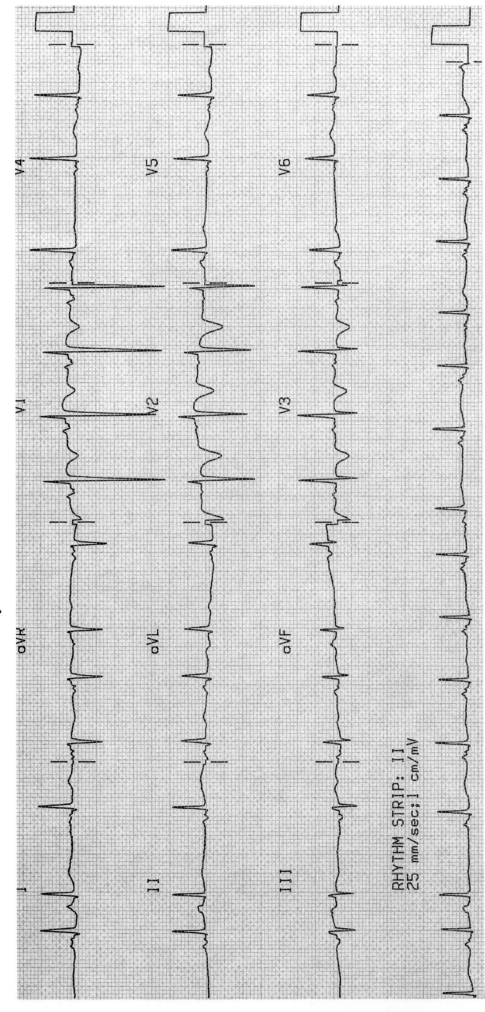

D-20

NARRATIVE INTERPRETATION

Rhythm:	**Sinus**
Rate:	**98**
Intervals:	**PR 0.16, QRS 0.08, QT 0.36**
Axis:	**0 degrees**

Abnormalities
R wave greater than S wave leads V1–V2. Flat T wave leads I, aVL.

Synthesis
Sinus rhythm. Tall R waves right precordial leads, probably within normal limits. Nonspecific T-wave abnormalities.

TEST ANSWERS: 1, 106.

Comment: The tall R waves in V1 and V2 in this example are normal, but require a careful differential diagnosis. The diagnoses to consider include RVH, posterior wall MI, and misplacement of the chest leads. Other conditions that may produce tall R waves in the right precordial leads are RBBB, dextrocardia, and preexcitation patterns.

In this example, the tall, narrow R waves in leads V1 and V2, without other abnormalities of axis or repolarization, are interpreted as a normal variant. This QRS pattern has an estimated prevalence in normal individuals of 1 percent in lead V1 and 10 percent in lead V2.

FURTHER READING

Zema MJ, Kligfield P: Electrocardiographic tall R waves in the right precordial leads: Vectorcardiographic and electrocardiographic distinction of posterior myocardial infarction from prominent anterior forces in normal subjects. *J Electrocardiol* 17:129–138, 1984.
Zema MJ: Electrocardiographic tall R waves in the right precordial leads. *J Electrocardiol* 23:147–156, 1990.

D-20

Clinical History

A 74-year-old asymptomatic woman scheduled for cataract surgery.

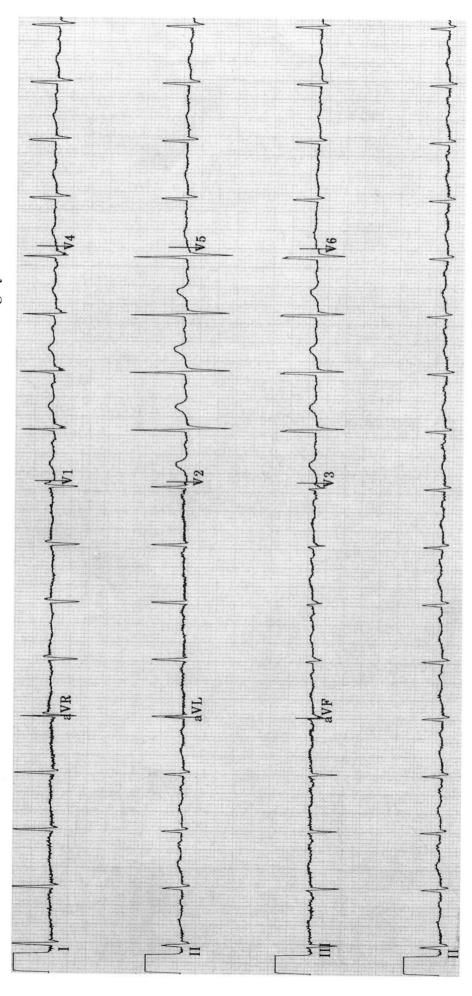

D-21

NARRATIVE INTERPRETATION

Rhythm:	**Sinus arrhythmia, AV junctional rhythm**
Rate:	**Sinus rate 65, AV junctional rate 63**
Intervals:	**PR 0.14, QRS 0.08, QT 0.40**
Axis:	**+15 degrees**

Abnormalities

Sinus rates vary by 0.16 s. AV dissociation. Junctional escape rhythm. Q wave leads II, III, aVF. ST elevation leads II, III, aVF, V5–V6. ST depression leads I, aVL. T-wave inversion leads II, III, aVF, V5–V6. R wave aVL greater than 11 mm. R wave aVL + S wave lead V3 greater than 28 mm in a man.

Synthesis

Sinus arrhythmia with AV junctional escape rhythm. Isorhythmic AV dissociation. Inferior wall MI with ST-T-wave abnormalities of acute myocardial injury. Additional ST abnormalities suggesting either reciprocal change or myocardial ischemia. LVH by voltage.

TEST ANSWERS: 2, 22, 53, 78, 91, 100, 101.

Comment: This patient is experiencing an acute inferior wall MI. Profound vagal influences are commonly seen in this situation which can produce a variety of rhythm disturbances including sinus bradyarrhythmias and varying degrees of AV block. In this example, the sinus rate periodically slows from a sinus arrhythmia, allowing a subsidiary pacemaker in the AV junction to emerge. A brief period of isorhythmic AV dissociation is seen where the sinus and junctional complexes occur nearly simultaneously, but are unrelated to each other. Eventually the sinus mechanism regains control.

D-21

Clinical History

A 44-year-old man with 2 h of chest discomfort and diaphoresis.

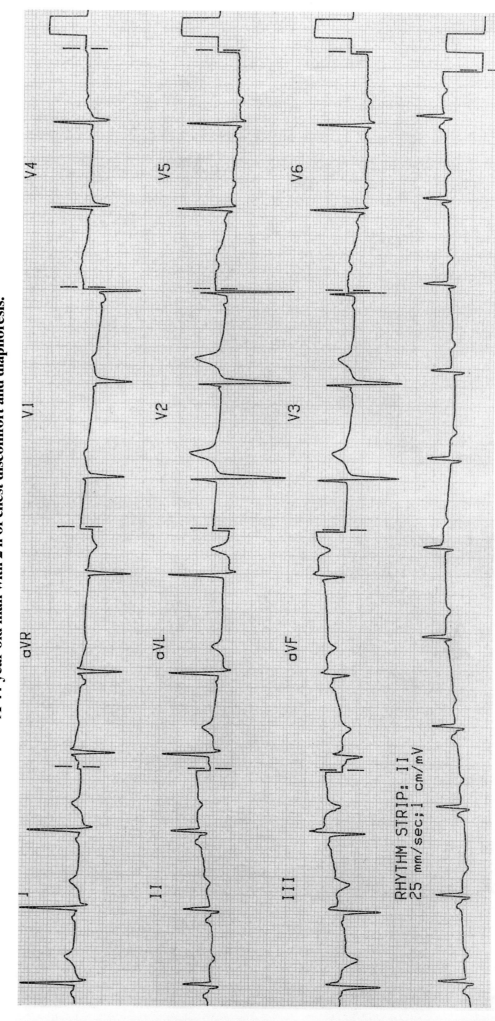

RHYTHM STRIP: II
25 mm/sec;1 cm/mV

D-22

NARRATIVE INTERPRETATION
(Interpret and synthesize abnormalities of right precordial leads only, V2R–V6R).

Abnormalities
Q wave leads V4R, V5R, V6R. ST elevation leads V4R, V5R, V6R.

Synthesis
ST elevation with Q waves in right precordial leads indicative of acute right ventricular MI.

TEST ANSWERS: Not applicable.

Comment: This tracing records the right-sided chest leads from the previous example. Obtaining right precordial leads is extremely useful for any patient with acute inferior wall MI and gives information regarding right ventricular infarction. In a patient with inferior wall MI, ST elevation in the right precordial leads (particularly V4R) of 1 mm or more suggests right ventricular involvement. A QS or QR pattern in V4R is another useful sign of RV infarction.

FURTHER READING

Lopez-Sendon J, Coma-Canella I, Alcasena S, et al: Electrocardiographic findings in acute right ventricular infarction: Sensitivity and specificity of electrocardiographic alterations in right precordial leads, V4R, V3R, V1, V2, and V3. *J Am Coll Cardiol* 6:1273–1279, 1985.

Robalino BD, Whitlow PL, Underwood DA, Salcedo EE: Electrocardiographic manifestations of right ventricular infarction. *Am Heart J* 118:138–144, 1989.

D-22

Clinical History

A 44-year-old man with 2 h of chest discomfort and diaphoresis. Right-sided precordial leads are presented for the patient in the previous ECG.

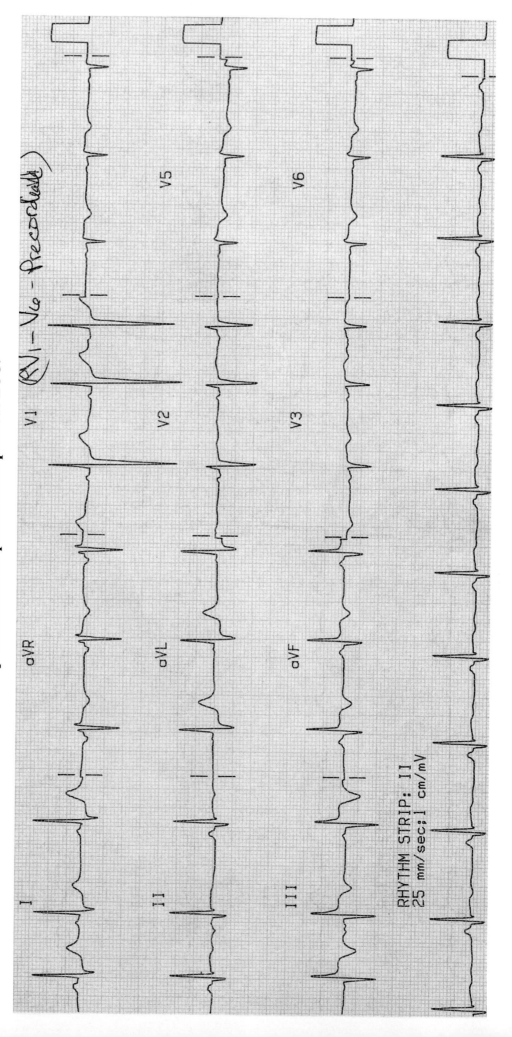

D-23

NARRATIVE INTERPRETATION

Rhythm:	**Atrial flutter with variable AV conduction**
Rate:	**Atrial 240, ventricular 64 (average)**
Intervals:	**PR −, QRS 0.08, QT −**
Axis:	**−15 degrees**

Abnormalities

Synthesis
Atrial flutter with variable AV conduction. Otherwise within normal limits.

TEST ANSWERS: 19, 51.

Comment: The differential diagnosis of this rhythm includes atrial tachycardia and atrial flutter. Atrial tachycardia is characterized by atrial rates of 150 to 250 bpm, upright P waves in leads II, III, and aVF and an isoelectric baseline between the P waves. Classic atrial flutter demonstrates characteristic "sawtooth" flutter waves in leads II, III, and aVF with an atrial rate generally between 250 and 350 bpm.

The correct rhythm diagnosis here is atrial flutter with a slower than expected atrial rate because of treatment with procainamide. AV conduction is suppressed by digoxin therapy. Low T-wave voltage is suggested, but cannot be accurately determined because of the superimposed flutter waves.

D-23

Clinical History

A 62-year-old man with palpitation. He is prescribed procainamide and digoxin.

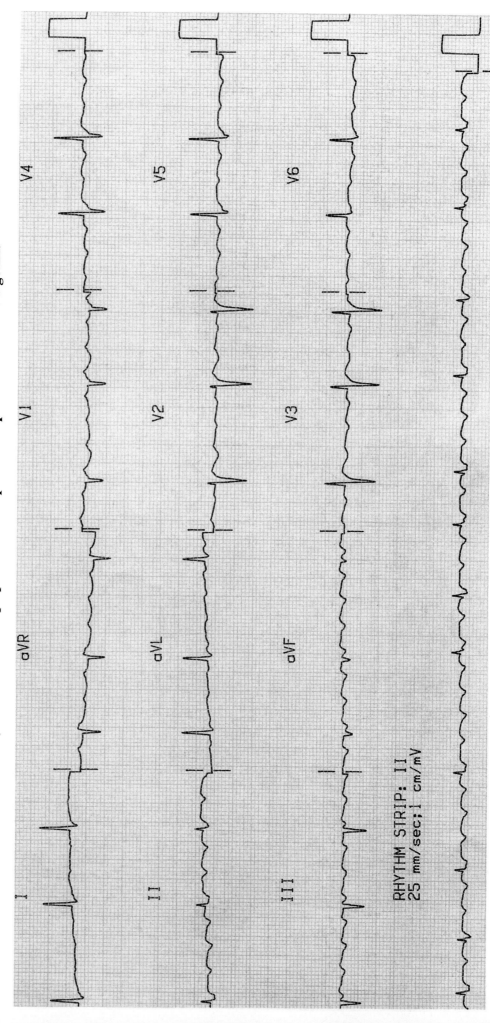

301

D-24

NARRATIVE INTERPRETATION

Rhythm:	**Atrial fibrillation**
Rate:	**63 (average)**
Intervals:	**PR –, QRS 0.12, QT 0.42**
Axis:	**–60 degrees**

Abnormalities
Limb lead voltage less than 5 mm. Precordial lead voltage less than 10 mm. Axis leftward of –30 degrees. QS wave leads II, III, aVF. Broad QRS and rSR' pattern with T-wave inversion lead V1.

Synthesis
Atrial fibrillation with a controlled ventricular response. Low voltage limb and precordial leads. Inferior wall MI of indeterminate age. Left-axis deviation (possible LAFB). RBBB with associated ST-T-wave abnormalities.

TEST ANSWERS: 20, 51, 64, 67, 68, 70, (72), 92, 104.

Comment: Low voltage may be caused by a number of entities including diffuse myocardial disease, pericardial effusion, myxedema, severe obesity, and chronic obstructive coronary disease. This patient had multiple reasons for low voltage including COPD, severe coronary heart disease with multiple prior myocardial infarctions, and a large anterior and posterior pericardial effusion.

He had a prior inferior wall MI, which resulted in QS waves in leads II, III, and aVF. The left-axis deviation is most likely related to the inferior wall MI. The low voltage and conduction abnormality in this example make it difficult to determine whether or not left anterior fascicular block is also present.

D-24

Clinical History

A 67-year-old man seen in preoperative evaluation.

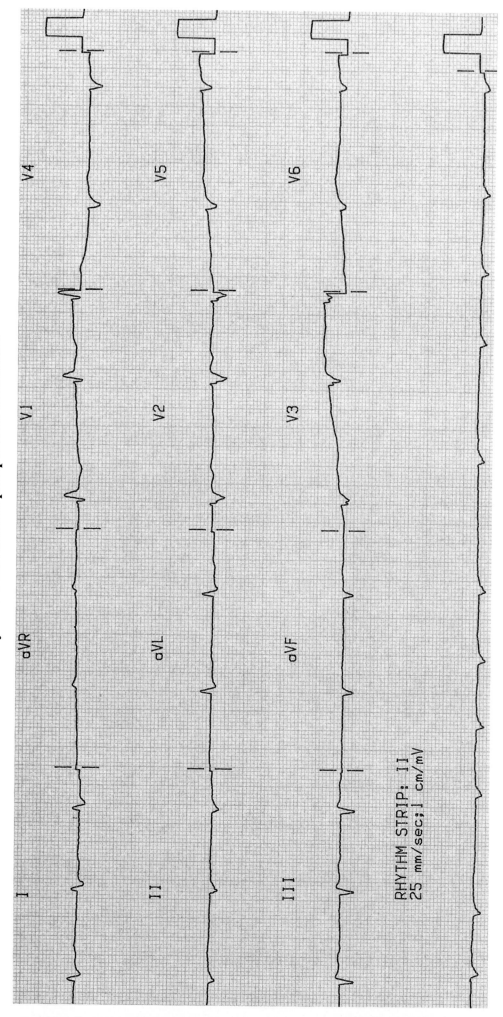

D-25

NARRATIVE INTERPRETATION

Rhythm:	**Sinus with SA exit block**
Rate:	**68**
Intervals:	**PR 0.14, QRS 0.08, QT 0.36**
Axis:	**+60 degrees**

Abnormalities
Gradual shortening of PP interval with abrupt lengthening of PP interval on rhythm strip. ST elevation leads III, aVF, V2–V4. Flat T wave leads II, V6. T-wave inversion leads V1–V4.

Synthesis
Sinus rhythm. Sinoatrial exit block. Nonspecific ST-T-wave abnormalities.

TEST ANSWERS: 1, 8, 106.

Comment: This is an interesting tracing in that normal sinus rhythm is seen only in the last three complexes of the rhythm strip. Prior to these complexes there are two sequences of four complexes that demonstrate shortening of the PP interval followed by a slight pause. The P-wave morphology and PR interval does not change. Therefore, the likely mechanism of this sequence is second-degree SA exit block, type I (SA Wenckebach).

D-25

Clinical History
An 86-year-old woman in the CCU.

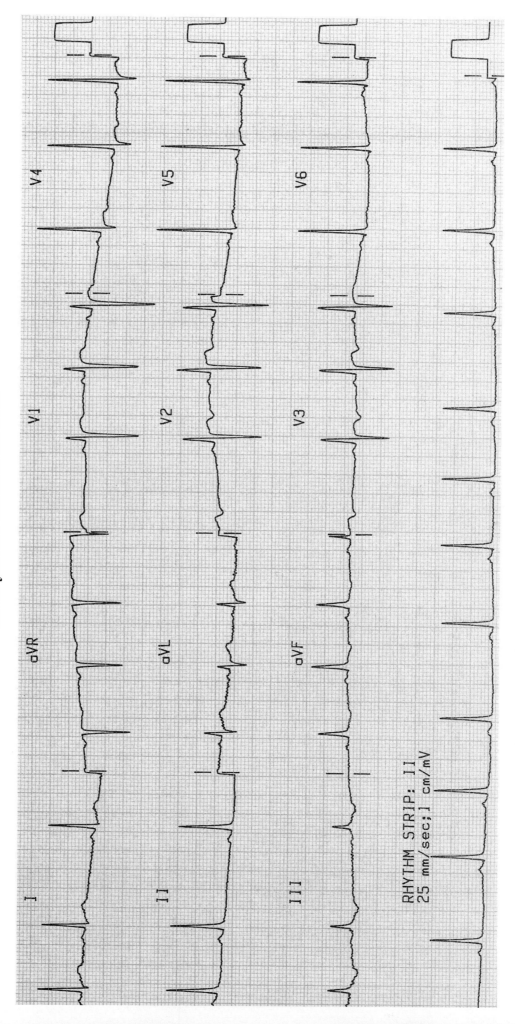

I

aVR

V1

V4

II

aVL

V2

V5

III

aVF

V3

V6

RHYTHM STRIP: II
25 mm/sec; 1 cm/mV

D-26

NARRATIVE INTERPRETATION

Rhythm:	**Sinus**
Rate:	**90**
Intervals:	**PR 0.16, QRS 0.10, QT 0.32**
Axis:	**+15 degrees**

Abnormalities
rSR' pattern with T-wave inversion leads V1–V2.

Synthesis
Sinus rhythm. Incomplete RBBB. Associated ST-T-wave abnormalities.

TEST ANSWERS: 1, 71, 104.

Comment: This tracing demonstrates an rSR' pattern in the right precordial leads. The diagnosis is *incomplete* RBBB because the QRS duration is less than 0.12 s. Incomplete RBBB may be seen in patients with atrial septal defect, but in most cases, this conduction abnormality is not associated with underlying cardiac disease. Although the likelihood of progression to complete RBBB is higher than that of the general population, studies indicate no increase in cardiac mortality in persons with incomplete RBBB.

FURTHER READING
Liao Y, Emidy LA, Dyer A, et al: Characteristics and prognosis of incomplete right bundle branch block: An epidemiologic study. *J Am Coll Cardiol* 7:492–499, 1986.

D-26

Clinical History

A 78-year-old asymptomatic man.

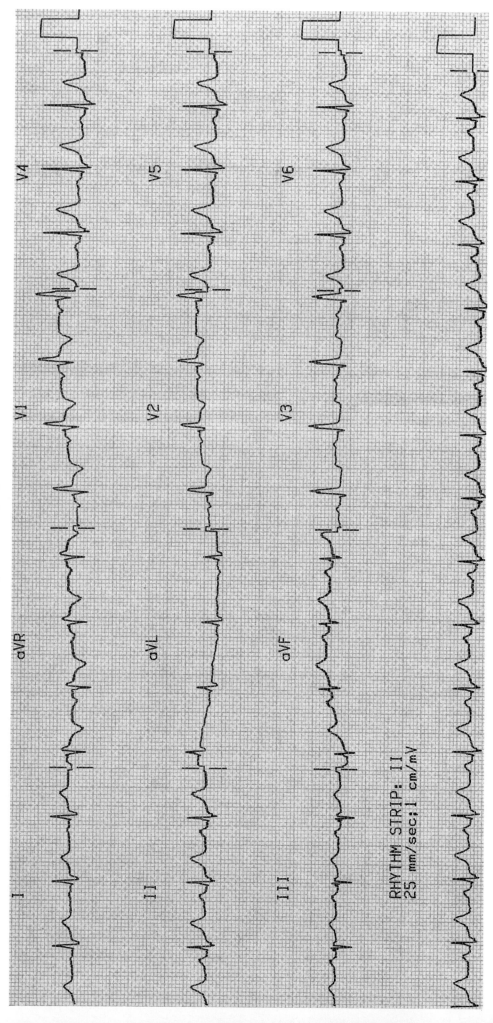

RHYTHM STRIP: II
25 mm/sec;1 cm/mV

D-27

NARRATIVE INTERPRETATION

Rhythm:	**Sinus**
Rate:	**68**
Intervals:	**PR 0.16, QRS 0.08, QT 0.46**
Axis:	**0 degrees**

Abnormalities

VPC. ST depression leads I, II, aVL, V3–V6. T-wave inversion leads II, III, aVF, V3–V6. Abnormal P terminal force lead V1. S wave lead V2 + R wave lead V5 greater than 35 mm. R wave lead aVL greater than 11 mm. R wave lead I + S wave lead III greater than 25 mm. R wave lead aVL + S wave lead V3 greater than 20 mm in a woman. QS lead III, with small Q waves leads II, aVF. Prolonged QTc.

Synthesis

Sinus rhythm. VPC. LVH. Left atrial abnormality. Probable inferior wall MI of indeterminate age. ST-T-wave abnormalities suggestive of myocardial ischemia. ST-T-wave abnormalities leads I, aVL likely asssociated with LVH. Prolongation of QTc interval.

TEST ANSWERS: 1, 26, 60, 78, 92, 102, 103, 109.

Comment: This patient had marked cardiomegaly and extensive coronary heart disease confirmed at cardiac catheterization. A prior inferior wall MI is suspected, although truly diagnostic inferior Q waves are not evident in this example. The small Q waves in leads II and aVF, accompanied by a QS in lead III, as well as the T-wave abnormalities in the inferior leads support this diagnosis. Some of the ST-T-wave findings in this patient were also likely related to LVH.

QT prolongation is also noted, a finding probably related to coronary heart disease.

FURTHER READING

Witham AC: VCG patterns of myocardial scarring in the absence of diagnostic Q waves. In: Schlant RC, Jurst JW (eds), *Advances in Electrocardiography*. New York, Grune & Stratton, 1972, pp. 349–365.

D-27

A 78-year-old woman admitted to the CCU with coronary heart disease and hypertension.

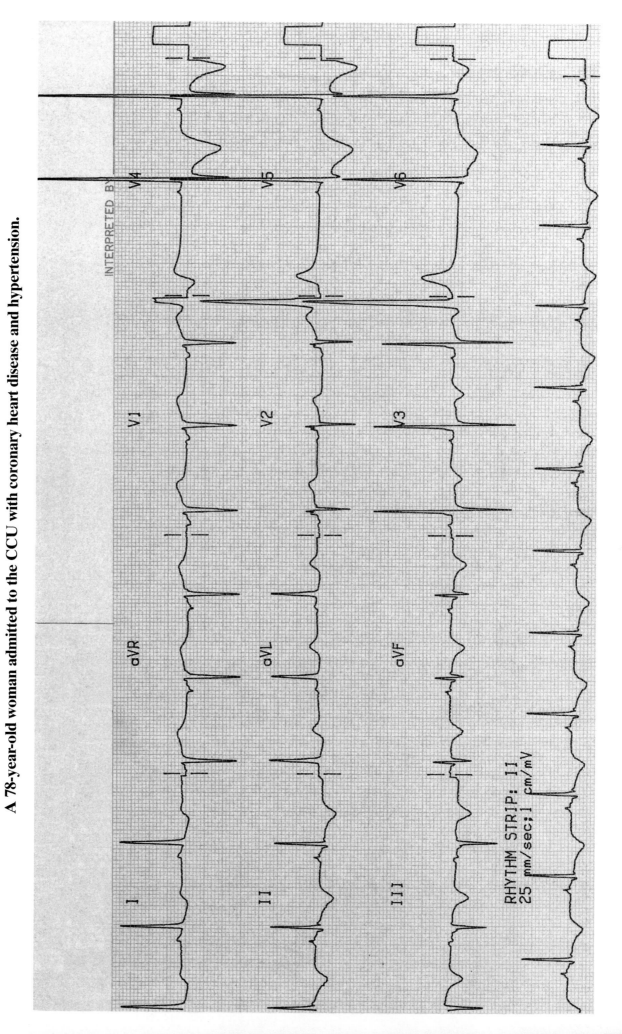

D-28

NARRATIVE INTERPRETATION

Rhythm:	**Multifocal atrial rhythm**
Rate:	98
Intervals:	PR variable, QRS 0.14, QT 0.34
Axis:	+105 degrees

Abnormalities

Irregular rhythm with variable P-wave morphologies. Axis rightward of +100 degrees. Broad QRS with rsR' pattern and T-wave inversion leads V1–V3.

Synthesis

Multifocal atrial rhythm. RBBB. Associated ST-T-wave changes. Right-axis deviation. Left posterior fascicular block.

TEST ANSWERS: 13, 65, 70, 73, 104.

Comment: This electrocardiogram demonstrates a chaotic, or multifocal, atrial rhythm. Note the differing P-wave morphologies and variable PR intervals. The rhythm is classified as *multifocal atrial rhythm* because the heart rate is less than 100 bpm. If faster, the rhythm would be classified as *multifocal atrial tachycardia.* The multifocal atrial rhythm in this tracing is distinguished from sinus rhythm with frequent APCs because there appears to be no clear sinus mechanism.

RBBB is evident in the right precordial leads. Note the marked right-axis deviation, which in the absence of RVH is indicative of left posterior fascicular block.

D-28

Clinical History
An 87-year-old woman with sepsis.

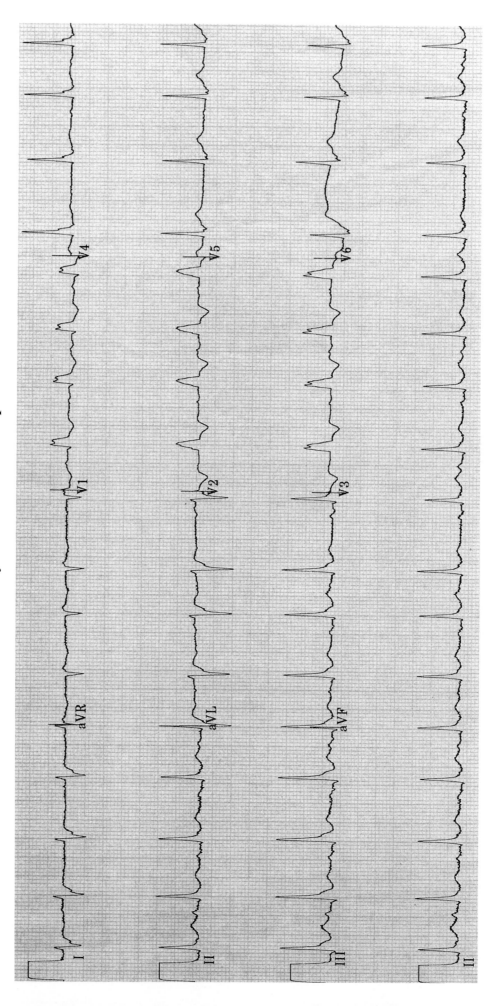

D-29

NARRATIVE INTERPRETATION

Rhythm:	**Sinus**
Rate:	**100**
Intervals:	**PR 0.20, QRS 0.18, QT 0.36**
Axis:	**−60 degrees**

Abnormalities
VPC. Prolonged QRS with broad, slurred R wave leads I, aVL, and ST depression and T-wave inversion leads I, aVL. Axis leftward of −30 degrees. (S wave lead V3 greater than 25 mm).

Synthesis
Sinus rhythm. VPC. LBBB with associated ST-T-wave abnormalities. Left-axis deviation. (Consider LVH).

TEST ANSWERS: 1, 26, 64, 74, (78), 104.

Comment: Many patients with LBBB also have LVH. Standard voltage criteria do not apply and most interpreters omit consideration of LVH in the presence of LBBB. There are however, clues to the diagnosis. One study found that the presence of an S wave in lead V3 greater than 25 mm was highly specific for LVH with LBBB. This criterion is present in this example.

At first glance, measuring the PR interval may have been difficult. The first beat after the VPC on the rhythm strip allows adequate visualization of the PR interval.

FURTHER READING
Kafka H, Burggraf GW, Milliken JA: Electrocardiographic diagnosis of left ventricular hypertrophy in the presence of left bundle branch block: An echocardiographic study. *Am J Cardiol* 55:103–106, 1985.

D-29

Clinical History
A 61-year-old woman with severe dyspnea.

I   aVR   V1   V4

II   aVL   V2   V5

III   aVF   V3   V6

RHYTHM STRIP: II
25 mm/sec; 1 cm/mV

313

D-30

NARRATIVE INTERPRETATION

Rhythm:	**Sinus bradycardia with first-degree AV block**
Rate:	**55**
Intervals:	**PR 0.21, QRS 0.16, QT 0.42**
Axis:	**0 degrees**

Abnormalities

Heart rate less than 60 bpm. Prolonged PR interval. Broad QRS complex with rSR' pattern and T-wave inversion leads V1–V3. VPC. Ventricular pacemaker firing on demand with appropriate capture, escape rate of 50 bpm (escape interval of 1200 ms), and pacing rate of 72 bpm (pacing interval of 833 1/3 ms).

Synthesis

Sinus bradycardia with first-degree AV block. RBBB with associated ST-T-wave changes. VPC. Ventricular pacemaker functioning on demand with appropriate sensing and pacing function. Pacing interval different from escape interval demonstrating hysteresis function.

TEST ANSWERS: 3, 26, 35, 42, 70, 104.

Comment: This is an excellent example of why it is mandatory to know the characteristics of a pacemaker before commenting on potential malfunction. If one were unaware of the hysteresis function (escape interval programmed at a longer interval than the pacing interval), it would be appropriate to consider a sensing malfunction of the pacemaker. Instead, this tracing demonstrates normal pacemaker function. When a VPC interrupts the sinus mechanism and produces a pause of at least 1200 ms (heart rate of 50 bpm), the pacemaker fires at a pacing rate of 72 bpm. Hysteresis is used to maintain AV synchrony for as long as possible, while pacing at a higher rate when the pacemaker engages.

FURTHER READING

Garson A Jr: Stepwise approach to the unknown pacemaker ECG. *Am Heart J* 119:924–941, 1990.

D-30

Clinical History

A 75-year-old man who is asymptomatic seen on routine examination. His pacemaker has a special programming function.

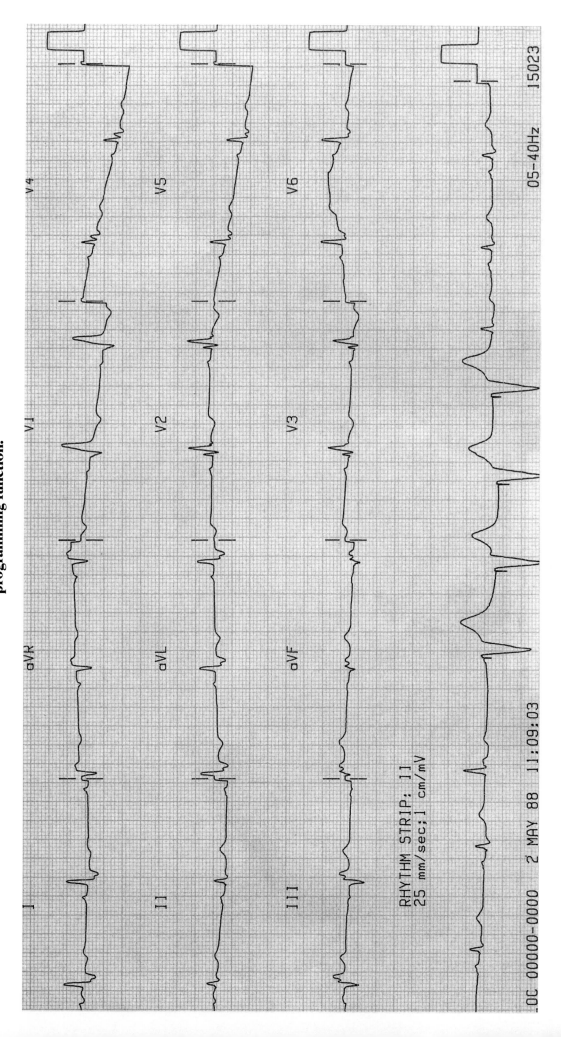

D-31

NARRATIVE INTERPRETATION

Rhythm:	**Sinus**
Rate	**68**
Intervals:	**PR 0.20, QRS 0.08, QT 0.36**
Axis:	**+15 degrees**

Abnormalities

ST elevation leads I, aVL, V2–V5. ST depression leads II, III, aVF. T-wave inversion lead V2–V5. Q wave leads V2–V3.

Synthesis

Sinus rhythm. Anteroseptal and lateral (anterolateral) wall MI, with ST-T-wave abnormalities suggesting acute myocardial injury. ST-T-wave abnormalities in leads II, III, aVF suggesting either reciprocal changes or myocardial ischemia.

TEST ANSWERS: 1, 81, (85), 89, 100, 101.

Comment: This patient sustained a large MI involving the anteroseptal and lateral (anterolateral) segments of the left ventricle. Note the additional ST depression in the inferior leads. The significance of this finding has not been resolved. Some investigators have found that reciprocal ST depression in anterior MI does not reflect additional inferior ischemia and is simply an electrical phenomenon. In contrast, others have determined that this finding reflects more extensive anterior infarction.

FURTHER READING

Ferguson DW, Pandian N, Kioschos JM, et al: Angiographic evidence that reciprocal ST-segment depression during acute myocardial infarction does not indicate remote ischemia: Analysis of 23 patients. *Am J Cardiol* 53:55–62, 1984.

Haraphongse M, Tanomsup S, Jugdutt BI: Inferior ST-segment depression during acute anterior myocardial infarction: Clinical and angiographic correlations. *J Am Coll Cardiol* 4:467–476, 1984.

D-31

Clinical History
A 73-year-old man with chest discomfort.

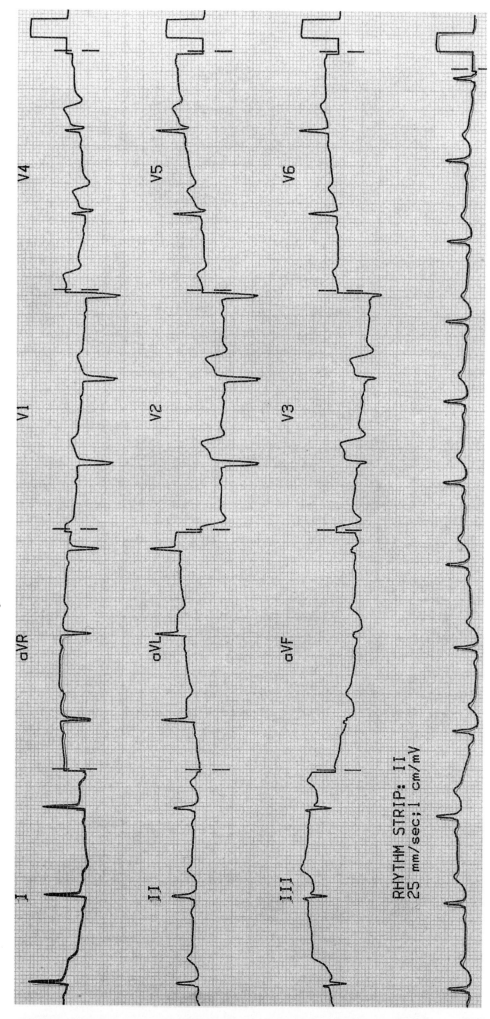

RHYTHM STRIP: II
25 mm/sec; 1 cm/mV

D-32

NARRATIVE INTERPRETATION

Rhythm:	**Sinus rhythm with complete AV block, AV junctional escape rhythm**
Rate:	**Atrial rate 74, junctional rate 36**
Intervals:	**PR −, QRS 0.08, QT 0.48**
Axis:	**+60 degrees**

Abnormalities

P waves fail to conduct to ventricles. ST elevation leads III, aVF. Straight ST segment lead II. ST depression leads I, aVL, V2–V6. T-wave inversion leads III, aVF.

Synthesis

Sinus rhythm with complete AV block. AV dissociation. AV junctional escape rhythm. Inferior wall MI with ST abnormalities suggestive of acute myocardial injury. ST abnormalities in leads I, aVL, V2–V6 consistent with myocardial ischemia or reciprocal changes.

TEST ANSWERS: 1, 22, 47, 53, 91, 100, 101.

Comment: The reader might initially mistake this tracing for sinus rhythm with some form of 2:1 AV block. However, the P waves that appear just before half of the QRS complexes are too close to be conducted. The sinus rate is approximately twice that of the AV junctional escape rate, giving the appearance of 2:1 AV conduction. In fact, there is AV dissociation.

Note that this patient has early ST changes of an acute inferior wall MI. Patients with inferior wall infarction may develop transient high-grade heart block due to profound vagotonia. In general, temporary pacemaker therapy is required only if the escape rate is so slow that there is hemodynamic compromise.

FURTHER READING

Berger PB, Ruocco NA Jr, Ryan TJ, et al: Incidence and prognostic implications of heart block complicating inferior myocardial infarction treated with thrombolytic therapy: Results from TIMI II. *J Am Coll Cardiol* 20:533–540, 1992.

Feigl D, Ashkenazy J, Kishon Y: Early and late atrioventricular block in acute inferior myocardial infarction. *J Am Coll Cardiol* 4:35–38, 1984.

D-32

Clinical History

A 71-year-old man with chest discomfort in the CCU.

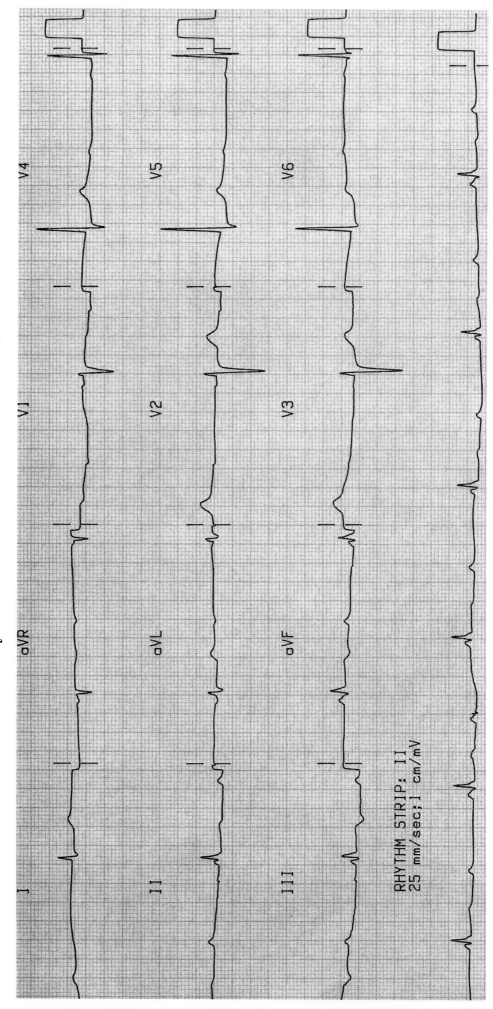

319

D-33

NARRATIVE INTERPRETATION

Rhythm:	**Atrial fibrillation**
Rate:	**75 (average)**
Intervals:	**PR –, QRS 0.08, QT 0.40**
Axis:	**+45 degrees**

Abnormalities
ST depression leads I, V4–V6. T-wave inversion leads I, aVL, V4–V5. Flat T wave lead V6. S wave lead V2 + R wave lead V5 greater than 35 mm.

Synthesis
Atrial fibrillation with a controlled ventricular response. LVH. Associated ST-T-wave abnormalities.

TEST ANSWERS: 20, 51, 78, 103.

Comment: Atrial fibrillation is an extremely common arrhythmia estimated to occur in 0.4 percent of the adult population. The prevalence rises with age, with atrial fibrillation present in approximately 4 percent of individuals over the age of 65, and 9 percent of those 80 years or older. Most patients with atrial fibrillation have organic heart disease. Causes include coronary heart disease, congestive heart failure, hypertensive heart disease, valvular heart disease, and hyperthyroidism. The Framingham study reported that the presence of LVH on the electrocardiogram was strongly associated with the development of atrial fibrillation. Initial therapy is directed at controlling the ventricular rate and preventing embolic events with anticoagulation. Additional therapeutic interventions may then be considered such as cardioversion via electrical or pharmacologic means (see following two tracings).

FURTHER READING
Falk RF: Atrial fibrillation. *N Engl J Med* 344:1067–1078, 2001.
Go AS, Hylek EM, Philips KA, et al: Prevalence of diagnosed atrial fibrillation in adults: National implications for rhythm management and stroke prevention. *JAMA* 285:2370–2375, 2001.
Kannel WB, Abbott RD, Savage DD, McNamara PM: Epidemiologic features of chronic atrial fibrillation: The Framingham study. *N Engl J Med* 306:1018–1022, 1982.

D-33

Clinical History
A 74-year-old woman with palpitations.

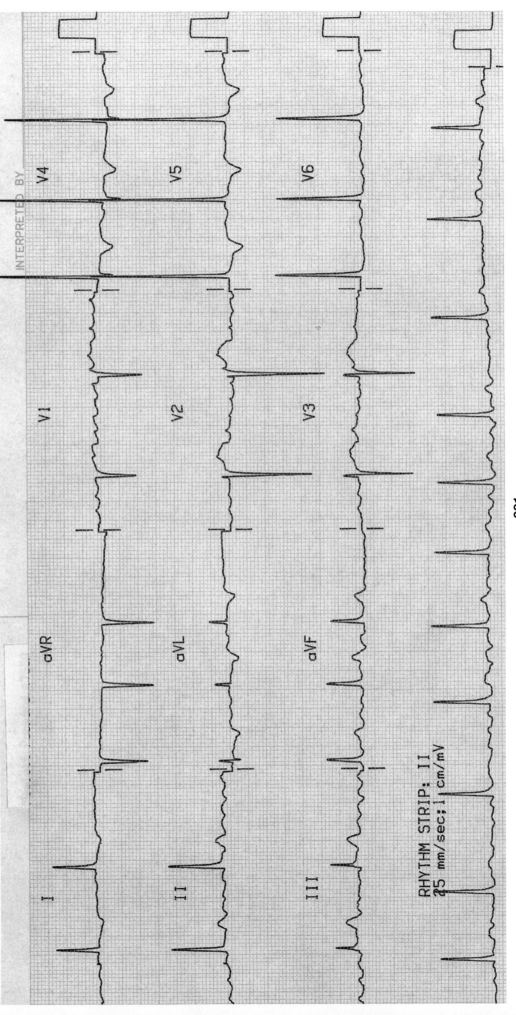

D-34

NARRATIVE INTERPRETATION

Rhythm:	**Sinus bradycardia**
Rate:	**54**
Intervals:	**PR 0.20, QRS 0.08, QT 0.42**
Axis:	**+60 degrees**

Abnormalities

Heart rate less than 60 bpm. Abnormal P terminal force lead V1. ST depression leads I, V5–V6. T-wave inversion leads I, aVL, V4–V6. Prominent U waves. S wave lead V2 + R wave lead V5 greater than 35 mm.

Synthesis

Sinus bradycardia. Left atrial abnormality. LVH by voltage criteria. Associated nonspecific ST-T-wave abnormalities. Prominent U waves.

TEST ANSWERS: 3, 60, 78, 103, (106), 110.

Comment: The patient in the previous tracing has converted to sinus rhythm after treatment with digoxin and quinidine. Note the prominent U waves with a normal QT interval. Prominent U waves are likely secondary to the effect of quinidine, but do not reflect quinidine toxicity.

Quinidine is a type I antiarrhythmic agent that acts on the fast sodium channel of the cell membrane. The drug affects the His-Purkinje system by depressing the action potential velocity and automaticity, decreasing conduction velocity, and prolonging the refractory period. This drug has the potential for life-threatening cardiotoxicity and is no longer commonly used to convert atrial fibrillation to sinus rhythm.

FURTHER READING

Lepeschkin E: The U wave of the electrocardiogram. *Mod Concepts Cardiovasc Dis* 38:39–45, 1969.

D-34

Clinical History

A 74-year-old woman in the CCU who has been treated with digoxin and quinidine.

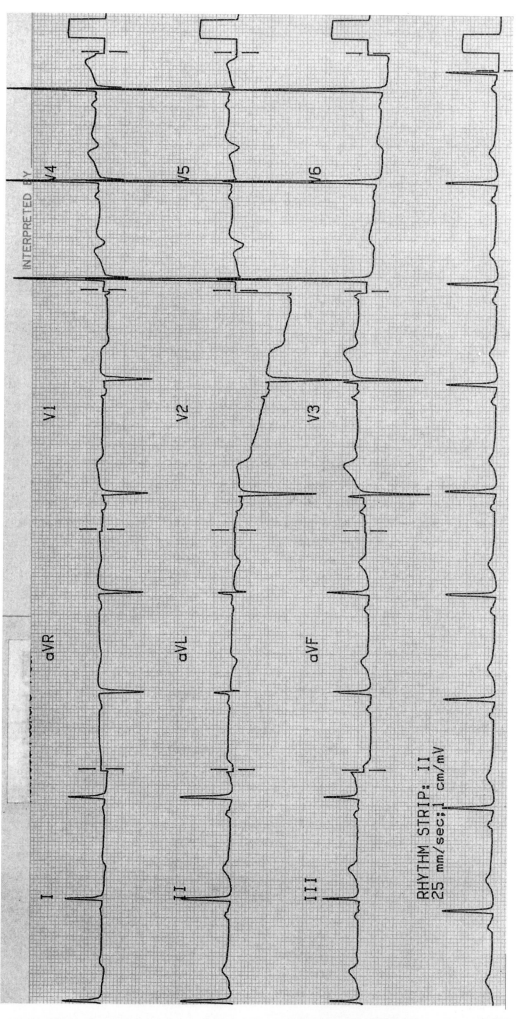

D-35

NARRATIVE INTERPRETATION

Rhythm:	**Sinus bradycardia**
Rate:	**47**
Intervals:	**PR 0.20, QRS 0.08, QT —**
Axis:	**+60 degrees**

Abnormalities

Heart rate less than 60 bpm. Abnormal P terminal force lead V1. ST depression leads I, II, aVL, aVF, V4–V6. S wave lead V2 + R wave lead V5 greater than 35 mm. QT-QU prolongation.

Synthesis

Sinus bradycardia. Left atrial abnormality. Prolonged QTc (QU) interval. LVH by voltage criteria. Diffuse, associated nonspecific ST-T-wave abnormalities.

TEST ANSWERS: 3, 60, 78, 103, (106), 109.

Comment: This tracing demonstrates many of the electrocardiographic effects of quinidine excess. Therapeutic quinidine doses normally produce T-wave flattening and slight prolongation of the QT interval. Prominent U waves may also be present. Marked QT prolongation however, reflects quinidine toxicity. Additional toxic effects may include widening of the QRS interval, atrial slowing, and AV block. Compared with the previous tracing, the QT interval now appears considerably more prolonged, with more prominent ST depression. The true QT interval is difficult to measure because it is merged with the U wave, but it is certainly more prolonged than in the previous example. It is important to recognize quinidine-induced QT prolongation because it may predispose to *torsades de pointes*.

FURTHER READING

Stratmann HG, Kennedy HL: Torsades de pointes associated with drugs and toxins: Recognition and management. *Am Heart J* 113:1470–1482, 1987.

D-35

A 74-year-old patient treated with digoxin and quinidine for control of paroxysmal atrial fibrillation.

I   aVR   V1   V4

II   aVL   V2   V5

III   aVF   V3   V6

RHYTHM STRIP: II
25 mm/sec; 1 cm/mV

D-36

NARRATIVE INTERPRETATION

Rhythm: Sinus
Rate: 72
Intervals: PR 0.16, QRS 0.12, QT 0.36
Axis: −45 degrees

Abnormalities

VPCs. Fusion complexes. Axis leftward of −30 degrees. Prolonged QRS duration. R wave aVL greater than 11 mm. R wave lead I + S wave lead III greater than 25 mm. R wave aVL + S wave lead V3 greater than 28 mm in a man. T-wave inversion leads I, aVL. R wave leads V1–V3 less than 3 mm.

Synthesis

Sinus rhythm. VPCs. Fusion complexes. Left-axis deviation. LAFB. LVH by voltage criteria. Poor R-wave progression. Nonspecific T-wave abnormalities associated with ventricular hypertrophy or conduction abnormality or both. Intraventricular conduction delay.

TEST ANSWERS: 1, 26, 56, 64, 66, 72, 76, 78, (103), (104), 106.

Comment: This tracing is a good example of fusion beats. Frequent VPCs are present on the rhythm strip. Because of slight variability of the relatively late coupling interval, some of the ventricular complexes are superimposed with the sinus impulse. The first and third wide complex beats of the rhythm strip demonstrate a morphology intermediate between the normal sinus configuration and that of the VPCs. Note that the third wide complex beat is the most narrow and similar to the native beat. This is because the ventricular depolarization occurs somewhat later than the previous fusion beat and demonstrates a longer PR interval. Thus, there is a greater opportunity for normal conduction prior to the ventricular ectopic depolarization.

The intraventricular conduction delay and poor R-wave progression are most likely secondary to the combination of LAFB and LVH. Left anterior fascicular block should be considered because this degree of left-axis deviation would not be expected with LVH alone.

D-36

Clinical History

A 68-year-old asymptomatic man with congestive heart failure.

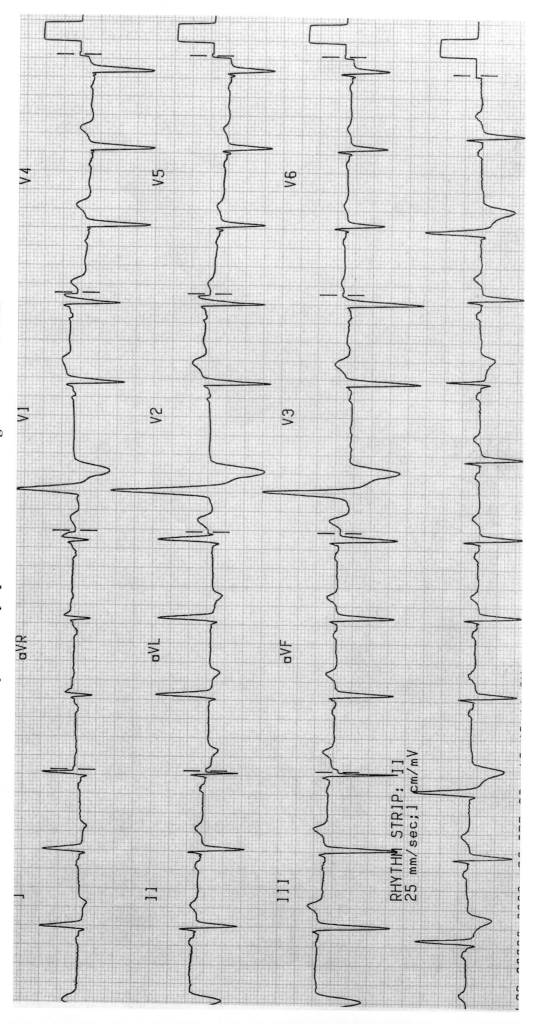

D-37

NARRATIVE INTERPRETATION

Rhythm:	**Sinus**
Rate:	**70**
Intervals:	**PR 0.16, QRS 0.10, QT 0.40**
Axis:	**−45 degrees**

Abnormalities

Axis leftward of −30 degrees. R wave lead aVL greater than 11 mm. R wave lead I + S wave lead III greater than 25 mm. R wave lead aVL + S wave lead V3 greater than 28 mm in a man. ST depression leads I, aVL. T-wave inversion leads I, aVL. QS wave leads V1–V3. APC.

Synthesis

Sinus rhythm. APCs. Left-axis deviation. Left anterior fascicular block. LVH by voltage criteria with associated ST-T-wave abnormalities. (Possible anteroseptal wall MI of indeterminate duration.)

TEST ANSWERS: 1, 10, 64, 72, (82), 103.

Comment: This patient had marked cardiomegaly secondary to a dilated cardiomyopathy. Precordial voltage criteria for LVH are absent because of the loss of R forces in the lateral precordial leads and left-axis deviation from the left anterior fascicular block. In contrast, multiple limb-lead voltage criteria for LVH are present.

The diagnosis of anteroseptal wall MI cannot be made definitively in the presence of LVH, particularly with coexistent LAFB. Both can produce a pseudoinfarction pattern. In general, anteroseptal MI should be avoided in this situation unless there is supporting clinical or electrocardiographic evidence. In the author's opinion, when QS waves are present in the right precordial leads in a patient with LVH, it is reasonable to comment on the potential diagnosis of anteroseptal MI.

FURTHER READING

Farnham DJ, Shah PM: Left anterior hemiblock simulating anteroseptal myocardial infarction. *Am Heart J* 92:363–367, 1976.

Gertsch M, Theler A, Foglia E: Electrocardiographic detection of left ventricular hypertrophy in the presence of left anterior fascicular block. *Am J Cardiol* 61:1098–1101, 1988.

Goldberger AL: ECG simulators of myocardial infarction. Part I. Pathophysiology and differential diagnosis of pseudoinfarct Q wave patterns. *PACE* 5:106–119, 1982.

D-37

Clinical History

A 59-year-old man with dyspnea.

aVR

aVL

aVF

I

II

III

V4

V5

V6

V1

V2

V3

RHYTHM STRIP: II
25 mm/sec 1 cm/mV

05-40Hz

22759

00:00000-0000 26 JAN 89 10:12:53

D-38

NARRATIVE INTERPRETATION

Rhythm:	**Atrial fibrillation**
Rate:	**75 (average)**
Intervals:	**PR −, QRS 0.12, QT 0.40**
Axis:	**−15 degrees**

Abnormalities

Prolonged QRS duration. R wave aVL greater than 11 mm. R wave lead I + S wave lead III greater than 25 mm. R wave aVL + S wave lead V3 greater than 20 mm in a woman. R-wave voltage V1–V3 less than 3 mm. Slight ST depression leads I, aVL, V6.

Synthesis

Atrial fibrillation with a controlled ventricular response. LVH. Intraventricular conduction delay. Poor R-wave progression. ST-T-wave abnormalities associated with LVH.

TEST ANSWERS: 20, 51, 66, 76, 78, 103.

Comment: This patient had marked cardiomegaly secondary to long-standing hypertension and mitral insufficiency. The increased limb-lead voltage, intraventricular conduction delay, and poor R-wave progression are all secondary to LVH. Incomplete LBBB cannot be diagnosed because of the persistence of septal Q waves in leads I and aVL. The axis is at the leftward limits of normal, but remains slightly positive in lead II and does not demonstrate left-axis deviation.

D-38

Clinical History

A 78-year-old woman admitted for elective colon surgery. She has a history of hypertension and congestive heart failure. Medications include digoxin, a diuretic, and ACE inhibitor.

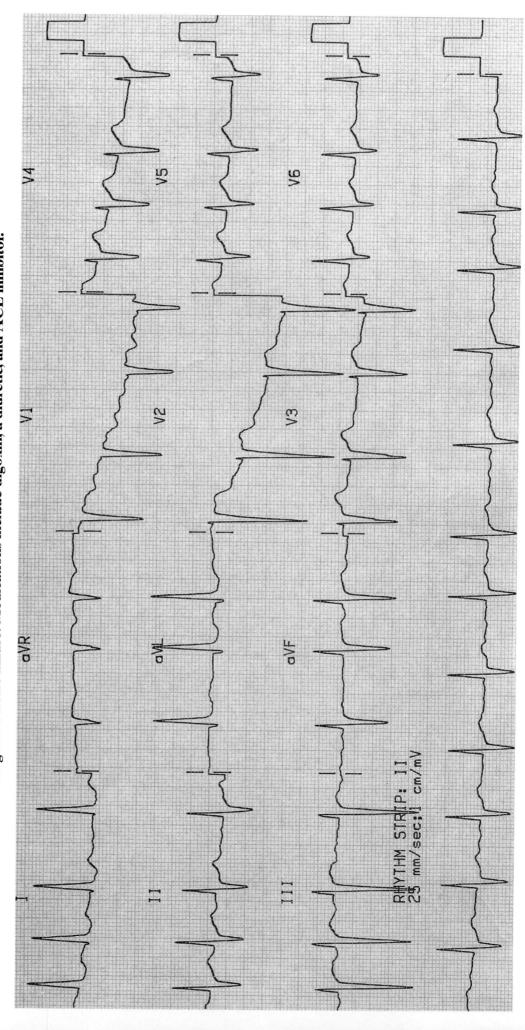

D-39

NARRATIVE INTERPRETATION

Rhythm:	**Sinus**
Rate:	**84**
Intervals:	**PR 0.20, QRS 0.08, QT 0.36**
Axis:	**−15 degrees**

Abnormalities
T-wave inversion leads I, II, III, aVL, aVF, V2–V6.

Synthesis
Sinus rhythm. T-wave inversion suggestive of myocardial ischemia.

TEST ANSWERS: 1, 102.

Comment: This patient presented with profound, diffuse T-wave inversion, a pattern that has anatomical significance. In patients with unstable angina, new T-wave inversion in the anterior precordial leads is found to predict a critical lesion in the proximal left anterior descending coronary artery. In the author's experience, when there is accompanying T-wave inversion in the inferior and lateral leads, the lesion is more distal and represents ischemia of the left ventricular apex.

FURTHER READING
de Zwaan C, Bar FWHM, Wellens HJJ: Characteristic electrocardiographic pattern indicating a critical stenosis high in left anterior descending coronary artery in patients admitted because of impending myocardial infarction. *Am Heart J* 103:730–737, 1982.

Haines DE, Raabe DS, Gundel WD, Wackers FJT: Anatomic and prognostic significance of new T-wave inversion in unstable angina. *Am J Cardiol* 52:14–18, 1983.

D-39

Clinical History

A 55-year-old man with severe chest discomfort.

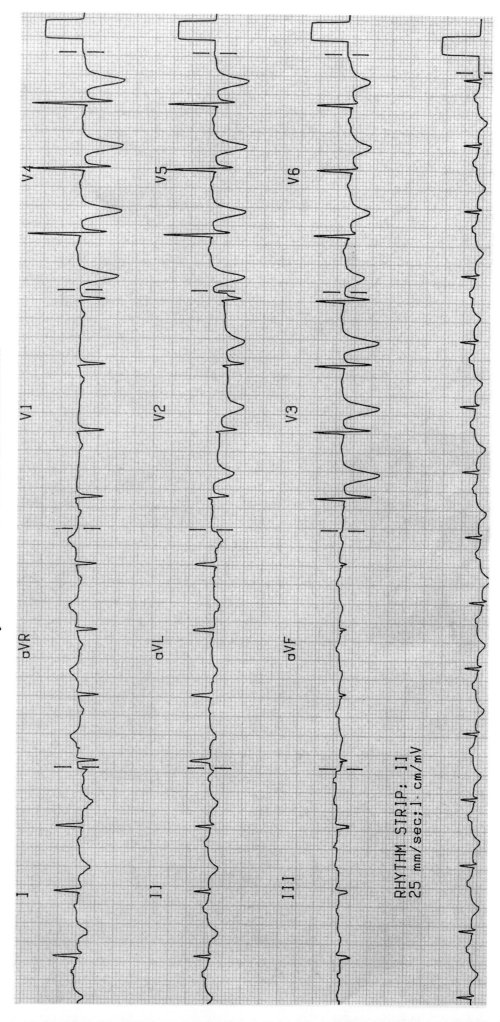

RHYTHM STRIP: II
25 mm/sec; 1 cm/mV

D-40

NARRATIVE INTERPRETATION

Rhythm:	Sinus
Rate:	65
Intervals:	PR 0.20, QRS 0.08, QT 0.40
Axis:	+45 degrees

Abnormalities
JPCs.

Synthesis
Sinus rhythm. JPCs. Otherwise within normal limits.

TEST ANSWERS: 1, 25.

Comment: Supraventricular premature complexes, either atrial or junctional, are frequently found in normal persons. Both atrial and junctional premature complexes generally have a constant coupling interval related to the previous sinus beat. Unlike ventricular premature complexes, a fully compensatory pause is usually absent because the sinus node is reset via retrograde conduction. In this example, junctional rather than atrial premature complexes are diagnosed because of absent P waves in the premature beats. The retrograde P wave is "buried" in the QRS. On close inspection, the ST segment of the premature beats is slightly elevated due to the influence of the retrograde P wave. Premature atrial or junctional complexes are generally benign, but may inititate reentrant supraventricular tachyarrhythmias in susceptible individuals.

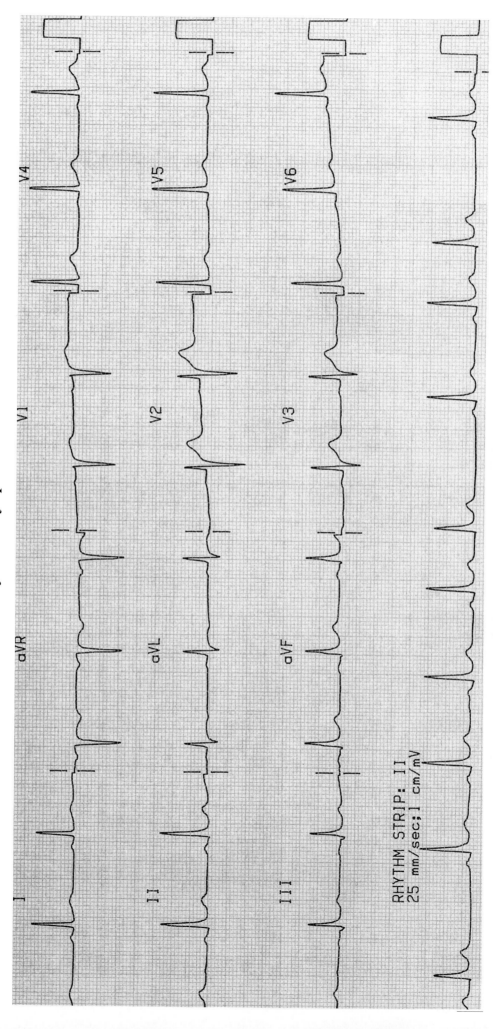

D-40

Clinical History
A 45-year-old asymptomatic man.

RHYTHM STRIP: II
25 mm/sec; 1 cm/mV

I aVR V1 V4

II aVL V2 V5

III aVF V3 V6

TEST E

NARRATIVE INTERPRETATION E-1

Rhythm:	**Wide complex tachycardia, probably supraventricular in origin**
Rate:	**158**
Intervals:	**PR –, QRS 0.13, QT 0.32**
Axis:	**–45 degrees**

Abnormalities

Axis leftwards of –30 degrees. Broad QRS with rsR' pattern and T-wave inversion leads V1–V3. Aberrantly conducted complex on rhythm strip.

Synthesis

Wide complex tachyarrhythmia, probably supraventricular in origin. (Possible atrial flutter with 2:1 AV conduction.) Aberrantly conducted complex on rhythm strip. RBBB with associated ST-T-wave changes. LAFB. Left-axis deviation.

TEST ANSWERS: 18, (19), 50, 64, 70, 72, 104.

Comment: The differentiation of ventricular tachycardia versus supraventricular tachycardia with aberrancy is one of the most challenging aspects of clinical electrocardiography. Analyzing a number of factors can assist in the diagnosis; but in this tracing, conflicting criteria appear. The RBBB pattern present in lead V1 suggests aberrancy, but the specific rsR' configuration is not classic. Conversely, the left axis favors ventricular ectopy. The rate of 158 somewhat favors ventricular tachycardia, but this finding is neither sensitive nor specific. The QRS duration of 0.13 s does not help to distinguish the origin of the tachyarrythmia.

Remember that a patient may have an underlying conduction abnormality to explain the wide complex. This indeed turns out to be the case in this patient (see next tracing). If one makes a very careful search in lead aVF, tiny, notched P waves can be seen before and after the QRS, suggesting that the rhythm is atrial flutter with 2:1 AV conduction. Without serial tracings or more information, it would be difficult to conclude this diagnosis.

FURTHER READING

Akhtar M, Shenasa M, Jazayeri M, et al: Wide QRS complex tachycardia. *Ann Intern Med* 109:905–912, 1988.
Tchou P, Young P, Mahmud R, et al: Useful clinical criteria for the diagnosis of ventricular tachycardia. *Am J Med* 84:53–56, 1988.
Wellens HJJ, Barr FWHM, Lie KI: The value of the electrocardiogram in the differential diagnosis of a tachycardia with a widened QRS complex. *Am J Med* 84:27–33, 1978.

E-1

Clinical History
A 77-year-old man with lightheadedness.

I

aVR

V1

V4

II

aVL

V2

V5

III

aVF

V3

V6

RHYTHM STRIP: II
25 mm/sec; 1 cm/mV

E-2

NARRATIVE INTERPRETATION

Rhythm:	**Atrial fibrillation, accelerated AV junctional rhythm**
Rate:	**82**
Intervals:	**PR −, QRS 0.13, QT 0.38**
Axis:	**−45 degrees**

Abnormalities
Axis leftward of −30 degrees. Broad QRS with rsR' pattern and T-wave inversion leads V1–V3.

Synthesis
Atrial fibrillation. Period of high-grade AV block with accelerated AV junctional rhythm. RBBB with associated ST-T-wave changes. Left anterior fascicular block. Left-axis deviation.

TEST ANSWERS: 20, 23, 46, 64, 70, 72, 104.

Comment: When comparing this tracing with the previous electrocardiogram, one can now determine that the wide complex tachyarrhythmia was secondary to an underlying conduction abnormality and not to ventricular tachycardia. The present electrocardiogram also demonstrates evidence of digoxin toxicity. The underlying rhythm is atrial fibrillation, seen only in the final three complexes of the rhythm strip. The remainder of the tracing demonstrates digoxin-induced suppression of AV conduction and an accelerated junctional rhythm. The degree of AV block is considered *high-grade* and not complete because there is evidence of intact AV conduction toward the end of the rhythm strip.

FURTHER READING

Kastor JA, Yurchak PM: Recognition of digitalis intoxication in the presence of atrial fibrillation. *Ann Intern Med* 67:1045–1054, 1967.

Kremers MS, Black WH, Wells PJ, Solodnya M: Effect of preexisting bundle branch block on the electrocardiographic diagnosis of ventricular tachycardia. *Am J Cardiol* 62:1208–1212, 1988.

E-2

Clinical History

A 77-year-old man with a history of atrial fibrillation and atrial flutter. He is treated with digoxin.

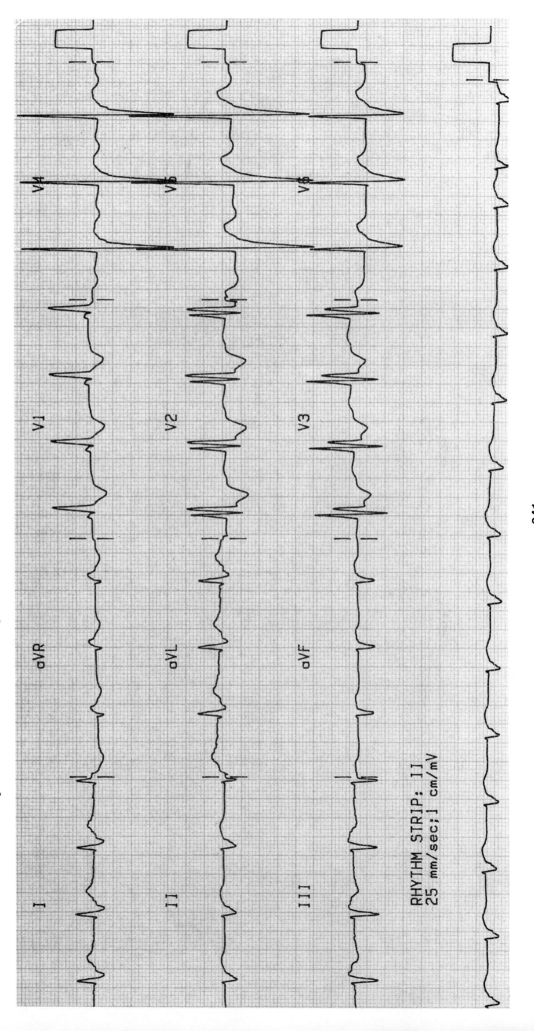

E-3

NARRATIVE INTERPRETATION

Rhythm: Sinus tachycardia
Rate: 110
Intervals: PR 0.14, QRS 0.08, QT 0.36
Axis: −15 degrees

Abnormalities

Heart rate greater than 100 bpm. ST elevation leads V1–V4. ST depression lead V6. T-wave inversion leads I, aVL. R wave leads V1–V3 less than 3 mm. S wave lead V2 + R wave lead V5 greater than 35 mm. R wave lead aVL + S wave lead V3 greater than 28 mm in a man.

Synthesis

Sinus tachycardia. Poor R-wave progression. Left ventricular hypertrophy. Possible anteroseptal wall MI of indeterminate age. Nonspecific ST-T-wave abnormalities. Possible ST-T-wave abnormalities of acute myocardial injury V1–V6. Possible ST-T-wave abnormalities associated with LVH.

TEST ANSWERS: 4, 66, 78, (82), (100), (101), (102), (103), 106.

Comment: This tracing illustrates the common need for serial tracings to accurately make an electrocardiographic diagnosis. The ST-T-wave abnormalities in the precordial leads are nonspecific, but could represent early, acute myocardial injury. LVH may also contribute to the ST-T-wave findings in these leads, as well as those seen in leads I and aVL. Until a more precise electrocardiographic diagnosis can be made, it is acceptable to categorize the ST-T-wave changes as nonspecific, while mentioning the potential for a more ominous condition.

Using the algorithm proposed by Zema, the poor R-wave progression suggests an anteroseptal wall MI. Remember that poor R-wave progression may also be due to LVH. A number of hours after admission, the diagnosis for this patient became clear (see next tracing).

FURTHER READING

James KB, Obarski TP, Underwood DA: Electrocardiographic criteria for anterior myocardial infarction. *Cleve Clin J Med* 57:618–621, 1990.

Zema MJ, Kligfield P: ECG poor R-wave progression. *Arch Intern Med* 142:1145–1148, 1982.

Clinical History

A 56-year-old man with profound diaphoresis and dyspepsia.

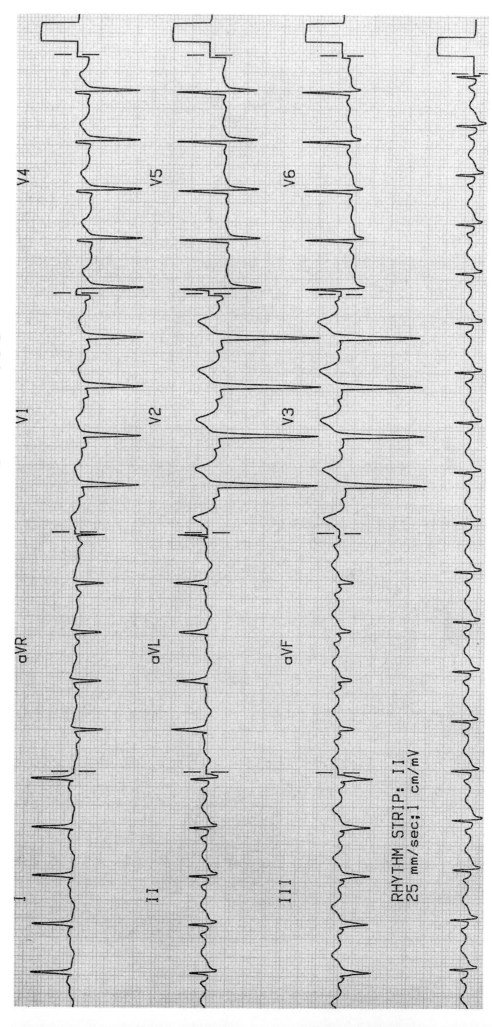

RHYTHM STRIP: II
25 mm/sec; 1 cm/mV

E-4

NARRATIVE INTERPRETATION

Rhythm:	**Sinus**
Rate:	**72**
Intervals:	**PR 0.16, QRS 0.08, QT 0.46**
Axis:	**−30 degrees**

Abnormalities

ST elevation leads V1–V4. ST depression leads V5–V6. T-wave inversion leads I, aVL, V3–V6. QS wave lead V1–V3. R wave lead aVL + S wave lead V3 greater than 28 mm in a man. QT prolongation for heart rate. S wave lead V2 + R wave lead V5 greater than 35 mm.

Synthesis

Sinus rhythm. Anterior (anteroseptal) wall MI with ST-T-wave abnormalities suggesting recent myocardial injury. ST-T-wave abnormalities in leads I, aVL, V5–V6, suggesting myocardial ischemia. Prolonged QTc interval. LVH.

TEST ANSWERS: 1, 78, (81), 83, 100, 101, 109.

Comment: Comparing this tracing with the previous example allows for a diagnosis of MI. The location may be considered anterior because of ST abnormalities and loss of the R wave in lead V4. The previous nonspecific ST-T-wave abnormalities now reflect the acute coronary process.

Note the prolonged QT interval, a frequent finding in myocardial ischemia. The actual QT interval is a bit difficult to determine because of superimposition of the U wave.

FURTHER READING

Al-Khatib SM, Allen LaPoint NMA, Kramer JM, et al: What clinicians should know about the QT interval. *JAMA:* 289:2120–2127, 2003.

Schweitzer P: The values and limitations of the QT interval in clinical practice. *Am Heart J* 124:1121–1126, 1992.

Simonson E, Cady LD, Woodbury M: The normal Q-T interval. *Am Heart J* 63:747–753, 1962.

E-4

Clinical History

A 56-year-old man admitted to the coronary care unit (CCU).

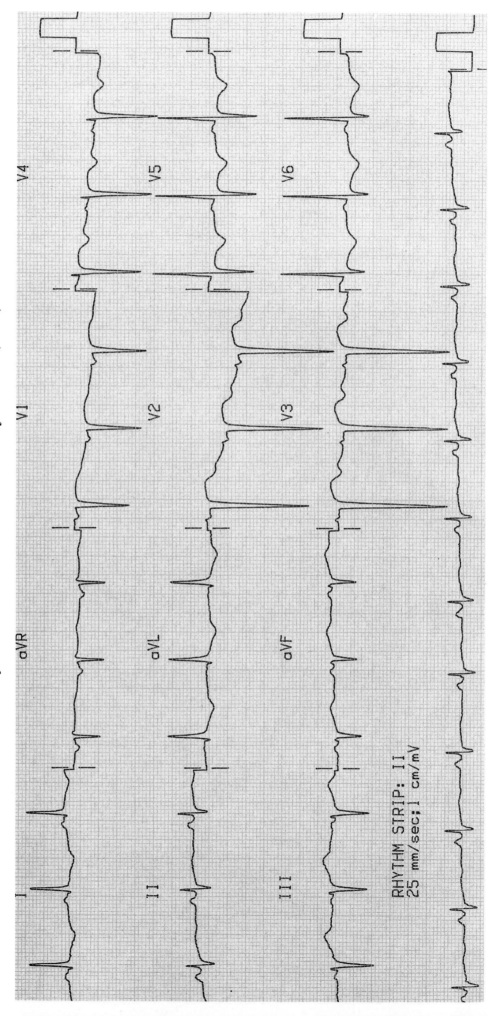

E-5

NARRATIVE INTERPRETATION

Rhythm:	**Sinus**
Rate	**92**
Intervals:	**PR 0.16, QRS 0.08, QT 0.36**
Axis:	**+40 degrees**

Abnormalities

JPCs. Biphasic P wave with tall initial component and abnormal P terminal force lead V1. ST depression leads I, II, III, aVF, V4–V6. T-wave inversion leads I, II, III, aVF, V5–V6. S wave lead V2 + R wave lead V5 greater than 35 mm. R wave lead aVL + S wave lead V3 greater than 20 mm in a woman.

Synthesis

Sinus rhythm. JPCs. LVH. Associated ST-T-wave abnormalities. Biatrial enlargement.

TEST ANSWERS: 1, 25, 61, 78, 103.

Comment: This patient had an idiopathic cardiomyopathy and four-chamber dilatation. LVH is evident, but RVH is not. Because left ventricular forces predominate, criteria for combined left and right ventricular hypertrophy are often absent on the electrocardiogram even in the presence of anatomic biventricular hypertrophy. Both left and right atrial enlargement are noted in lead V1.

FURTHER READING

Saunders JL, Calatayud JB, Schulz KJ, et al: Evaluation of ECG criteria for P-wave abnormalities. *Am Heart J* 74:757–765, 1967.

Thomas PM, DeJong D: The P wave in the electrocardiogram in the diagnosis of heart disease. *Br Heart J* 16:241–254, 1954.

E-5

Clinical History

A 66-year-old woman seen in routine follow-up for chronic dyspnea.

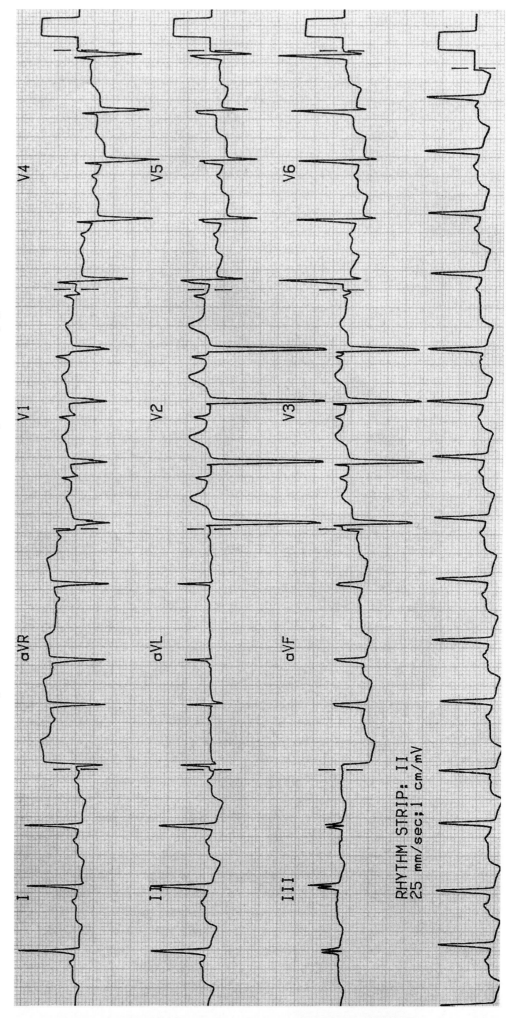

E-6

NARRATIVE INTERPRETATION

Rhythm:	**Ectopic atrial rhythm**
Rate:	**84**
Intervals:	**PR 0.20, QRS 0.08, QT 0.32**
Axis:	**+60 degrees**

Abnormalities
Inverted P waves leads II, III, aVF. VPCs. Interpolated VPC. ST depression leads I, II III, aVL, aVF, V2–V6.

Synthesis
Ectopic atrial rhythm. VPCs. Interpolated VPC. Nonspecific ST abnormalities.

TEST ANSWERS: 9, 26, 58, 106.

Comment: On careful inspection, inverted P waves can be seen in leads II, III, and aVF, implicating an origin for the rhythm outside the sinus node. It cannot be determined with certainty if this focus is AV junctional with considerable antegrade block, or whether it is from an ectopic atrial site. It would be unusual however, for an accelerated AV junctional rhythm to have a PR interval of 0.20 s.

This tracing may represent a "dig toxic" rhythm. Digoxin toxicity may present with suppression of normal pacemakers and enhancement of others. The most common digitalis-induced arrhythmias are ventricular in origin. Frequent VPCs are present, one of which is interpolated between two supraventricular complexes.

FURTHER READING
Fisch C, Knoebel SB: Digitalis cardiotoxicity. *J Am Coll Cardiol* 5:91A–98A, 1985.
Saner HE, Lange HW, Pierach CA, Aeppli DM: Relation between serum digoxin concentration and the electrocardiogram. *Clin Cardiol* 11:752–756, 1988.
Smith TW, Antman EM, Friedman PL, et al: Digitalis glycosides: Mechanisms and manifestations of toxicity. *Prog Cardiovasc Dis* 27:21–56, 1984.

E-6

Clinical History

A 61-year-old woman with a history of mitral valve replacement and atrial fibrillation. She is prescribed digoxin.

I aVR V1 V4

II aVL V2 V5

III aVF V3 V6

INTERPRETED BY

RHYTHM STRIP: II
25 mm/sec; 1 cm/mV

E-7

NARRATIVE INTERPRETATION

Rhythm:	**Sinus tachycardia, multifocal atrial tachycardia (MAT)**
Rate:	**Sinus rate 104, rate of MAT 180**
Intervals:	**PR 0.16, QRS 0.08, QT 0.34**
Axis:	**+15 degrees**

Abnormalities

Heart rate greater than 100 bpm. APCs. VPCs, multiform. Paired VPCs. S wave lead V2 + R wave lead V5 greater than 35 mm. R wave lead aVL + S wave lead V3 greater than 20 mm in a woman.

Synthesis

Sinus tachycardia. APCs. VPCs multiform. Paired VPCs. Multifocal atrial tachycardia on rhythm strip. LVH by voltage criteria.

TEST ANSWERS: 4, 10, 14, 27, 28, 78, 103.

Comment: A number of rhythm abnormalities are evident in this tracing. A run of MAT begins the rhythm strip. It is initially difficult to differentiate this from atrial fibrillation. However, there are deformities of the T waves that suggest superimposed P waves rather than fibrillatory waves. Frequent VPCs are noted on the rhythm strip, both multiform and in pairs. APCs are present in the 5th and 15th beats of the 12-lead tracing.

Do not overlook that the chest leads are recorded at one-half standard. One might easily miss the increased voltage for LVH.

E-7

Clinical History
A 92-year-old woman with dyspnea.

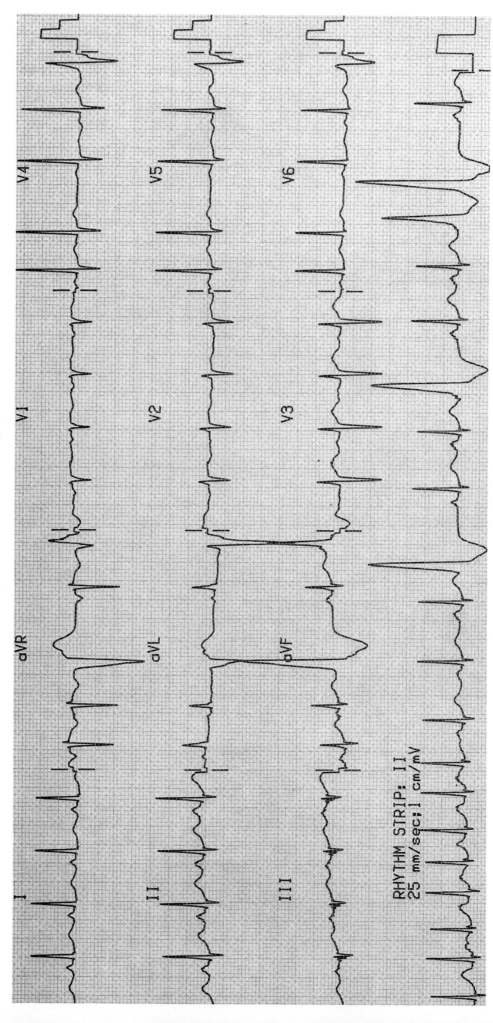

E-8

NARRATIVE INTERPRETATION

> **Rhythm:** Atrial tachycardia with variable AV conduction
> **Rate:** Atrial 210, ventricular 62 (average)
> **Intervals:** PR –, QRS 0.10, QT 0.40
> **Axis:** –15 degrees

Abnormalities
Rapid atrial rate with variable conduction.

Synthesis
Atrial tachycardia with variable AV conduction. Otherwise within normal limits.

TEST ANSWERS: 17, 51.

Comment: Atrial tachycardia with block is considered a characteristic arrhythmia of digitalis toxicity. This arrhythmia may also result from pulmonary, coronary, or valvular heart disease. Atrial tachycardia with block should be differentiated from atrial flutter with block. The atrial rate in atrial tachycardia is between 150 and 250, whereas the atrial rate in atrial flutter is usually greater than 250. Atrial flutter should also demonstrate characteristic flutter waves that are inverted in leads II, III, and aVF. In contrast, atrial tachycardia has an isoelectric baseline between the P waves.

Remember that at atrial rates greater than 200, 2:1 AV conduction is an expected, physiologic response of the AV node. Conduction ratios greater than 2:1 imply a nonphysiologic response secondary to either intrinsic conduction disease or the effect of pharmacologic agents.

FURTHER READING
Ganz LI, Friedman PL: Supraventricular tachycardia. *N Engl J Med* 332:162–173, 1995.

E-8

Clinical History

A 79-year-old man with palpitations and lightheadedness. He takes no medications.

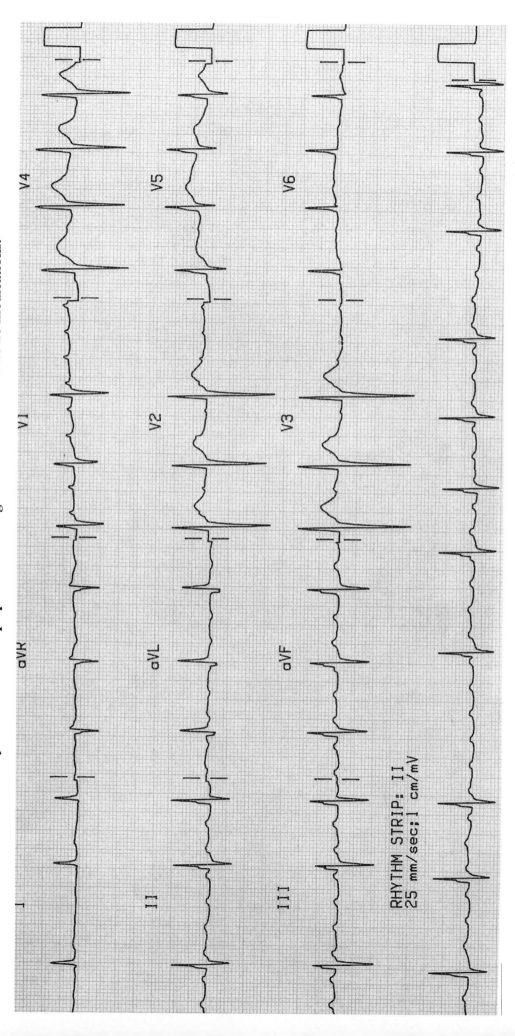

RHYTHM STRIP: II
25 mm/sec;1 cm/mV

E-9

NARRATIVE INTERPRETATION

Rhythm:	**Sinus tachycardia**
Rate:	**105**
Intervals:	**PR 0.18, QRS 0.08, QT 0.30**
Axis:	**+75 degrees**

Abnormalities

Heart rate greater than 100 bpm. Q wave leads I, aVL, V1–V6. ST elevation leads I, aVL, V1–V6. Slight ST depression leads III, aVF.

Synthesis

Sinus tachycardia. Extensive anterior and lateral MI with ST abnormalities of acute myocardial injury. ST depression in leads III, aVF suggesting myocardial ischemia.

TEST ANSWERS: 4, 87, 89, 100, 101.

Comment: This patient suffered an extensive MI secondary to occlusion of the proximal left anterior descending coronary artery. The abnormalities in the lateral leads reflect occlusion of this artery proximal to a large diagonal vessel that supplied the lateral wall of the left ventricle. The rapid heart rate is likely a compensatory mechanism to maintain cardiac output in the presence of extensive loss of functioning myocardium.

E-9

Clinical History

A 60-year-old man in the CCU.

I

aVR

V1

V4

II

aVL

V2

V5

III

aVF

V3

V6

RHYTHM STRIP: II
25 mm/sec; 1 cm/mV

E-10

NARRATIVE INTERPRETATION

Rhythm:	**Sinus**
Rate:	**82**
Intervals:	**PR 0.20, QRS 0.10, QT 0.32**
Axis:	**+60 degrees**

Abnormalities

QS leads V1–V2. Q wave leads V3–V4. ST depression leads I, II, III, aVF, V4–V6. ST elevation leads V1–V3. T-wave inversion leads aVL, V3. Biphasic T wave leads I, V4–V6. S wave lead V2 + R wave lead V5 greater than 35 mm.

Synthesis

Sinus rhythm. LVH. Anterior wall MI of indeterminate age. ST elevation suggestive of ventricular aneurysm (cannot exclude ST abnormalities of acute myocardial injury). Nonspecific ST-T-wave abnormalities.

TEST ANSWERS: 1, 78, (82), 84, 95, (100), (103), 106.

Comment: This tracing demonstrates the coexistence of LVH and prior anterior MI. LVH may produce poor R-wave progression or even a QS pattern in leads V1–V3 and mimic anteroseptal MI. The QR pattern in lead V3 in this tracing, however, cannot be ascribed to LVH alone and points to the additional diagnosis of anterior wall infarction. It is difficult to confirm whether the septum is involved.

When combined with the clinical history, the ST elevation seen in leads V1–V3 suggests formation of a ventricular aneurysm. Comparison with a prior tracing is required to exclude acute injury. The additional, diffuse ST-T-wave abnormalities are likely to be from a combination of factors including, LVH, anterior wall MI, and digitalis effect and are therefore listed as nonspecific. The effect of digitalis is also suggested by a relatively short QT interval.

E-10

Clinical History

An 84-year-old man seen in a clinic with chronic dyspnea on exertion. Medications include digitalis, diuretics, and an ACE inhibitor.

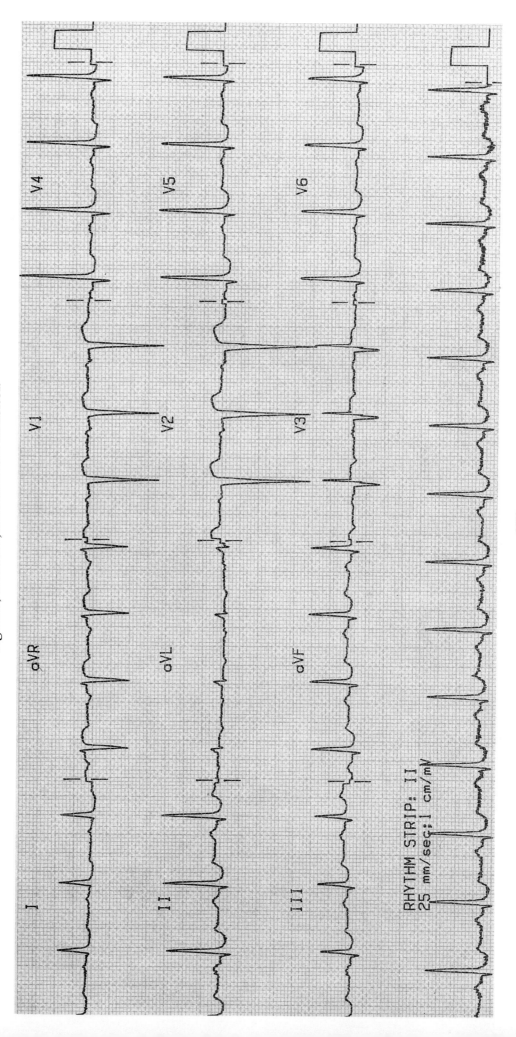

357

E-11

NARRATIVE INTERPRETATION

Rhythm:	**Sinus bradycardia with first-degree AV block**
Rate:	**58**
Intervals:	**PR 0.24, QRS 0.08, QT 0.38**
Axis:	**0 degrees**

Abnormalities
Heart rate less than 60 bpm. Prolonged PR interval.

Synthesis
Sinus bradycardia. First-degree AV block. Otherwise within normal limits.

TEST ANSWERS: 3, 42.

Comment: First-degree AV block is diagnosed when the PR interval is prolonged beyond 0.20 s. This may be observed in completely healthy persons. In a review of a number of series, the overall prevalence of first-degree AV block in healthy servicemen was 0.6 percent. One study analyzed the long-term prognosis of first-degree AV block in 3983 healthy men. In the 30 years of followup, there was no difference in mortality compared with individuals without first-degree AV block.

A number of medications may prolong the PR interval, including beta-blockers, digoxin, verapamil, and diltiazem. Acute prolongation of the PR interval may also be seen in inferior wall MI, acute rheumatic fever, or Lyme carditis.

FURTHER READING
Barrett PA, Peter CT, Swan HJC, et al: The frequency and prognostic significance of electrocardiographic abnormalities in clinically normal individuals. *Prog Cardiovasc Dis* 23:299–319, 1981.

Mymin D, Matewson FAL, Tate RB, Manfreda J: The natural history of primary first-degree atrioventricular heart block. *N Engl J Med* 315:1183–1187, 1986.

E-11

Clinical History

A 60-year-old asymptomatic man seen for an insurance physical. He takes no medications.

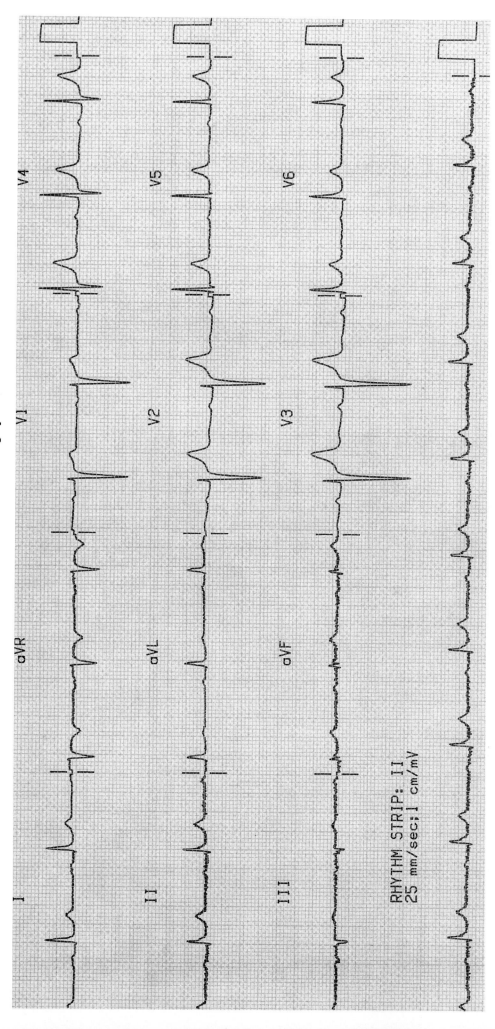

E-12

NARRATIVE INTERPRETATION

> **Rhythm:** Sinus bradycardia, junctional escape rhythm
> **Rate:** 55 (sinus bradycardia), 46 (junctional escape rhythm)
> **Intervals:** PR 0.16, QRS 0.08, QT 0.44
> **Axis:** +45 degrees

Abnormalities
Heart rate less than 60 bpm. Sinus pause. Junctional escape beats. Two-beat junctional escape rhythm on rhythm strip. ST depression leads I, II, aVF, V4–V6.

Synthesis
Sinus bradycardia with sinus pause. Junctional escape beats and brief junctional escape rhythm. Nonspecific ST-segment abnormalities.

TEST ANSWERS: 3, 7, 22, 24, 106.

Comment: The basic rhythm is sinus bradycardia with periodic sinus pauses. The intrinsic sinus rate is approximately 55 bpm and the rate of the escape rhythm is approximately 46 bpm. The sixth complex of the rhythm strip is a single junctional escape beat.

The differential diagnosis of this tracing includes sinus arrhythmia with wandering atrial pacemaker to the AV junction. This is unlikely because of the rather abrupt pause in the sinus rate on the rhythm strip and the lack of significant variation in the PP interval. SA block should also be considered, however the junctional escape beats interrupt the sinus mechanism and preclude further analysis. The likely cause of this patient's rhythm disturbance was digoxin, which was also responsible for the non-specific ST changes.

E-12

Clinical History
A 91-year-old man with congestive heart failure.

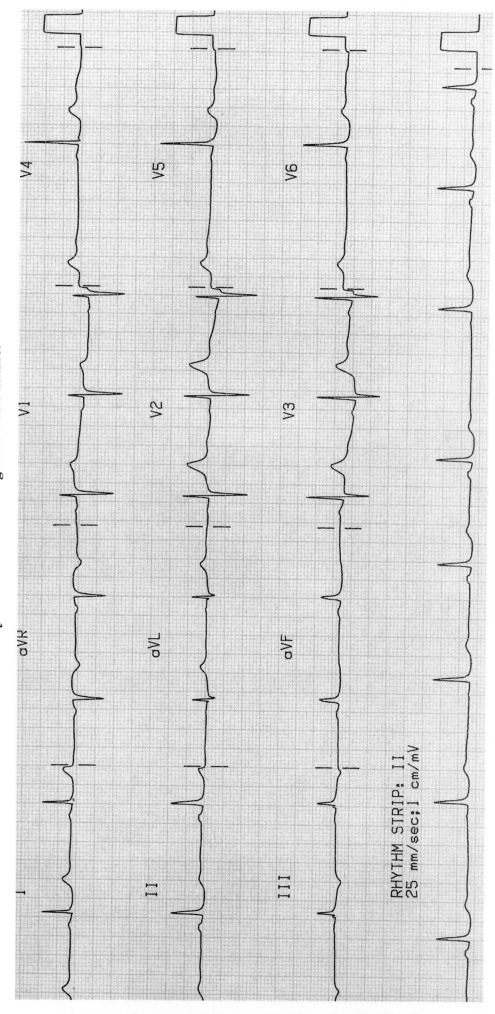

NARRATIVE INTERPRETATION E-13

Rhythm:	**Atrial fibrillation**
Rate:	**75 (average)**
Intervals:	**PR −, QRS 0.08, QT 0.38**
Axis:	**−15 degrees**

Abnormalities

Q wave leads II, III, aVF. ST elevation leads II, III, aVF. T-wave inversion leads II, III, aVF, V4–V6. Tall R wave with R greater than S and upright T wave lead V2. Pacemaker complexes at rate of 60 bpm with no relationship to QRS complex. Pacemaker fails to depolarize ventricle.

Synthesis

Atrial fibrillation with a controlled ventricular response. Acute inferior wall and posterior wall MI with ST-T-wave abnormalities of acute myocardial injury. Pacemaker malfunction, failure to sense QRS complex. Pacemaker malfunction, failure to capture ventricle.

TEST ANSWERS: 20, 39, 40, 51, 91, 93, 100.

Comment: This electrocardiogram demonstrates an acute inferior and probable posterior wall MI. The Q waves and ST-T-wave abnormalities of the acute inferior wall are fairly obvious; however, the posterior wall involvement is more subtle. Note the tall R wave in lead V2 with slight ST depression. In the presence of a concomitant inferior wall infarction, these findings suggest posterior wall MI as well.

Two separate forms of pacemaker malfunction are present in this electrocardiogram. The pacemaker clearly fails to sense the native rhythm and is firing at a set rate of 60 bpm. Failure to capture is easily diagnosed on the rhythm strip. The first, fifth, and seventh pacemaker stimuli occur far enough outside the refractory period of the ventricle to produce capture. It is conceivable that the other pacemaker complexes fall in the refractory period and might not produce ventricular capture. In this patient, a temporary pacemaker lead had slipped out of position.

FURTHER READING

Chaitman BR: Posterior myocardial infarction revisited. *J Am Coll Cardiol* 12:1167–1168, 1988.

Huey BL, Beller GA, Kaiser DL, Gibson RS: A comprehensive analysis of myocardial infarction due to left circumflex artery occlusion: Comparison with infarction due to right coronary artery and left anterior descending artery occlusion. *J Am Coll Cardiol* 12:1156–1166, 1988.

Nestico PF, Hakki A-Hamid, Iskandrian AS, Anderson GJ: Electrocardiographic diagnosis of posterior myocardial infarction revisited: A new approach using a multivariate discriminant analysis and thallium-201 myocardial scintigraphy. *J Electrocardiol* 19:33–40, 1986.

E-13

Clinical History

A 58-year-old man in the CCU with recurrent chest pain. A temporary ventricular pacemaker was placed earlier in his hospital course for symptomatic bradyarrhythmias.

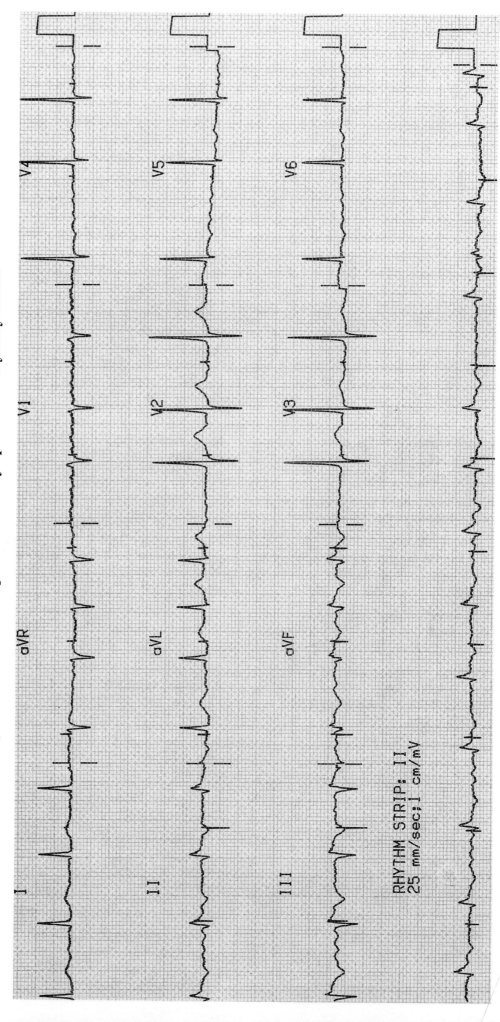

RHYTHM STRIP: II
25 mm/sec; 1 cm/mV

E-14

NARRATIVE INTERPRETATION

Rhythm:	**Sinus**
Rate:	**82**
Intervals:	**PR 0.18, QRS 0.12, QT 0.38**
Axis:	**−15 degrees**

Abnormalities
Broad, slurred QRS leads I, aVL, V5–V6. ST depression leads I, aVL, V4–V6. T-wave inversion leads I, aVL. Biphasic T wave leads V5, V6. (S wave lead V2 + R wave lead V5 greater than 45 mm.)

Synthesis
Sinus rhythm. LBBB. Associated ST-T-wave abnormalities (consider LVH).

TEST ANSWERS: 1, 74, (78), 104.

Comment: The diagnosis of LVH in the presence of LBBB is problematic and should generally be avoided. However, a substantial number of patients with LBBB have anatomic LVH. One of the more reliable criterion to diagnose LVH with LBBB is the S wave in lead V2 + R wave lead V5 greater than 45 mm. This was reported in one study to have a sensitivity of 86 percent and a specificity of 100 percent. This patient indeed had marked LVH secondary to aortic stenosis.

FURTHER READING
Klein RC, Vera Z, DeMaria JA, Mason DT: Electrocardiographic diagnosis of left ventricular hypertrophy in the presence of left bundle branch block. *Am Heart J* 108:502–506, 1984.

E-14

Clinical History
A 72-year-old man with a harsh systolic murmur.

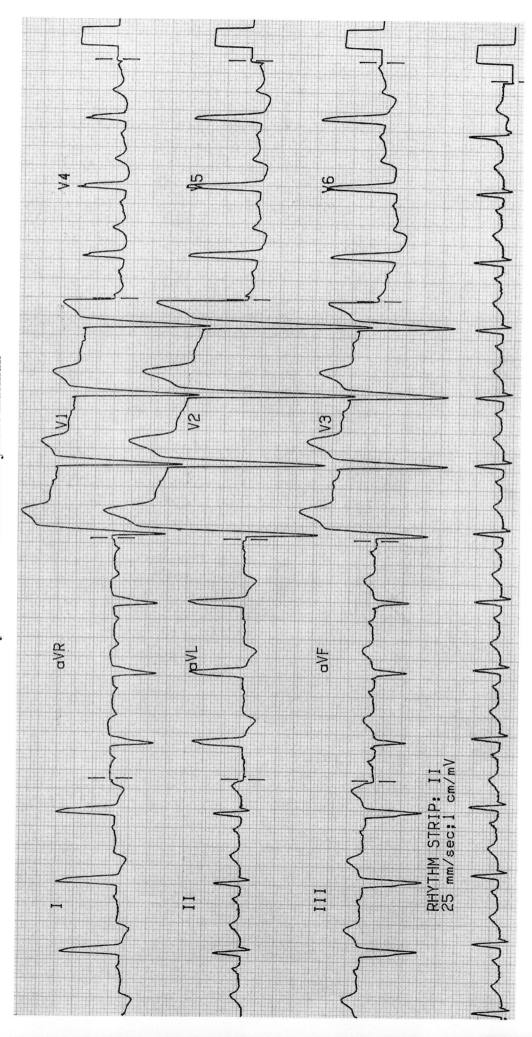

RHYTHM STRIP: II
25 mm/sec; 1 cm/mV

E-15

NARRATIVE INTERPRETATION

Rhythm:	**Sinus**
Rate:	**72**
Intervals:	**PR 0.16, QRS 0.08, QT 0.40**
Axis:	**+60 degrees**

Abnormalities
Slight ST depression leads II, aVF, V6.

Synthesis
Sinus rhythm. Nonspecific ST abnormalities.

TEST ANSWERS: 1, 106.

Comment: Patients may have extensive coronary heart disease with only subtle or no abnormalities on the resting electrocardiogram. The ST abnormalities in this tracing are quite minor. Nevertheless, this patient had severe, diffuse coronary disease on angiography. The presence of ST-T-wave abnormalities has prognostic relevance in patients with coronary heart disease. One large study of nearly 10,000 patients found that in patients with coronary heart disease, the presence of ST-T-wave abnormalities was an independent predictor of reduced survival. In patients without coronary disease, ST-T-wave abnormaltities had no independent effect on prognosis.

FURTHER READING

Crenshaw JH, Mirvis DM, El-Zeky F, et al: Interactive effects of ST-T-wave abnormalities on survival of patients with coronary artery disease. *J Am Coll Cardiol* 18:413–420, 1991.

Daviglus ML, Liao Y, Greenland P, et al: Association of nonspecific minor ST-T abnormalities with cardiovascular mortality. *JAMA* 281:530–536, 1999.

Joy M, Trump DW: Significance of minor ST segment and T wave changes in the resting electrocardiogram of asymptomatic subjects. *Br Heart J* 45:48–55, 1981.

E-15

Clinical History

A 59-year-old diabetic woman admitted to the CCU.

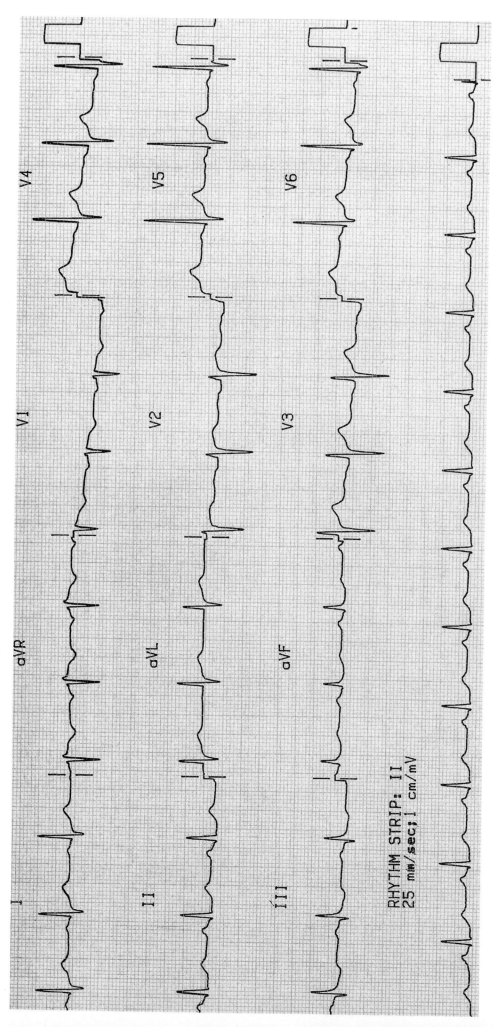

aVR

V1

V4

II

aVL

V2

V5

III

aVF

V3

V6

RHYTHM STRIP: II
25 mm/sec; 1 cm/mV

NARRATIVE INTERPRETATION E-16

Rhythm:	**Sinus with second-degree AV block, Mobitz type I**
Rate:	**75**
Intervals:	**PR variable, QRS 0.08, QT 0.40**
Axis:	**−45 degrees**

Abnormalities

Variable PR intervals with periodic failure to conduct. Atrial escape complex on rhythm strip. Axis leftward of −30 degrees. R wave less than 3 mm leads V1–V3 with small R wave lead V4. Q wave leads V5–V6. S wave lead V2 + R wave lead V5 greater than 35 mm. R wave lead aVL + S wave lead V3 greater than 28 mm in a man. T-wave inverted leads I, aVL, V5–V6. ST depression leads aVL, V5–V6. Prolonged QTc interval.

Synthesis

Sinus rhythm. Second-degree AV block, Mobitz type I (Wenckebach). Atrial escape complex on rhythm strip. Poor (reverse) R-wave progression. Left-axis deviation. Left anterior fascicular block. LVH. Associated ST-T-wave abnormalities. Anterolateral wall MI of indeterminate age. Possible anterior wall MI of indeterminate age. Possible inferior wall MI of indeterminate age. Prolonged QTc.

TEST ANSWERS: 1, 43, 64, 66, 72, 78, (84), 86, (92), 103, 109.

Comment: The rhythm is easily identified as sinus with a Wenckebach pattern. Note that the ninth P wave on the rhythm strip has a different configuration than the others and is likely a *low* atrial escape complex.

Left-axis deviation with LAFB is present. A possible concomitant inferior MI is suggested by the notched S wave in lead II. A small Q wave in lead II appears in some of the complexes, while in others a "micro" R wave remains.

The Q waves in the left precordial leads suggest a previous anterolateral MI. Prior anterior wall MI is also possible on the basis of reverse R-wave progression in leads V1–V4. This is difficult to confirm in the presence of LVH and left-axis deviation.

FURTHER READING

DePace NL, Colby J, Hakki A, et al: Poor R-wave progression in the precordial leads: Clinical implications for the diagnosis of myocardial infarction. *J Am Coll Cardiol* 2:1073–1079, 1983.

Warner RA, Reger M, Hill NE, et al: Electrocardiographic criteria for the diagnosis of anterior myocardial infarction: Importance of the duration of precordial R waves. *Am J Cardiol* 52:690–692, 1983.

Zema MJ, Kligfield P: Electrocardiographic poor R-wave progression. I. Correlation with the Frank vectorcardiogram. *J Electrocardiol* 12:3–10, 1979.

Zema MJ, Kligfield P: Electrocardiographic poor R-wave progression. II. Correlation with angiography. *J Electrocardiol* 12:11–15, 1979.

E-16

Clinical History
A 74-year-old man with lightheadedness.

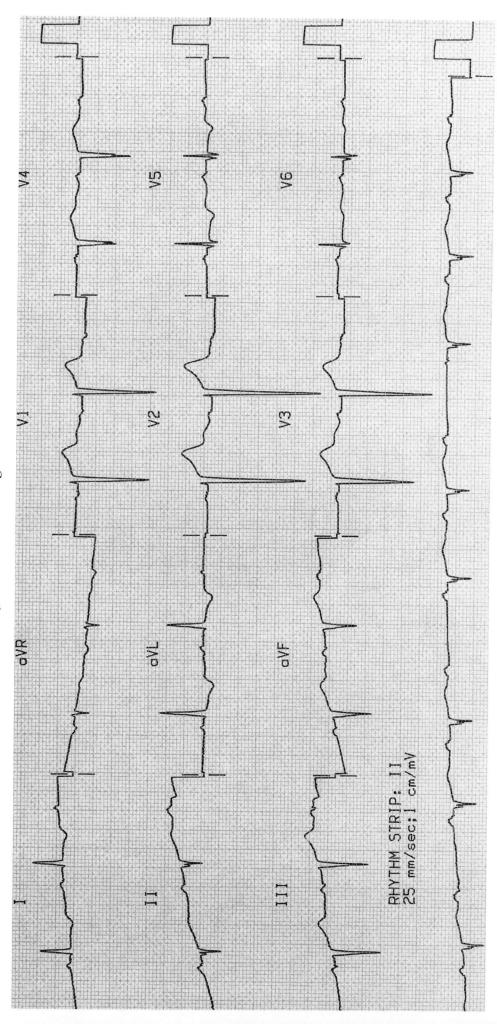

E-17

NARRATIVE INTERPRETATION

Rhythm: AV junctional rhythm
Rate: 65
Intervals: PR 0.11, QRS 0.08, QT 0.36
Axis: −15 degrees

Abnormalities
Inverted P wave leads II, III, aVF with short PR interval.

Synthesis
AV junctional rhythm (possibly accelerated). Otherwise within normal limits.

TEST ANSWERS: 21, (23).

Comment: This patient had suppression of the sinus node induced by verapamil, allowing a subsidiary pacemaker in the AV junctional tissue to emerge. Without first knowing the intrinsic sinus rate, it is not possible to determine whether this rhythm is an escape rhythm induced by sinus node depression or whether the AV junctional rhythm usurps control because of enhanced automaticity. For this reason, this example is simply characterized as *AV junctional rhythm* rather than *accelerated* or *escape* rhythm. It would not be unreasonable to classify this rhythm as *accelerated* because the rate is slightly faster than is normally expected for the AV junction.

E-17

Clinical History

A 67-year-old man taking verapamil for hypertension.

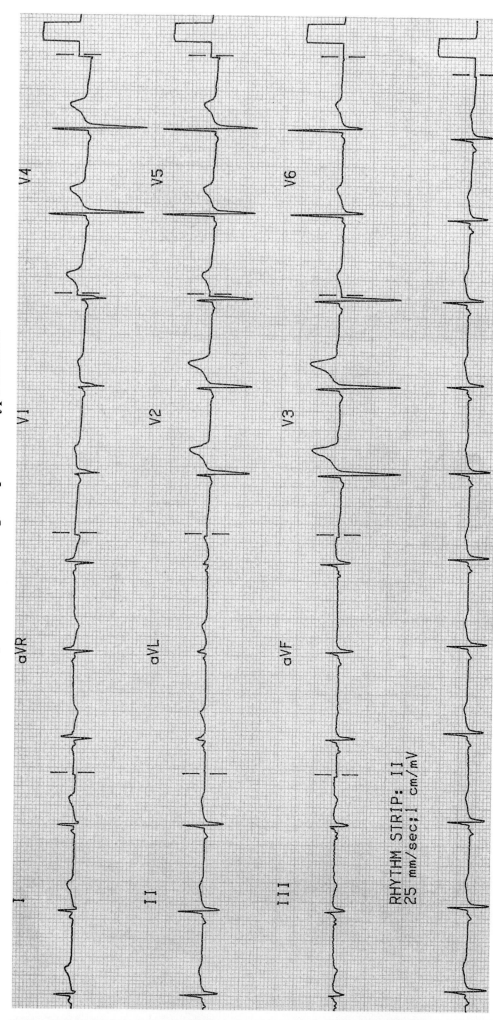

RHYTHM STRIP: II
25 mm/sec; 1 cm/mV

E-18

NARRATIVE INTERPRETATION

Rhythm:	**Sinus**
Rate:	**84**
Intervals:	**PR 0.16, QRS 0.08, QT 0.38**
Axis:	**+110 degrees**

Abnormalities
Axis rightward of +90 degrees. Abnormal P terminal force lead V1. Tall R wave leads V1–V2.

Synthesis
Sinus rhythm. Left atrial abnormality. Right-axis deviation. RVH.

TEST ANSWERS: 1, 60, 65, 79.

Comment: This electrocardiogram demonstrates the characteristic findings of a patient with long-standing mitral stenosis. There is a markedly abnormal P terminal force in V1 and a broad, notched P wave in lead II. Right-axis deviation and tall R waves in the right precordial leads are indicative of RVH, the result of the increased right-sided pressures seen in critical mitral stenosis.

E-18

Clinical History

A 29-year-old woman with a history of rheumatic fever.

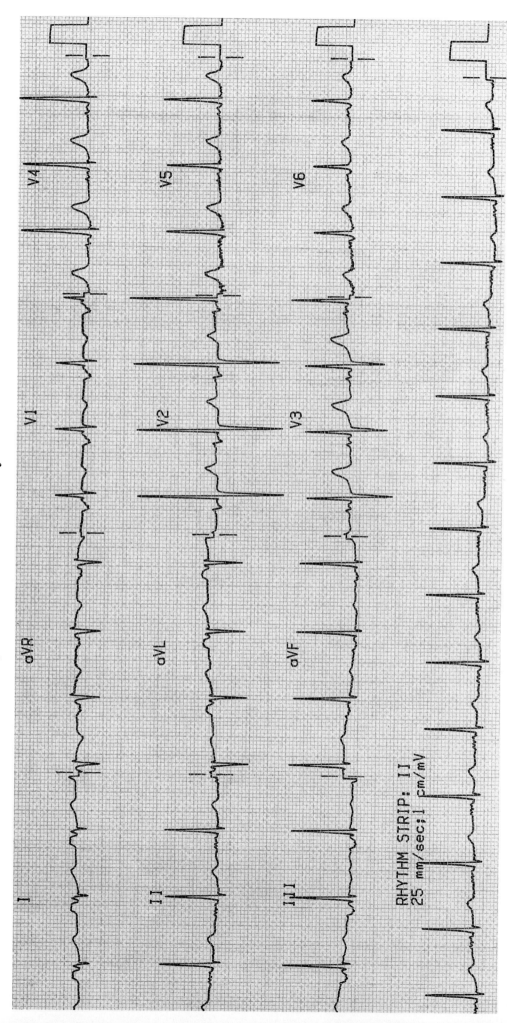

RHYTHM STRIP: II
25 mm/sec; 1 cm/mV

E-19

NARRATIVE INTERPRETATION

Rhythm:	**Sinus with complete AV block, accelerated AV junctional rhythm**
Rate:	**Atrial rate 88, AV junctional rate 74**
Intervals:	**PR –, QRS 0.13, QT 0.40**
Axis:	**–45 degrees**

Abnormalities

P waves fail to conduct to ventricles. Axis leftward of –30 degrees. R wave lead aVL greater than 11 mm. R wave aVL + S wave lead V3 greater than 20 mm in a woman. Prolonged QRS with rSR' and T-wave inversion leads V1–V2. VPC. Alteration and reset of sinus and AV junctional cycle post-VPC.

Synthesis

Sinus rhythm with complete AV block. Accelerated AV junctional rhythm. AV dissociation. VPC. Left-axis deviation. LAFB. RBBB with associated ST-T-wave abnormalities. LVH. (Cycle alteration probably secondary to retrograde atrial activation from ventricular depolarization.)

TEST ANSWERS: 1, 23, 26, 47, 53, (55), 64, 70, 72, 78, 104.

Comment: This is a complex ECG. Notice first that despite a sinus mechanism, there is no constant relationship between the P waves and QRS complexes. The P waves "march through" characteristic of AV dissociation. Several of the sinus beats fail to conduct to the ventricles when expected; therefore, complete AV block is present.

An accelerated AV junctional rhythm has become the dominant pacemaker. Note that the relatively high rate of the AV junctional rhythm characterizes it as *accelerated* and not as an *escape* mechanism.

An interesting finding on the rhythm strip occurs after the VPC. Note that both the junctional complex and nonconducted P wave occur earlier than expected. This is usually seen when the dominant rhythm is other than sinus and a VPC depolarizes the underlying pacemaker in the AV junction. The P wave following the VPC occurs early, also secondary to retrograde conduction and a resetting of the sinus cycle.

Remember that with complete RBBB, the first 0.06 s of the complex may be interpreted in a normal fashion. Criteria for LVH and LAFB are present.

E-19

Clinical History

An 89-year-old woman with congestive heart failure. Medications include digoxin.

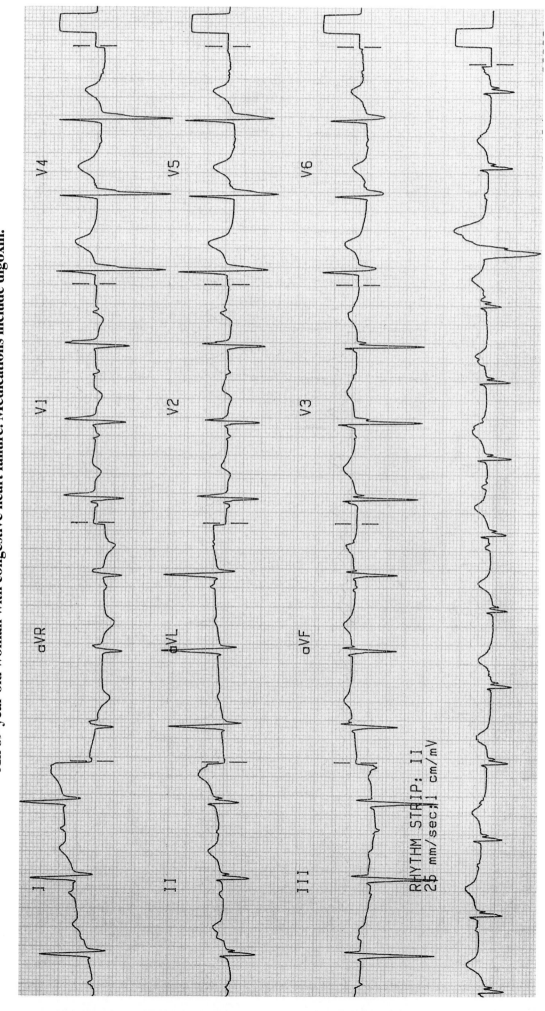

E-20

NARRATIVE INTERPRETATION

Rhythm:	**Atrial tachycardia with variable (predominantly 2:1) AV conduction**
Rate:	**Atrial rate 250, ventricular rate 125**
Intervals:	**PR 0.28, QRS 0.08, QT 0.28**
Axis:	**–30 degrees**

Abnormalities

R-wave amplitude less than 3 mm leads V1–V3. Slight ST depression leads V4–V6. T-wave inversion lead aVL. VPC.

Synthesis

Atrial tachycardia with predominantly 2:1 AV conduction (brief period of variable AV conduction). Poor R-wave progression. Nonspecific ST-segment abnormalities. VPC.

TEST ANSWERS: 17, 26, 50, (51), 66, 106.

Comment: On initial examination, the reader might mistakenly interpret this rhythm as sinus tachycardia. However, a brief period of variable AV conduction is evident prior to the first complex of the precordial leads, exposing the P waves of atrial tachycardia. This tracing is difficult to interpret because the reader might also mistake the rhythm for atrial flutter. Note the isoelectric baseline between the P waves, best seen in lead V1, as well as the absence of true flutter waves. These characteristics help to distinguish this rhythm as atrial tachycardia with 2:1 AV conduction rather than atrial flutter. Like atrial flutter, the AV node conducts in a 2:1 fashion when presented with an atrial rate of 250; therefore, the 2:1 ratio does not actually represent AV block. The 2:1 conduction is a physiologic property of the AV node. Higher ratios of conduction however, are not physiologic (seen here only briefly).

376

E-20

Clinical History

A 67-year-old woman with palpitations.

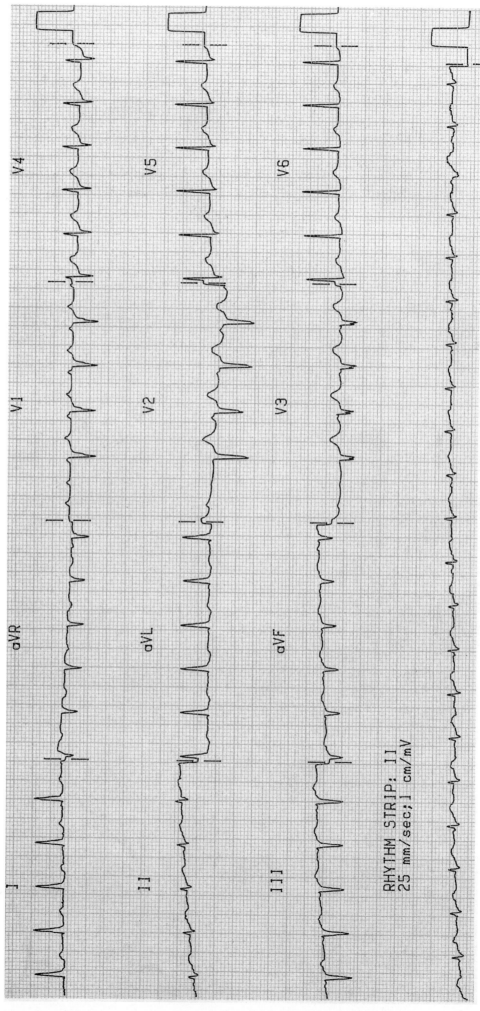

RHYTHM STRIP: II
25 mm/sec;1 cm/mV

E-21

NARRATIVE INTERPRETATION

Rhythm:	**Sinus tachycardia**
Rate:	**120**
Intervals:	**PR 0.16, QRS 0.10, QT 0.28**
Axis:	**−30 degrees**

Abnormalities

Heart rate greater than 100 bpm. VPCs. ST-segment elevation at J point leads V1–V4. T-wave inversion leads I, aVL, V5–V6. S wave lead V2 + R wave lead V5 greater than 35 mm. R wave lead aVL + S wave lead V3 greater than 28 mm in a man.

Synthesis

Sinus tachycardia. VPCs. Fusion complex (on rhythm strip). LVH by voltage criteria. Associated ST-T-wave abnormalities. (Clinical correlation required to exclude myocardial injury.)

TEST ANSWERS: 4, 26, 56, 78, (100), 103.

Comment: This patient had an idiopathic dilated cardiomyopathy with left ventricular dilatation. The ST configuration in leads V1–V3, and especially V4, is suspicious for myocardial injury. Review of old tracings however, revealed that the ST findings were chronic and due to LVH. In the absence of serial tracings, one should at least consider the potential of myocardial injury.

The different morphologies of the VPCs seen on the rhythm strip are caused by fusion with conduction from the sinus mechanism. This phenomenon is clearest in the third-from-last beat on the rhythm strip.

E-21

Clinical History
A 50-year-old man with dyspnea.

RHYTHM STRIP: II
25 mm/sec; 1 cm/mV

I aVR V1 V4

II aVL V2 V5

III aVF V3 V6

379

E-22

NARRATIVE INTERPRETATION

Rhythm:	**Sinus**
Rate:	**90**
Intervals:	**PR 0.14, QRS 0.11, QT 0.36**
Axis:	**−15 degrees**

Abnormalities

Abnormal P terminal force V1. S wave lead V2 + R wave lead V5 greater than 35 mm. R wave lead aVL greater than 11 mm. R wave aVL + S wave lead V3 greater than 20 mm in a woman. R wave lead I + S wave lead III greater than 25 mm. ST depression leads I, aVL, V6. T-wave inversion leads I, aVL, V6. QS leads V1–V2. "Micro" R wave lead V3. Prolonged QRS duration.

Synthesis

Sinus rhythm. Left atrial abnormality. Left ventricular hypertrophy with associated ST-T-wave abnormalities. Intraventricular conduction delay (cannot exclude prior anteroseptal myocardial infarction).

TEST ANSWERS: 1, 60, 76, 78, (82), 103.

Comment: Note that a *pseudoinfarction* pattern is present in leads V1–V3. The diagnosis of anteroseptal MI is difficult in the presence of LVH. The transitional zone is commonly shifted leftward in patients with LVH and may produce either poor R-wave progression, or as in this example, a QS pattern in the right precordial leads. Although an anteroseptal MI cannot be excluded, there should be additional supporting evidence with either clinical data or serial electrocardiograms to support this diagnosis.

FURTHER READING

Goldberger AL: ECG simulators of myocardial infarction. Part I. Pathophysiology and differential diagnosis of pseudoinfarct Q-wave patterns. *PACE* 5:106–119, 1982.

E-22

Clinical History

A 77-year-old woman admitted with pneumonia.

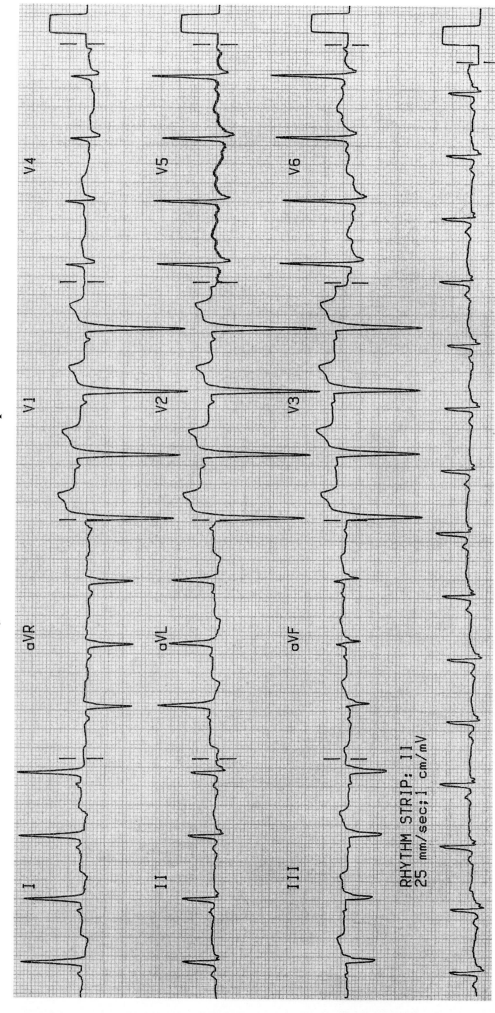

E-23

NARRATIVE INTERPRETATION

Rhythm:	Sinus bradycardia, sinus pause
Rate:	52
Intervals:	PR 0.16, QRS 0.08, QT 0.40
Axis:	+60 degrees

Abnormalities

Heart rate less than 60 bpm. Sinus pause with AV junctional escape complexes. Limb lead voltage less than 5 mm. S wave lead V2 + R wave lead V5 greater than 35 mm. R wave aVL + S wave lead V3 greater than 20 mm in a woman. R wave leads V1–V3 less than 3 mm. ST depression leads V4–V6. Low T-wave voltage in limb leads. T-wave biphasic leads V5–V6.

Synthesis

Sinus bradycardia with sinus pause. AV junctional escape complexes. Low voltage in limb leads. Poor R-wave progression. LVH. Associated nonspecific ST-T-wave abnormalities.

TEST ANSWERS: 3, 7, 24, 66, 67, 78, 103.

Comment: This tracing demonstrates sinus bradycardia with a periodic sinus pause and AV junctional escape beats. Note that the intrinsic sinus bradycardia rate is around 52 bpm, whereas the AV junctional escape rate is about 42 bpm.

This patient has the interesting combination of low voltage in the limb leads secondary to chronic pulmonary disease and increased voltage in the precordial leads secondary to long-standing hypertension.

E-23

Clinical History

A 79-year-old woman with long-standing COPD.

INTERPRETED BY

I aVR V1 V4

II aVL V2 V5

III aVF V3 V6

RHYTHM STRIP: II
25 mm/sec; 1 cm/mV

E-24

NARRATIVE INTERPRETATION

> **Rhythm:** **Sinus**
> **Rate:** **87**
> **Intervals:** **PR 0.16, QRS 0.08, QT 0.36**
> **Axis:** **−45 degrees**

Abnormalities

APCs, normally conducted. Nonconducted APC. VPCs. Paired, multiform VPCs. Echo complexes. Axis leftward of −30 degrees. R wave lead aVL + S wave lead V3 greater than 20 mm in a woman. R wave leads V1–V3 less than 3 mm. ST depression leads I, aVL. ST elevation leads III, aVF, V2–V5. T-wave inversion leads I, aVL.

Synthesis

Sinus rhythm. VPCs. Paired, multifocal VPCs. VPC with echo beat and retrograde atrial activation. APCs (possible JPC). Nonconducted APC. Left-axis deviation. Left anterior fascicular block. Poor R-wave progression. LVH. Associated ST-T-wave abnormalities. Probable anterior wall MI of indeterminate age (cannot exclude ST abnormalities of recent myocardial injury or ischemia).

TEST ANSWERS: 1, 10, 12, (25), 26, 27, 28, 54, 55, 64, 66, 72, 78, 84, (100), (102), 103.

Comment: A multitude of ectopic complexes are present on this tracing. The basic sinus mechanism is seen only in the first two complexes of the rhythm strip and the first three complexes in leads V4–V6. Frequent VPCs and APCs are present. The seventh complex of the rhythm strip is a "late" VPC, that occurs just after the P wave. The T wave of this complex is tall secondary to a retrograde P wave and ventriculoatrial conduction. This retrograde P wave is then conducted back to the ventricles as an *echo* beat. The negative P wave of the ninth complex of the rhythm strip also suggests one more cycle of retrograde atrial activation with a more prolonged V-A interval. A junctional or atrial premature beat is also possible. The sinus mechanism resumes with the next complex. The 13th complex of the rhythm strip is a normally conducted APC. A second, nonconducted APC follows immediately afterward.

An anterior wall MI is suggested by the poor (reverse) R-wave progression. These were unchanged from prior tracings. The ST changes were longstanding and likely due to LVH rather than ischemia or injury. Serial tracings are required to confirm this diagnosis.

384

E-24

Clinical History

A 78-year-old woman in the ICU with gastrointestinal bleeding. She has a history of multiple myocardial infarctions (MIs).

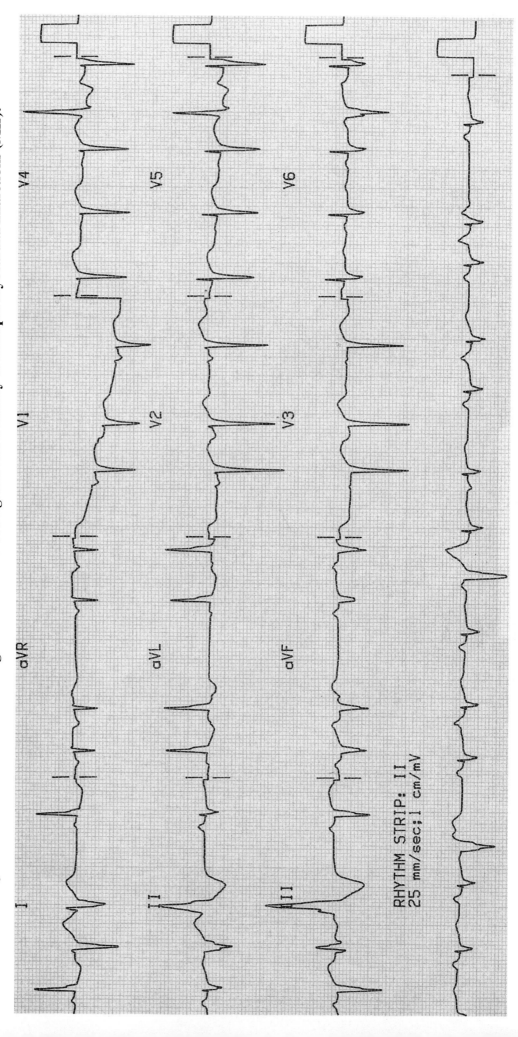

RHYTHM STRIP: II
25 mm/sec; 1 cm/mV

E-25

NARRATIVE INTERPRETATION

Rhythm:	**Sinus**
Rate:	**74**
Intervals:	**PR 0.20, QRS 0.10, QT 0.40**
Axis:	**+15 degrees**

Abnormalities

ST depression leads V4–V6. T-wave inversion leads I, II, aVL, aVF, V3–V6. S wave lead V2 + R wave lead V5 greater than 35 mm. R wave aVL + S wave lead V3 greater than 20 mm in a woman. R wave less than 3 mm leads V1–V3.

Synthesis

Sinus rhythm. LVH by voltage criteria. ST-T-wave abnormalities associated either with LVH or secondary to myocardial ischemia, or both. Poor R-wave progression.

TEST ANSWERS: 1, 66, 78, 102, 103.

Comment: At first glance, there appears to be a left bundle branch pattern in lead aVL; however, criteria for LBBB are absent in view of a QRS duration of only 0.10 s. Incomplete LBBB is a consideration, but there is no significant slurring of the R wave in the left precordial leads or delay in the intrinsicoid deflection. There is loss of the septal Q waves in the left precordial leads, a finding in incomplete LBBB and in septal fibrosis.

The poor R-wave progression is likely secondary to LVH; however, a prior anteroseptal wall MI cannot be excluded. The ST-T-wave abnormalities appear more pronounced than those normally seen in LVH alone and suggest the diagnosis of coronary heart disease.

FURTHER READING

Romanelli R, Willis WH Jr, Mitchell WA, Boucek RJ: Coronary arteriograms and myocardial scintigrams in the electrocardiographic syndrome of septal fibrosis. *Am Heart J* 100:617–621, 1980.

Clinical History

A 72-year-old woman seen on routine follow-up.

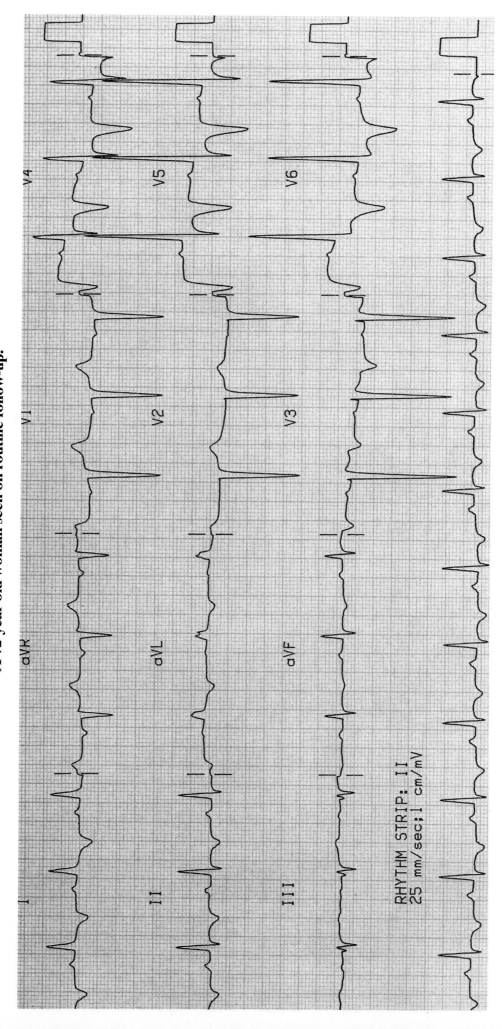

RHYTHM STRIP: II
25 mm/sec; 1 cm/mV

E-26

NARRATIVE INTERPRETATION

Rhythm:	**Sinus**
Rate:	**61**
Intervals:	**PR 0.18, QRS 0.08, QT 0.36**
Axis:	**Uninterpretable**

Abnormalities
Electrode reversal. Tracing uninterpretable.

Synthesis
Sinus rhythm. Right arm and right leg limb electrode reversal.

TEST ANSWERS: 1, 112.

Comment: This tracing demonstrates the characteristic findings of a reversal of the right arm and right leg electrodes. The P wave and QRS complex are negative in leads I and aVL and are positive in lead aVR. Lead II appears as isoelectric because this lead now records the electrical potential between the right and left legs, which is virtually zero. Remember that apparent asystole in a single lead of the electrocardiogram may be artifactual because of incorrect electrode placement. More than one monitoring lead is always desirable.

E-26

Clinical History

A 38-year-old asymptomatic man.

RHYTHM STRIP: II
25 mm/sec; 1 cm/mV

389

E-27

NARRATIVE INTERPRETATION

Rhythm:	**Atrial fibrillation with complete AV block, AV junctional escape rhythm**
Rate:	**45**
Intervals:	**PR −, QRS 0.08, QT 0.38**
Axis:	**+105 degrees**

Abnormalities
Axis rightward of +90 degrees. Limb-lead voltage less than 5 mm. R wave leads V1–V3 less than 3 mm. ST depression leads V3–V6. T-wave inversion leads II, III, aVF, V4–V6.

Synthesis
Atrial fibrillation with complete AV block. AV junctional escape rhythm. Low-voltage limb leads. Right-axis deviation. Nonspecific ST-T-wave abnormalities. Poor R-wave progression.

TEST ANSWERS: 20, 22, 47, 65, 66, 67, 106.

Comment: This patient developed renal insufficiency from marked dehydration. As a result, digoxin accumulated to toxic levels. A "regularized" rhythm in a patient with atrial fibrillation should raise the suspicion of digitalis toxicity. Electronic filtering of an electrocardiogram, present in this electrocardiogram, may make interpretation more difficult by obscuring the fibrillatory waves. Look closely in lead V2, where atrial fibrillation can be identified as the underlying rhythm. Confirmation is best made after examining prior tracings.

Additional items in this electrocardiogram are findings suggestive of chronic pulmonary disease. A mean QRS axis of +105 degrees is unusual in older individuals. Low voltage and poor R-wave progression are also characteristic of emphysema.

FURTHER READING
Fisch C, Knoebel SB: Digitalis cardiotoxicity. *J Am Coll Cardiol* 5:91A–98A, 1985.
Smith TW, Antman EM, Friedman PL, et al: Digitalis glycosides: Mechanisms and manifestations of toxicity. *Prog Cardiovasc Dis* 27:21–56, 1984.

E-27

Clinical History

A 75-year-old man with chronic atrial fibrillation with nausea and dehydration. Medications include digoxin. He is a long-time smoker.

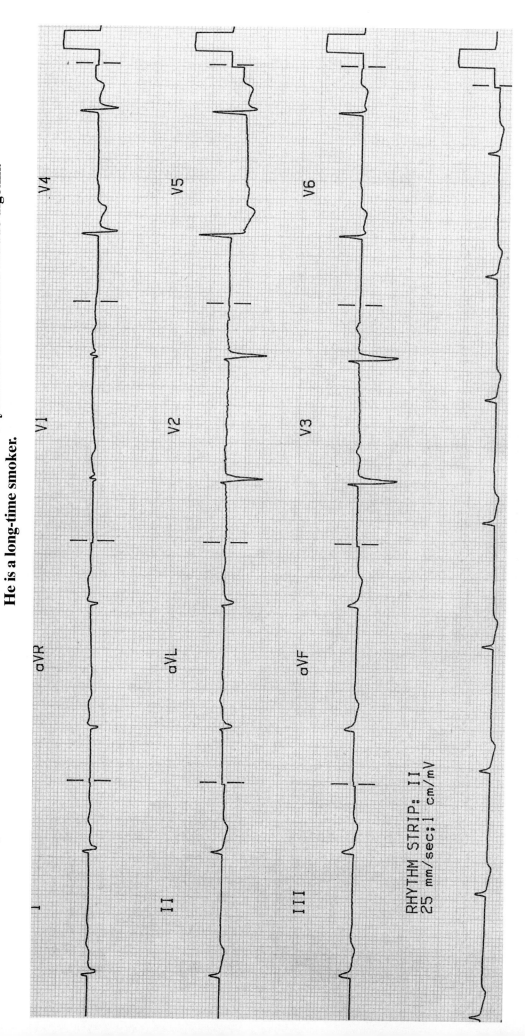

E-28

NARRATIVE INTERPRETATION

Rhythm:	**Sinus**
Rate:	**76**
Intervals:	**PR 0.12, QRS 0.08, QT 0.38**
Axis:	**+225 (or −135) degrees**

Abnormalities

Marked right-axis deviation (or marked left superior axis deviation). Q wave leads I, aVL. "Micro" R waves with RS pattern leads V1–V6. ST elevation leads I, aVL, V5–V6. ST depression leads II, III, aVF. T-wave inversion leads I, II, III, aVF, V4–V6. Abnormal P terminal force lead V1.

Synthesis

Sinus rhythm. Extreme right-axis deviation (or extreme left superior axis deviation). Left anterior fascicular block. Left atrial abnormality. Extensive anterior MI. Lateral wall MI. ST-T-wave abnormalities suggesting myocardial ischemia. ST-T-wave abnormalities suggesting aneurysm formation. (Serial tracings required to exclude acute myocardial injury and related ischemia.)

TEST ANSWERS: 1, 60, (64), 65, 72, 88, 90, 95, (100), (101), 102.

Comment: This patient has evidence of extensive myocardial necrosis. There is loss of R forces across the entire precordium with concomitant infarction of the lateral wall. In an asymptomatic person, the persistent ST elevation in the lateral leads seen here suggests aneurysm formation. Without serial tracings or clinical correlation, one cannot distinguish the chronic ST elevation from that of recent myocardial injury.

Lateral wall MI will often produce extreme right-axis deviation (extreme left superior axis deviation). The marked superior and rightward axis shift in this example is likely secondary to left anterior fascicular block combined with a lateral and anterior infarction.

FURTHER READING

Milliken JA: Isolated and complicated left anterior fascicular block: A review of suggested electrocardiographic criteria. *J Electrocardiol* 16:199–212, 1983.

392

E-28

Clinical History

A 59-year-old asymptomatic man seen in the clinic 1 month following a CCU admission.

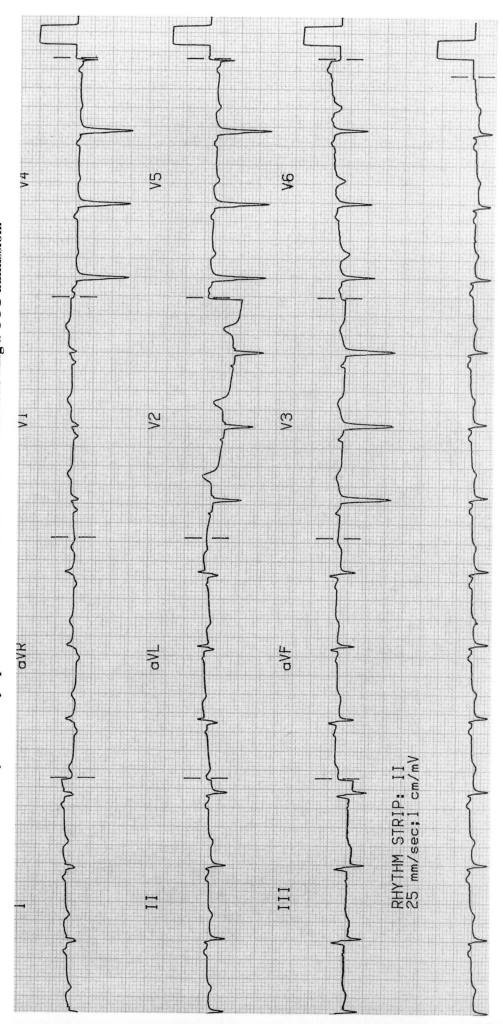

RHYTHM STRIP: II
25 mm/sec; 1 cm/mV

E-29

NARRATIVE INTERPRETATION

Rhythm:	**Sinus**
Rate	**90**
Intervals:	**PR 0.16, QRS 0.08, QT 0.32**
Axis:	**+15 degrees**

Abnormalities

S wave lead V2 + R wave lead V5 greater than 45 mm. ST depression leads I, II, aVL, aVF, V5–V6. T-wave inversion leads I, aVL, V6. Biphasic T waves leads II, V5.

Synthesis

Sinus rhythm. LVH. Associated ST-T-wave abnormalities.

TEST ANSWERS: 1, 78, 103.

Comment: This patient had LVH on the basis of congenital aortic valve disease with chronic aortic insufficiency. Patients with aortic regurgitation often have massive left ventricular enlargement. The precordial voltage criterion of 45 mm rather than 35 mm is used for the diagnosis of LVH because of the patient's young age.

FURTHER READING

Kannel WB, Dannenberg AL, Levy D: Population implications of electrocardiographic left ventricular hypertrophy. *Am J Cardiol* 60:85I–93I, 1987.

Manning GW, Smiley JR: QRS voltage criteria for left ventricular hypertrophy in a normal male population. *Circulation* 29:224–230, 1964.

Walker CHM, Rose RL: Importance of age, sex, and body habitus in the diagnosis of left ventricular hypertrophy from the precordial electrocardiogram in childhood and adolescence. *Pediatrics* 28:705–711, 1961.

Clinical History
A 31-year-old man with dyspnea on exertion.

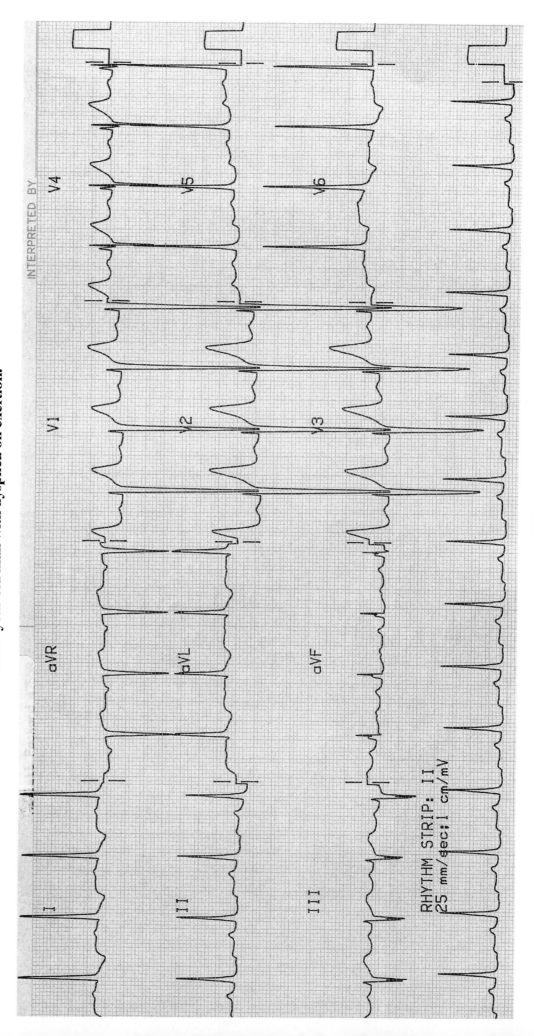

E-30

NARRATIVE INTERPRETATION

Rhythm:	**Supraventricular tachycardia**
Rate:	**135**
Intervals:	**PR −, QRS 0.08, QT 0.28**
Axis:	**+60 degrees**

Abnormalities
Rapid heart rate. ST-segment elevation at J point leads II, III, aVF, V3–V6.

Synthesis
Supraventricular tachycardia. Nonspecific ST-segment abnormalities. Normal variant, J-point elevation.

TEST ANSWERS: 18, 96, 106.

Comment: This tracing may represent an orthodromic AV reciprocating tachycardia that involves the AV node as the antegrade limb and an AV nodal bypass tract as the retrograde limb. This is the second most common mechanism of supraventricular tachycardia (second only to AV nodal reentrant tachycardia). A clue for involvement of an accessory pathway in the retrograde limb of the reentry circuit is a P wave seen after the QRS complex. With careful examination, an inverted P wave may be seen in lead I, and is also suggested in leads II, III, and aVF.

FURTHER READING
Ganz LI, Friedman PL: Supraventricular tachycardia. *N Engl J Med* 332:162–173, 1995.

E-30

Clinical History

A 28-year-old woman with palpitations seen in the emergency department.

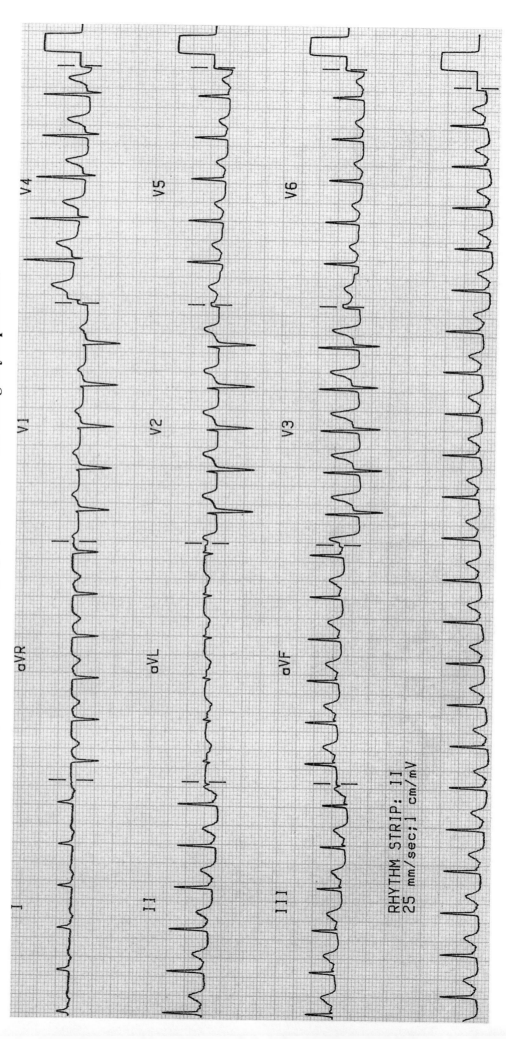

E-31

NARRATIVE INTERPRETATION

Rhythm:	**Sinus with first-degree AV block**
Rate:	**100**
Intervals:	**PR 0.24, QRS 0.08, QT 0.34**
Axis:	**+90 degrees**

Abnormalities
Prolonged PR interval. Q wave leads II, III, aVF. ST elevation leads II, III, aVF. ST depression leads I, aVL, V2–V6. T-wave inversion leads III, aVF, V4–V6. R wave leads V1–V3 less than 3 mm. VPC.

Synthesis
Sinus rhythm. First-degree AV block. VPC. Inferior wall MI with ST-T-wave abnormalities suggestive of acute myocardial injury. ST abnormalities in leads I, aVL, V2–V6 suggestive of either myocardial ischemia or reciprocal changes. Poor R-wave progression.

TEST ANSWERS: 1, 26, 42, 66, 91, 100, 101.

Comment: This patient is suffering an obvious inferior wall MI. It is controversial whether the presence of concomitant anterior ST-segment depression represents myocardial ischemia in a different coronary distribution or is simply a reciprocal electrical phenomenon.

FURTHER READING
Croft CH, Woodward W, Nicod P, et al: Clinical implications of anterior S-T-segment depression in patients with acute inferior myocardial infarction. *Am J Cardiol* 50:428–436, 1982.

Schweitzer P: The electrocardiographic diagnosis of acute myocardial infarction in the thrombolytic era. *Am Heart J* 119:642–654, 1990.

Shah PK: New insights into the electrocardiogram of acute myocardial infarction. In: Gersh BJ, Rahimtoola SH (eds), *Acute Myocardial Infarction.* New York, Elsevier, 1991, pp. 128–143.

E-31

Clinical History

A 63-year-old man with chest discomfort.

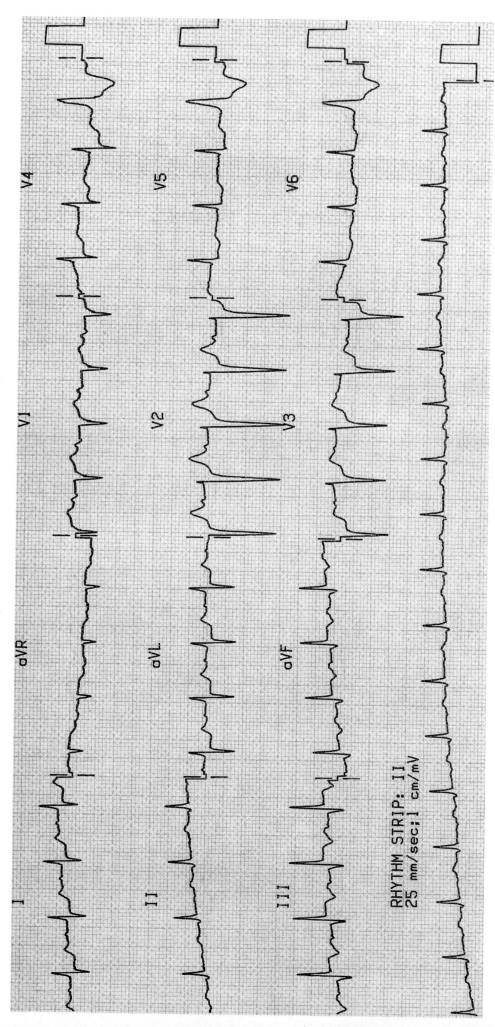

E-32

NARRATIVE INTERPRETATION

Rhythm:	**Sinus**
Rate:	**96**
Intervals:	**PR 0.20, QRS 0.08, QT 0.30**
Axis:	**−30 degrees**

Abnormalities

Abnormal P terminal force lead V1. ST depression leads I, II, aVL, aVF, V5, V6. T-wave inversion leads I, aVL, V4–V6. Biphasic T wave leads II, aVF, V2, V3. R wave lead aVL + S wave lead V3 greater than 20 mm in a woman. R-wave voltage less than 3 mm leads V1–V3. APC.

Synthesis

Sinus rhythm. APC. Left atrial abnormality. LVH. Associated ST-T-wave abnormalities. Poor R-wave progression.

TEST ANSWERS: 1, 10, 60, 66, 78, 103.

Comment: Note that left ventricular hypertrophy is diagnosed only by the newer Cornell criteria. None of the traditional limb lead or precordial criteria allow for this diagnosis. This patient did have mild cardiomegaly secondary to long-standing mitral insufficiency.

Left atrial abnormality is easily appreciated in lead V1. Remember to look carefully at the entire tracing and not overlook the single APC (fourth complex of the right precordial leads).

FURTHER READING

Casale PN, Devereux RB, Kligfield P, et al: Electrocardiographic detection of left ventricular hypertrophy: Development and prospective validation of improved criteria. *J Am Coll Cardiol* 6:572–580, 1985.
Romhilt DW, Estes EH: A point score system for the ECG diagnosis of left ventricular hypertrophy. *Am Heart J* 75:752–758, 1968.
Romhilt DW, Bove KE, Norris RJ, et al: A critical appraisal of the electrocardiographic criteria for the diagnosis of left ventricular hypertrophy. *Circulation* 40:185–195, 1969.
Surawicz B: Electrocardiographic diagnosis of chamber enlargement. *J Am Coll Cardiol* 8:711–724, 1986.

E-32

Clinical History

A 68-year-old woman admitted to the CCU for dyspnea.

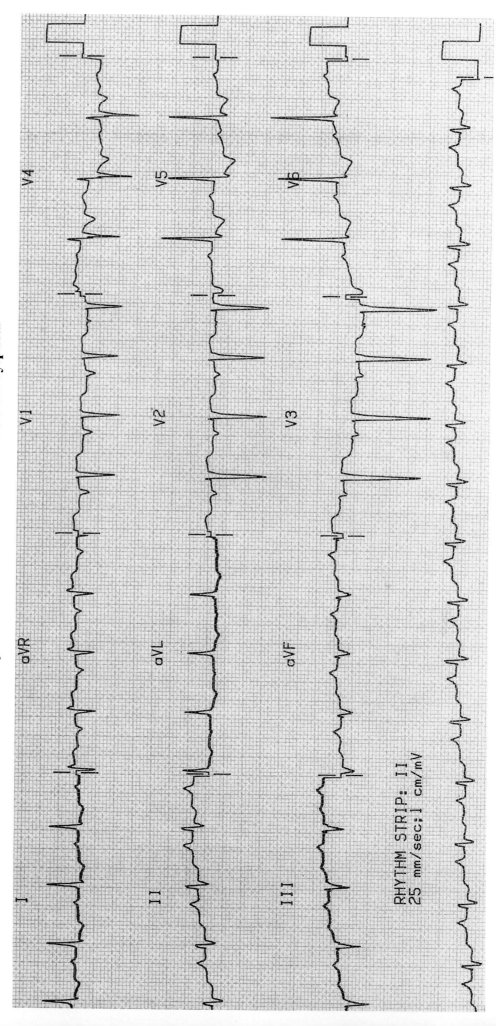

E-33

NARRATIVE INTERPRETATION

Rhythm:	**Accelerated ectopic atrial rhythm**
Rate:	**105**
Intervals:	**PR 0.16, QRS 0.08, QT 0.36**
Axis:	**+60 degrees**

Abnormalities

Rapid heart rate. Inverted P wave leads II, III, aVF. PR elevation leads II, III, aVF. APCs. Q wave aVL, V6 (with "micro" Q wave lead I). ST elevation leads aVL, V5–V6. ST depression leads V2–V4.

Synthesis

Ectopic atrial rhythm, accelerated (or accelerated junctional rhythm with antegrade block). APCs. Lateral wall MI with ST-segment abnormalities suggestive of acute myocardial injury. ST depression in leads V2–V4 suggestive of either myocardial ischemia or reciprocal change. PR elevation suggestive of atrial injury.

TEST ANSWERS: 9, 10, (23), 89, 100, 101.

Comment: The rhythm disturbance of this tracing is difficult to define exactly. Options include an accelerated ectopic atrial rhythm. One must characterize the ectopic focus as *accelerated* because the rate is greater than 100 bpm. Another option is an accelerated AV junctional rhythm, however one must postulate antegrade block to explain the normal PR interval.

A lateral wall MI is present with abnormal Q waves and ST elevation in leads aVL and V6. A tiny Q wave is seen in the small lead I complex, but this finding is not truly diagnostic of an MI. This patient did go on to develop a lateral wall MI with positive cardiac enzymes. The rhythm disturbance also resolved with resolution of the acute myocardial injury.

An interesting aspect of this tracing is the PR elevation in the inferior limb leads, a finding that suggests atrial injury. Atrial arrhythmias often accompany atrial infarction.

FURTHER READING

Gardin JM, Singer DH: Atrial infarction. *Arch Intern Med* 141:1345–1348, 1981.
Lazar EJ, Goldberger J, Peled H, et al: Atrial infarction: Diagnosis and management. *Am Heart J* 116:1058–1063, 1988.

E-33

Clinical History
An 80-year-old man admitted to the ICU.

I aVR V1 V4

II aVL V2 V5

III aVF V3 V6

RHYTHM STRIP: II
25 mm/sec;1 cm/mV

INTERPRETED BY

E-34

NARRATIVE INTERPRETATION

Rhythm:	**Sinus rhythm, accelerated AV junctional rhythm**
Rate:	**Sinus rate 68, AV junctional rate 74**
Intervals:	**PR −, QRS 0.08, QT 0.38**
Axis:	**+45 degrees**

Abnormalities

Failure of P waves to conduct to ventricles. Isorhythmic dissociation. Sinus capture beat with prolonged PR interval. ST depression leads I, II, aVF, V2–V6. Diffuse low T voltage.

Synthesis

Sinus rhythm with accelerated AV junctional rhythm. Isorhythmic AV dissociation. Sinus capture with prolonged PR interval. Nonspecific ST-T-wave abnormalities.

TEST ANSWERS: 1, 23, 53, 57, 106.

Comment: This is an example of two supraventricular mechanisms occurring simultaneously. The AV junction has accelerated secondary to digitalis toxicity and usurped control of the normally slower sinus node. The two heart rates are nearly identical and manifest as P waves and QRS complexes that appear together, but are unrelated. Although AV dissociation is present, complete heart block is not, as proved by the ventricular capture beat (eighth complex on the rhythm strip). Additional signs of the effects of digitalis are the generalized ST-segment depression and low T-wave voltage.

FURTHER READING

Fisch C, Knoebel SB: Digitalis cardiotoxicity. *J Am Coll Cardiol* 5:91A–98A, 1985.
Saner HE, Lange HW, Pierach CA, Aeppli DM: Relation between serum digoxin concentration and the electrocardiogram. *Clin Cardiol* 11:752–756, 1988.

E-34

Clinical History

A 70-year-old woman seen in the emergency department for nausea. She is prescribed digoxin and diuretics for congestive heart failure.

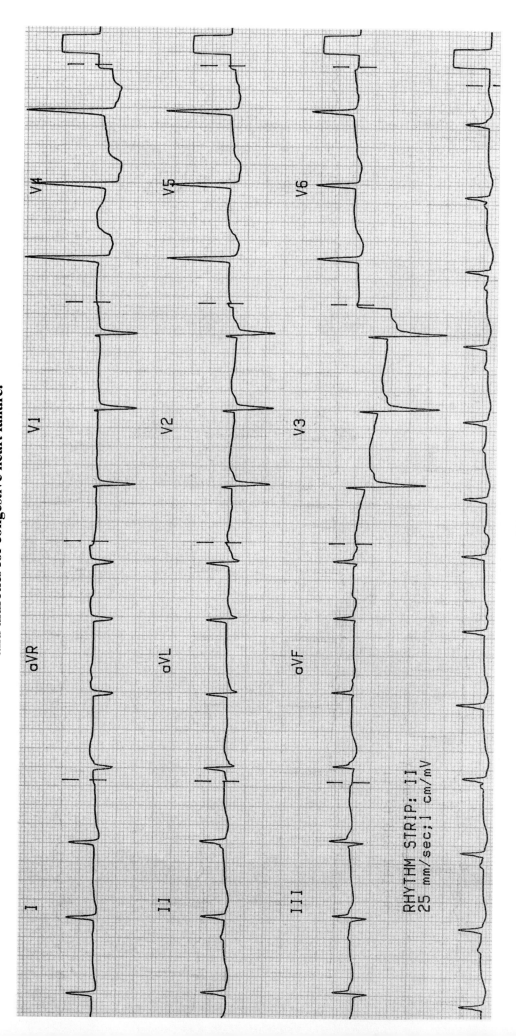

E-35

NARRATIVE INTERPRETATION

Rhythm:	**Sinus**
Rate:	**80**
Intervals:	**PR 0.12, QRS 0.12, QT 0.36**
Axis:	**−45 degrees**

Abnormalities
APC. Axis leftward of −30 degrees. Broad QRS with rsR' leads V1–V3 and T-wave inversion leads V1–V2.

Synthesis
Sinus rhythm. APC. RBBB. Associated ST-T-wave abnormalities. Left-axis deviation. Left anterior fascicular block.

TEST ANSWERS: 1, 10, 64, 70, 72, 104.

Comment: This tracing is from an asymptomatic patient with *bifascicular block.* Although patients with bifascicular block have excess mortality over patients without such findings, the causes of death are related to underlying cardiac disease and not to advanced heart block. Accordingly, prophylactic permanent pacing is not indicated in asymptomatic patients.

Note that the PR interval is at the lower limits of normal, but does not have characteristics that suggest an ectopic or AV junctional focus.

FURTHER READING
McAnulty JH, Rahimtoola SH, Murphy E, et al: Natural history of *high risk* bundle branch block. *N Engl J Med* 307:137–143, 1982.

E-35

Clinical History
An 81-year-old asymptomatic man.

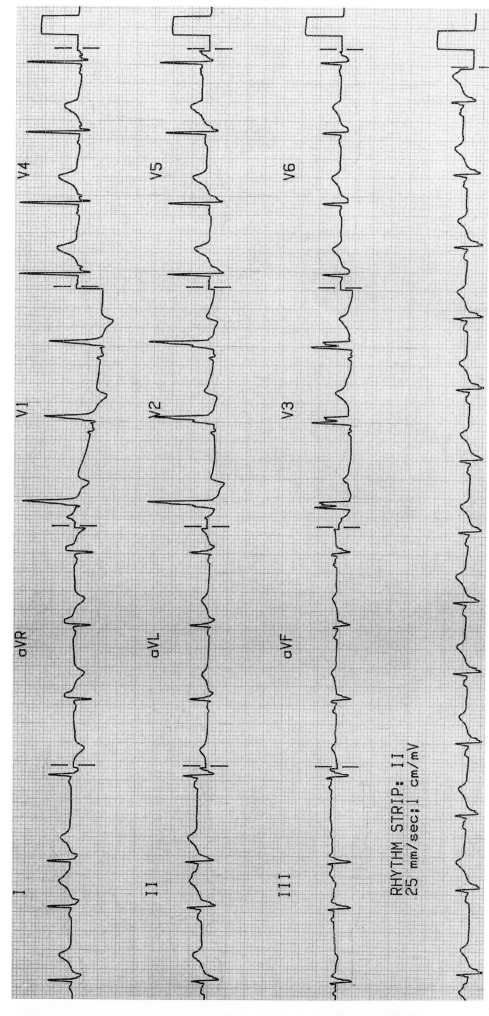

RHYTHM STRIP: II
25 mm/sec; 1 cm/mV

407

E-36

NARRATIVE INTERPRETATION

Rhythm:	**Sinus**
Rate:	**100**
Intervals:	**PR 0.16, QRS 0.08, QT 0.36**
Axis:	**+60 degrees**

Abnormalities

Temporary abrupt pauses in sinus rate. S wave lead V2 + R wave lead V5 greater than 35 mm. Biphasic T waves V5–V6. VPC on rhythm strip.

Synthesis

Sinus rhythm with sinus pauses. VPC. LVH. Nonspecific T-wave abnormality.

TEST ANSWERS: 1, 7, 26, 78, 106.

Comment: A series of sinus pauses follows the fifth complex in the limb leads. One might initially suspect a form of SA block to explain the pauses, but on further scrutiny, the pattern does not meet criteria for either type I or type II second-degree SA block.

Note the prolonged postectopic interval after the VPC on the rhythm strip. This appears to represent another sinus pause. The next sinus complex has a relatively short PR interval, possibly due to facilitated AV conduction following the pause.

E-36

Clinical History
A 90-year-old asymptomatic man.

RHYTHM STRIP: II
25 mm/sec; 1 cm/mV

E-37

NARRATIVE INTERPRETATION

Rhythm:	**Sinus**
Rate:	**90**
Intervals:	**PR 0.16, QRS 0.08, QT 0.34**
Axis:	**−15 degrees**

Abnormalities

ST depression leads I, aVL, V4–V6. T-wave inversion leads I, aVL, V4–V6. S wave lead V2 + R wave V5 greater than 35 mm. R wave lead aVL + S wave lead V3 greater than 28 mm in a man. VPC.

Synthesis

Sinus rhythm. VPC. LVH by voltage criteria with associated ST-T-wave abnormalities.

TEST ANSWERS: 1, 26, 78, 103.

Comment: This patient had aortic insufficiency with marked cardiac enlargement. There are characteristic findings for LVH with increased precordial voltage. Additional findings include ST depression with an asymmetrically inverted T wave. The ST- and T-wave abnormalities have been called the left ventricular *strain* pattern. It is interesting to note that despite obvious criteria for LVH in the precordial leads, the QRS voltage in the limb leads is quite low. This is because the major forces of the QRS vector in this patient are perpendicular to the frontal plane.

E-37

Clinical History

An 88-year-old man with a history of a diastolic murmur.

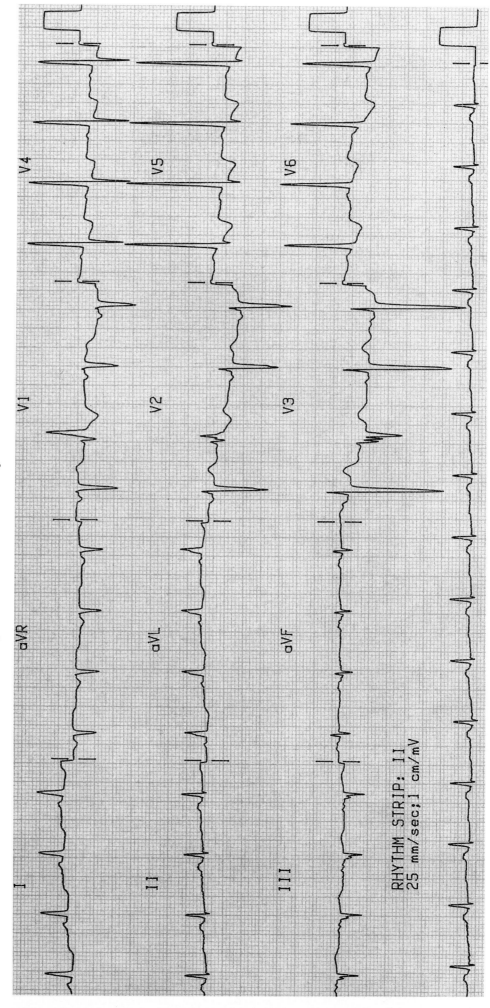

411

E-38

NARRATIVE INTERPRETATION

Rhythm:	**Sinus tachycardia**
Rate:	**126**
Intervals:	**PR 0.14, QRS 0.06, QT 0.30**
Axis:	**+30 degrees**

Abnormalities
Heart rate greater than 100 bpm. Slight ST depression leads I, II, aVF, V4–V6.

Synthesis
Sinus tachycardia. Nonspecific ST-segment abnormalities.

TEST ANSWERS: 4, 106.

Comment: The only significant abnormality of this electrocardiogram is the rapid heart rate. The minor, nonspecific ST abnormalities are likely associated with the sinus tachycardia and are not indicative of underlying cardiac disease. Remember that sinus tachycardia at rest is generally secondary to some other medical condition. Therapy should be directed to the primary disorder, not to the tachycardia itself. Conditions that frequently cause sinus tachycardia include hypotension, hypovolemia, hypoxia, fever, pain, and anxiety. Endocrine disorders such as hyperthyroidism or pheochromocytoma may also present with unexplained sinus tachycardia.

E-38

Clinical History

A 35-year-old man seen in the emergency department.

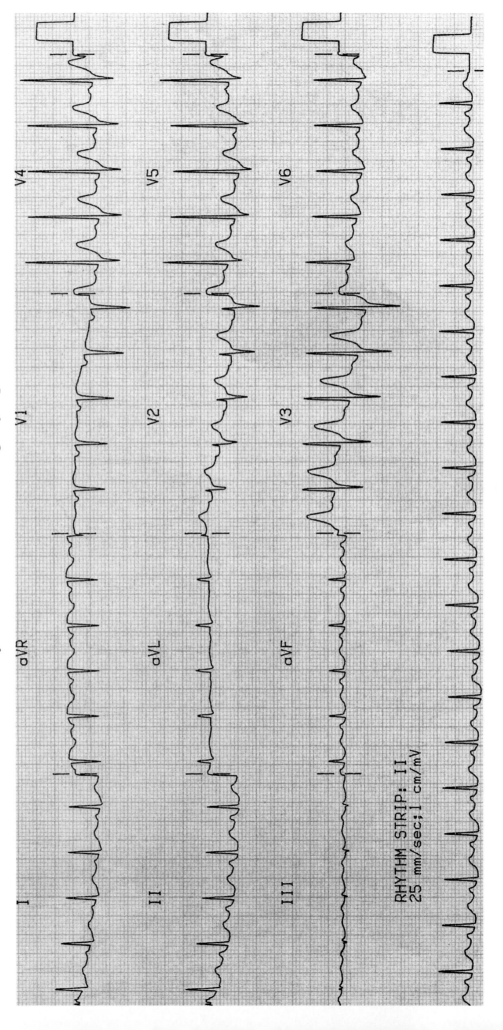

I

aVR

V1

V4

II

aVL

V2

V5

III

aVF

V3

V6

RHYTHM STRIP: II
25 mm/sec; 1 cm/mV

413

E-39

NARRATIVE INTERPRETATION

Rhythm:	**Sinus**
Rate:	**86**
Intervals:	**PR 0.19, QRS 0.08, QT 0.36**
Axis:	**−30 degrees**

Abnormalities
Slight ST elevation with downward concavity (coved) leads V5–V6. T-wave inversion leads I, aVL, V6. VPC. APC.

Synthesis
Sinus rhythm. VPC. APC. ST-T-wave abnormalities in leads V5–V6 suggesting myocardial injury. Nonspecific ST-T-wave abnormalities in leads I and aVL.

TEST ANSWERS: 1, 10, 26, 100, (102), 106.

Comment: The ST-T-wave abnormalities in this example are nondiagnostic but are somewhat worrisome. The "coved," or concave downward, ST elevation in leads V5 and V6 may represent myocardial injury and appear a bit more significant than just "nonspecific" findings. Indeed, this patient did eventually develop more significant EKG abnormalities and an anterolateral wall MI.

Remember to carefully check the rhythm strip of each tracing. The VPCs are easily seen on the 12-lead tracing. However, the seventh complex of the rhythm strip is an APC that might be overlooked by the casual interpreter.

414

E-39

Clinical History

A 75-year-old man with mild indigestion.

I aVR V1 V4

II aVL V2 V5

III aVF V3 V6

RHYTHM STRIP: II
25 mm/sec; 1 cm/mV

415

E-40

NARRATIVE INTERPRETATION

Rhythm:	**Sinus bradycardia**
Rate:	**50**
Intervals:	**PR 0.20, QRS 0.08, QT 0.42**
Axis:	**Unable to be determined**

Abnormalities
Heart rate less than 60 bpm. VPCs with retrograde atrial activation. Junctional escape complexes.

Synthesis
Sinus bradycardia. VPCs with retrograde atrial activation. Junctional escape complexes.

TEST ANSWERS: 3, 24, 26, 55.

Comment: The basic rhythm is sinus bradycardia interrupted by VPCs. On close inspection, inverted P waves can be appreciated in the ST segment of the VPCs. The sinus node is depolarized in a retrograde fashion and the sinus bradycardia cycle is reset. But before the sinus mechanism resumes, a subsidiary pacemaker in the AV junction emerges. The intrinsic rate of the AV junction is slower than the normal sinus rate and the sinus node quickly regains control in the following complex.

E-40

Clinical History
A 62-year-old woman in the CCU.

I

aVR

V1

V4

II

aVL

V2

V5

III

aVF

V3

V6

RHYTHM STRIP: II
25 mm/sec; 1 cm/mV

417

Index for Electrocardiographic Diagnoses